ORAL AND MAXILLOFACIAL SURGERY CLINICS
of North America

Management of the Pediatric Maxillofacial Patient

MARK A. EGBERT, DDS and
BONNIE L. PADWA, DMD, MD, FACS
Guest Editors

RICHARD H. HAUG, DDS
Consulting Editor

November 2005 • Volume 17 • Number 4

SAUNDERS
An Imprint of Elsevier, Inc.
PHILADELPHIA LONDON TORONTO MONTREAL SYDNEY TOKYO

W.B. SAUNDERS COMPANY
A Division of Elsevier Inc.

1600 John F. Kennedy Blvd., Suite 1800, Philadelphia, PA 19103-2899

http://www.oralmaxsurgery.theclinics.com

ORAL AND MAXILLOFACIAL SURGERY
CLINICS OF NORTH AMERICA   Volume 17, Number 4
November 2005   ISSN 1042-3699
Editor: John Vassallo   ISBN 1-4160-2842-0

Copyright © 2005 Elsevier Inc. All rights reserved. No part of this publication may be reproduced or transmitted in any form or by any means, electronic or mechanical, including photocopy, recording, or any information retrieval system, without written permission from the Publisher.

Single photocopies of single articles may be made for personal use as allowed by national copyright laws. Permission of the Publisher and payment of a fee is required for all other photocopying, including multiple or systematic copying, copying for advertising or promotional purposes, resale, and all forms of document delivery. Special rates are available for educational institutions that wish to make photocopies for non-profit educational classroom use. Permissions may be sought directly from Elsevier's Rights Department in Philadelphia, PA, USA: phone: (+1) 215 239 3804, fax: (+1) 215 239 3805, e-mail: healthpermissions@elsevier.com. Requests may also be completed on-line via the Elsevier homepage (http://www.elsevier.com/locate/permissions). In the USA, users may clear permissions and make payments through the Copyright Clearance Center, Inc., 222 Rosewood Drive, Danvers, MA 01923, USA; phone: (978) 750-8400, fax: (978) 750-4744, and in the UK through the Copyright Licensing Agency Rapid Clearance Service (CLARCS), 90 Tottenham Court Road, London W1P 0LP, UK; phone: (+44) 171 436 5931; fax: (+44) 171 436 3986. Other countries may have a local reprographic rights agency for payments.

Reprints. For copies of 100 or more, of articles in this publication, please contact the Commercial Reprints Department, Elsevier Inc., 360 Park Avenue South, New York, New York 10010-1710. Tel. (212) 633-3813 Fax: (212) 462-1935 email: reprints@elsevier.com

The ideas and opinions expressed in *Oral and Maxillofacial Surgery Clinics of North America* do not necessarily reflect those of the Publisher. The Publisher does not assume any responsibility for any injury and/or damage to persons or property arising out of or related to any use of the material contained in this periodical. The reader is advised to check the appropriate medical literature and the product information currently provided by the manufacturer of each drug to be administered to verify the dosage, the method and duration of administration, or contraindications. It is the responsibility of the treating physician or other health care professional, relying on independent experience and knowledge of the patient, to determine drug dosages and the best treatment for the patient. Mention of any product in this issue should not be construed as endorsement by the contributors, editors, or the Publisher of the product or manufacturers' claims.

Oral and Maxillofacial Surgery Clinics of North America (ISSN 1042-3699) is published quarterly by W.B. Saunders Company. Corporate and editorial offices: Elsevier, Inc., 1600 John F. Kennedy Blvd., Suite 1800, Philadelphia, PA 19103-2899. Accounting and circulation offices: 6277 Sea Harbor Drive, Orlando, FL 32887-4800. Periodicals postage paid at Orlando, FL 32862, and additional mailing offices. Subscription prices are $195.00 per year for US individuals, $295.00 per year for US institutions, $90.00 per year for US students and residents, $225.00 per year for Canadian individuals, $345.00 per year for Canadian institutions, $245.00 per year for international individuals, $345.00 per year for international institutions and $115.00 per year for Canadian and foreign students/residents. To receive student/resident rate, orders must be accompanied by name or affiliated institution, date of term, and the *signature* of program/residency coordinator on institution letterhead. Orders will be billed at individual rate until proof of status is received. Foreign air speed delivery is included in all *Clinics* subscription prices. All prices are subject to change without notice. POSTMASTER: Send address changes to *Oral and Maxillofacial Surgery Clinics of North America*, W.B. Saunders Company, Periodicals Fulfillment, Orlando, FL 32887-4800. **Customer Service: 1-800-654-2452 (US). From outside of the US, call 1-407-345-4000.**

Printed in the United States of America.

MANAGEMENT OF THE PEDIATRIC MAXILLOFACIAL PATIENT

CONSULTING EDITOR

RICHARD H. HAUG, DDS, Professor of Oral and Maxillofacial Surgery; and Executive Associate Dean, University of Kentucky College of Dentistry, Lexington, Kentucky

GUEST EDITORS

MARK A. EGBERT, DDS, Associate Professor, Oral and Maxillofacial Surgery, University of Washington; and Chief, Oral and Maxillofacial Surgery, Children's Hospital and Regional Medical Center, Seattle, Washington

BONNIE L. PADWA, DMD, MD, FACS, Associate Professor, Oral and Maxillofacial Surgery, Harvard School of Dental Medicine and Harvard Medical School, Children's Hospital, Boston, Massachusetts

CONTRIBUTORS

JAIME S. BRAHIM, DDS, MS, Senior Oral and Maxillofacial Surgeon, National Institutes of Health, National Institute of Dental and Craniofacial Research, Bethesda, Maryland

ROBERT P. CARMICHAEL, MDM, MSc, FRCDC, Assistant Professor and Coordinator of Prosthodontics, The Hospital for Sick Children and Bloorview MacMillan Children's Centre; and Department of Oral and Maxillofacial Surgery, Mount Sinai Hospital, Toronto, Ontario, Canada

RADHIKA CHIGURUPATI, BDS, DMD, Assistant Clinical Professor, Department of Oral and Maxillofacial Surgery, University of California–San Francisco, San Francisco, California

BERNARD J. COSTELLO, DMD, MD, Chief, Division of Craniofacial and Cleft Surgery, Department of Oral and Maxillofacial Surgery, University of Pittsburgh School of Dental Medicine; and Chief, Division of Pediatric Oral and Maxillofacial Surgery, Children's Hospital of Pittsburgh, Pittsburgh, Pennsylvania

JOHN DASKALOGIANNAKIS, DDS, MSc, FRCDC, Assistant Professor, University of Toronto; and Staff Orthodontist, The Hospital for Sick Children and Bloorview MacMillan Children's Medical Centre, Toronto, Ontario, Canada

THOMAS B. DODSON, DMD, MPH, Associate Professor and Visiting Oral and Maxillofacial Surgeon, Department of Oral and Maxillofacial Surgery, Massachusetts General Hospital, Harvard School of Dental Medicine, Boston, Massachusetts

SEAN P. EDWARDS, DDS, MD, Fellow, Craniofacial Surgery, Department of Oral and Maxillofacial Surgery, University of Pittsburgh School of Dental Medicine, Pittsburgh, Pennsylvania

KENNETH W. FELDMAN, MD, Clinical Professor, Department of Pediatrics, Division of General Pediatrics, University of Washington School of Medicine, Children's Hospital and Regional Medical Center, Seattle, Washington

ANDREW A. HEGGIE, MBBS, MDSc, FFDRCS, FRACDS(OMS), Associate Professor and Head, Oral and Maxillofacial Surgery Unit, Department of Plastic and Maxillofacial Surgery, The Royal Children's Hospital of Melbourne, Melbourne, Victoria, Australia

LEONARD B. KABAN, DMD, MD, Walter C. Guralnick Professor and Chairman, Department of Oral and Maxillofacial Surgery, Massachusetts General Hospital, Harvard School of Dental Medicine, Boston, Massachusetts

GEORGE M. KUSHNER, DMD, MD, Associate Professor and Program Director, Oral and Maxillofacial Surgery, Department of Surgical and Hospital Dentistry, School of Dentistry, University of Louisville, Louisville, Kentucky

NINA A. MAHMUD, BS, Research Assistant, Oral and Maxillofacial Surgery, Oregon Health and Science University, Portland, Oregon

ROBERT W.T. MYALL, BDS, FRCD, FDS, MD, Professor, Oral and Maxillofacial Surgery, Oregon Health and Science University, Portland, Oregon

IAIN A. NISH, DDS, FRCDC, Associate in Dentistry, University of Toronto; Staff Pediatric Oral and Maxillofacial Surgeon, The Hospital for Sick Children, Toronto; and Lakeridge Medical Centre, Oshawa, Ontario, Canada

DOLPHINE ODA, BDS, MSc, Professor, Department of Oral and Maxillofacial Surgery, University of Washington, Seattle, Washington

MARIA E. PAPADAKI, DDS, MD, AO-ASIF/Synthes Fellow in Pediatric Oral and Maxillofacial Surgery, Department of Oral and Maxillofacial Surgery, Massachusetts General Hospital, Harvard School of Dental Medicine, Boston, Massachusetts

RAMON L. RUIZ, DMD, MD, Division of Pediatric Craniofacial Surgery, Department of Oral/Maxillofacial Surgery, Southwest Florida Oral and Facial Surgery; and Attending Surgeon, Children's Hospital of Southwest Florida, Fort Myers, Florida

GEORGE K.B. SÁNDOR, MD, DDS, PhD, Dr Habil, FRCDC, FRCSC, FACS, Professor and Director, Graduate Program in Oral and Maxillofacial Surgery and Anesthesia, University of Toronto; Coordinator of Pediatric Oral and Maxillofacial Surgery, The Hospital for Sick Children and Bloorview MacMillan Children's Centre; Staff Oral, Maxillofacial, Plastic, and Craniofacial Surgeon, Mount Sinai Hospital; Toronto, Ontario, Canada; and Docent in Oral and Maxillofacial Surgery, University of Oulu, Oulu, Finland

WILLY SERLO, MD, PhD, Professor of Pediatric Surgery, University of Turku, Turku; and Head, Department of Pediatric Surgery, Oulu University Hospital, Oulu, Finland

JOCELYN M. SHAND, MBBS, MDSc, FDSRCS, FRACDS(OMS), Consultant, Oral and Maxillofacial Surgery Unit, Department of Plastic and Maxillofacial Surgery, The Royal Children's Hospital of Melbourne, Melbourne, Victoria, Australia

NAOMI F. SUGAR, MD, Clinical Associate Professor, Department of Pediatrics, Division of General Pediatrics, University of Washington School of Medicine, Harborview Medical Center, Seattle, Washington

PAUL S. TIWANA, DDS, MD, MS, Assistant Professor and Chief, Pediatric Oral and Maxillofacial Surgery, Kosair Children's Hospital; and Department of Surgical and Hospital Dentistry, School of Dentistry, University of Louisville, Louisville, Kentucky

MARIA J. TROULIS, DDS, MSc, Associate Professor, Department of Oral and Maxillofacial Surgery; and Director of Minimally Invasive OMFS Program, Massachusetts General Hospital, Harvard School of Dental Medicine, Boston, Massachusetts

TIMOTHY A. TURVEY, DDS, Professor and Chair, Department of Oral and Maxillofacial Surgery, University of North Carolina at Chapel Hill, Chapel Hill, North Carolina

BRETT A. UEECK, DMD, MD, Assistant Professor, Oral and Maxillofacial Surgery, Oregon Health and Science University, Portland, Oregon

LEENA P. YLIKONTIOLA, DDS, PhD, Assistant Professor, Department of Oral and Maxillofacial Surgery, Institute of Dentistry, University of Oulu; and Coordinator of Cleft Lip and Palate Surgery, Oulu University Hospital, Oulu, Finland

CONTENTS

Preface xi
Mark A. Egbert and Bonnie L. Padwa

Management of Impacted Teeth in Children 365
Paul S. Tiwana and George M. Kushner

> Ankylosis remains one of the major complications associated with impacted teeth in children. Orthodontically-assisted eruption of an ankylosed tooth may intrude or displace the adjacent teeth. Children who undergo orthodontically assisted eruption should be followed closely to ensure that movement of an impacted tooth is occurring. In general, the removal or assisted eruption of impacted teeth in children requires a thoughtful interdisciplinary evaluation between the surgeon and orthodontist/primary dental care provider. Factors that must be considered include operative feasibility, orthodontic management, future growth, and psychosocial considerations. The use of emerging technology, such as cone beam CT and skeletal anchorage, should better equip surgeons to navigate the anatomy three-dimensionally and provide assistance in management of difficult cases.

Dental Implants in Children 375
Jaime S. Brahim

> Some children and adolescents have anodontia, partial anodontia, congenitally missing teeth, and lost teeth as a result of trauma, and they may benefit from early placement of dental implants. Clinicians should have an understanding of the potential risks involved in placing implants in jaws that are still growing and developing and consider the effect that implants have on craniofacial growth. Implants may act as ankylotic teeth and fail to move together with the surrounding structures, which produces an infraocclusion that leads to difficulties with prosthetics. Young patients may require general anesthesia for the procedure and there may be limited cooperation in maintaining good oral hygiene.

Soft-Tissue Lesions in Children 383
Dolphine Oda

> This article reviews some of the benign and malignant oral soft-tissue swellings that occur in children, with an emphasis on their clinical presentation, etiology, histopathology, and treatment. These lesions include single and multiple nodules, reactive lesions, and benign and malignant neoplasms. Diseases discussed include reactive gingival swellings, generalized gingival fibromatosis, melanotic neuroectodermal tumor of infancy, fibromas, vascular

lesions, salivary gland lesions, and infantile rhabdomyoma. Also covered are lesions that may present in multiples, such as neuromas, multiple endocrine neoplasia type 2b, neurofibromatosis, and human papilloma virus–related benign epithelial lesions. Benign but locally aggressive and malignant neoplasms are discussed, such as aggressive fibromatosis, myofibromatosis, fibrosarcoma, and rhabdomyosarcoma.

Cysts of the Jaws and Advances in the Diagnosis and Management of Nevoid Basal Cell Carcinoma Syndrome 403
Jocelyn M. Shand and Andrew A. Heggie

Cysts of the jaws are a relatively commonly encountered pathologic condition, and a full spectrum of these lesions may present in pediatric patients. Most cystic lesions are of odontogenic origin, as seen in adult patients, and a range of surgical approaches are available for their management. These approaches are based on the clinical and radiologic features and the behavioral and histologic characteristics of each cyst. Advances in imaging techniques and laboratory investigations, such as immunocytochemistry and genetic analysis, will continue to facilitate improved diagnoses, patient management, and clinical outcomes.

Advances in Diagnosis and Management of Fibro-Osseous Lesions 415
Maria E. Papadaki, Maria J. Troulis, and Leonard B. Kaban

Fibro-osseous lesions are benign mesenchymal skeletal tumors in which mineralized tissue, blood vessels, and giant cells, in varying proportions, replace normal bone. Included in this group are fibrous dysplasia, cherubism, ossifying fibromas, and osteoblastoma, with fibrous dysplasia being the most common entity. Although fibro-osseous lesions have similar histologic and radiographic features, they may exhibit a wide range of biologic behaviors. Because the histologic appearance does not predict the rate of growth or prognosis, treatment is based on the clinical and biologic behavior of the tumor. The purpose of this article is to describe advances in diagnosis and management of fibro-osseous lesions.

Oral Surgical Aspects of Child Abuse and Neglect 435
Naomi F. Sugar and Kenneth W. Feldman

Oral trauma is a frequent manifestation of child abuse. Injuries to the oral hard and soft tissues are common in active children, but any oral injury in a young pre-ambulatory infant should raise concern for abuse. Oral-facial trauma may be the primary presenting injury, or may accompany other severe inflicted injuries such as head injury, fractures, or abdominal trauma. Some congenital or acquired medical disorders may be mistaken for abuse or neglect. The oral surgeon is a critical participant in the collaborative management of child abuse cases.

Condyle and Ramus-Condyle Unit Fractures in Growing Patients: Management and Outcomes 447
Thomas B. Dodson

Controversy exists regarding the best management of ramus-condyle unit fractures. Treatment recommendations include observation (with or without physiotherapy or use of functional appliances), maxillomandibular fixation (for varying durations of time), and open reduction internal fixation (with varying degrees of maxillomandibular fixation postoperatively). Some unique complications also may occur after ramus-condyle unit fractures, including asymmetric mandibular growth and temporomandibular joint ankylosis. The purpose of this article is to review the evaluation and management of ramus-condyle unit fractures in growing patients with an emphasis on treatment outcomes.

Pediatric Mandibular Hypomobility: Current Management and Controversies 455
Bernard J. Costello and Sean P. Edwards

Limited range of motion of the pediatric mandible (eg, mandibular hypomobility) presents many challenges. Untreated or recurrent hypomobility can cause problems with mastication, oral hygiene, speech, growth, and the airway. Treatments for ankylosis or adhesions include coronoidectomy, gap arthroplasty, costochondral rib reconstruction, prosthetic joint replacement, and transport distraction osteogenesis. There are many different causes of mandibular hypomobility in young patients, including idiopathic (congenital), post-traumatic, infectious, inflammatory, neoplastic, and iatrogenic. A detailed evaluation and diagnosis of the limited range of motion are critical to developing an appropriate treatment strategy. This article outlines evaluation, differential diagnosis, and the current operative approaches for treating hypomobility in young patients. Controversies related to timing of various procedures and the uses of various treatment options are discussed.

Dealing with the Effects of Juvenile Rheumatoid Arthritis in Growing Children 467
Brett A. Ueeck, Nina A. Mahmud, and Robert W.T. Myall

Juvenile rheumatoid arthritis is a chronic childhood disease that has a multiplicity of effects on the growth and development of the facial skeleton. An understanding of the disease in general and its therapy is necessary for successful surgical-orthodontic care.

Mandibular Distraction Osteogenesis in Children 475
Ramon L. Ruiz, Timothy A. Turvey, and Bernard J. Costello

Distraction osteogenesis is currently considered a useful treatment option for the correction of specific facial skeletal deformities. Although it is apparent that distraction may have significant potential and broader application in the management of maxillofacial problems, very few comprehensive scientific data exist, making it difficult to describe its exact role in the reconstructive oral and maxillofacial surgeon's armamentarium. This article reviews the biologic basis for distraction osteogenesis, potential applications, and current surgical approaches for mandibular distraction in children.

Distraction Osteogenesis of the Midface 485
George K.B. Sándor, Leena P. Ylikontiola, Willy Serlo, Robert P. Carmichael, Iain A. Nish, and John Daskalogiannakis

Distraction osteogenesis has become an important part of pediatric oral and maxillofacial surgery. It is especially useful in the midface to overcome the perturbations of growth caused by congenital malformations, benign and malignant tumors, and traumatic injuries. Midfacial distraction osteogenesis can take various forms, depending on the exact anatomic site where it is applied in the midfacial skeleton. This article reviews the various locations in the midface in which distraction techniques might be useful and highlights the important differences in application at these sites.

Orthognathic Surgery for Secondary Cleft and Craniofacial Deformities 503
Radhika Chigurupati

Orthognathic surgery is a critical component of surgical management of craniofacial deformities such as cleft lip and palate, craniofacial dysostoses, and mandibulofacial dysostoses. These operations can correct discrepancy in jaw relationship and malocclusion, relieve airway obstruction, correct facial asymmetry, optimize facial aesthetics, improve speech articulation, improve ability to masticate, and enhance psychological development and social interaction. Oral and maxillofacial surgeons who treat these deformities should be part of a craniofacial team to provide interdisciplinary care for patients. Distraction osteogenesis is a useful technique in the management of severe craniofacial deformities but does not replace conventional orthognathic surgery, which is safe and predictable. Recent advances in three-dimensional imaging and planning tools have made it possible to plan surgery more accurately and predictably.

Cumulative Index 2005   **519**

FORTHCOMING ISSUES

February 2006

    Perioperative Management of the OMS Patient, Part I
    Harry Dym, DDS, *Guest Editor*

May 2006

    Perioperative Management of the OMS Patient, Part II
    Harry Dym, DDS, *Guest Editor*

August 2006

    Surgical Management of the Temporomandibular Joint
    A. Thomas Indresano, DMD, *Guest Editor*

PREVIOUS ISSUES

August 2005

    The Role of the Oral and Maxillofacial Surgeon in Wartime, Emergencies, and Terrorist Attacks
    David B. Powers, DMD, MD, *Guest Editor*

May 2005

    Diagnosis and Management of Skin Cancer
    Michael S. Goldwasser, DDS, MD, and
    Jonathan S. Bailey, DMD, MD, FACS, *Guest Editors*

February 2005

    Minimally Invasive Cosmetic Facial Surgery
    Joseph Niamtu III, DMD, *Guest Editor*

THE CLINICS ARE NOW AVAILABLE ONLINE!

Access your subscription at:
www.theclinics.com

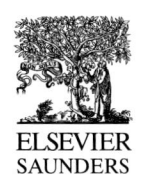

Preface

Management of the Pediatric Maxillofacial Patient

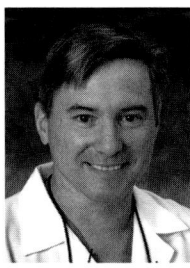

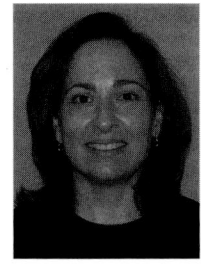

Mark A. Egbert, DDS   Bonnie L. Padwa, DMD, MD, FACS
Guest Editors

In the preface to the February 1994 issue of the *Oral and Maxillofacial Surgery Clinics of North America* entitled "Oral and Maxillofacial Surgery in Children and Adolescents," Dr. Leonard Kaban wrote:

> Oral and maxillofacial surgery (OMFS) is an anatomically defined specialty. Hence, clinicians treat at least a few patients of all ages, without emphasis on any particular group. In many OMFS training programs, the number of pediatric patients encountered is low. Therefore, graduating residents often view general oral and maxillofacial surgical management of children as an area of weakness in their training.

This description of the state of pediatric training in OMFS, with few exceptions, remains the same today. Training programs in OMFS have an obligation to provide a reasonable training and a basic exposure to a breadth of pediatric oral and maxillofacial surgery to their residents. Accreditation standards ensuring a pediatric component for training programs are lenient, but remain a challenge for many programs for a variety of reasons. As a specialty, organized oral and maxillofacial surgery continues to recognize the importance of childhood health, and the maintenance of at least a minimal standard for our trainees. Perhaps the best evidence of this commitment is the inclusion of a pediatric section within each and every component of our specialties' published *Parameters of Care* document.

To date, there is one well-recognized comprehensive text on pediatric oral and maxillofacial surgery. This issue is not intended to compete with that text. Rather, a variety of articles devoted to topics of perpetual interest, and areas of evolving contemporary thought or controversy are presented to educate, and hopefully, to stimulate continued advancement and renewed awareness of pediatric oral health issues.

The subject of managing impacted teeth in children leads off this collection and should be of interest to all practicing oral and maxillofacial surgeons (Tiwana and Kushner). Dentoalveolar reconstruction follows with an update on the use of dental implants in the growing patient (Brahim).

Pathology is the next focus for review, with updates on soft tissue lesions in children (Oda), followed by a review of cysts of the jaws in children and the current treatment of basal cell nevoid syndrome (Heggie and Shand). These are followed by an article on advances in the diagnosis and management of fibro-osseous lesions in children by Drs. Kaban, Troulis, and Papadaki. The application of adjuvant chemotherapy augmenting and enhancing surgical outcomes is a very exciting development in the man-

1042-3699/05/$ – see front matter © 2005 Elsevier Inc. All rights reserved.
doi:10.1016/j.coms.2005.10.001

oralmaxsurgery.theclinics.com

agement of these often locally aggressive and deforming, yet "benign" entities.

A heightened awareness regarding the prevalence and potential signs of child abuse and neglect is provided by an article devoted to the role of the oral and maxillofacial surgeon in confronting and managing this problem. Although disturbing to read, we hope the impact of this article by Drs. Sugar and Feldman will stimulate reflection and increase the collective awareness of this most important and damaging scourge.

Problems afflicting the cranio-mandibular articulation in the growing patient are the focus of the next three articles. These problems can be acquired (eg, trauma, infection, pathology, systemic disease), congenital (eg, congenital absence, syngnathia), or they can be iatrogenic (eg, poor fracture management, failed costochondral grafts). These problems always challenge the clinician to understand the relationship between morphologic form and function regarding both mobility and growth. Dr. Dodson begins with an excellent article discussing and presenting condylar fracture management in the growing patient. This is followed by Drs. Costello and Edwards' article discussing mandibular hypomobility and ankylosis including some of the controversies currently argued. The focus on the cranio-mandibular articulation continues with an article contributed by Drs. Myall, Ueeck, and Mahmud discussing the management of juvenile rheumatoid arthritis and its effects on the growing patient.

Certainly, no more current topic of interest exists than that of distraction osteogenesis, and this is also true for its applications in the growing patient. Distraction osteogenesis is discussed in separate articles for the mandible (Ruiz, Turvey, and Costello) and for midfacial applications (Sándor). To balance the enthusiasm for the new, with a review of the tried and true, finally, an excellent article devoted to the orthognathic correction of secondary deformities in the cleft and craniofacial patients is provided by Dr. Chigurupati.

All of these articles provide a resource of information to educate and to stimulate further thought and reflection on the often unique issues encountered in the management of pediatric and growing patients.

We wish to thank all of these authors for their considerable efforts in producing this issue. We also wish to thank John Vassallo for his help, guidance, and unending patience in bringing this issue to press.

Mark A. Egbert, DDS
Children's Hospital and Regional Medical Center
4800 Sand Point Way, NE
Box 5371/4E-2
Seattle, WA 98105-0371, USA
E-mail address: mark.egbert@seattlechildrens.org

Bonnie L. Padwa, DMD, MD, FACS
Division of Plastic and Oral Surgery
Children's Hospital
300 Longwood Avenue
Boston, MA 02115, USA
E-mail address: bonnie.padwa@childrens.harvard.edu

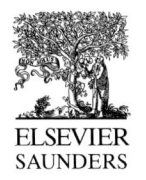

Management of Impacted Teeth in Children

Paul S. Tiwana, DDS, MD, MS*, George M. Kushner, DMD, MD

Department of Surgical and Hospital Dentistry, School of Dentistry, University of Louisville, 501 South Preston Street, Louisville, KY 40292, USA

The contemporary oral and maxillofacial surgeon is frequently confronted with dentoalveolar surgical problems in childhood, such as impacted teeth. This increase is likely the result of better dental health awareness among parents and a push from the dental profession in general to improve access to care for children. Management of impactions for this group of patients demands not only technical skill but also proficiency in outpatient anesthetic techniques. An appreciation by surgeons of the implications of future growth, dental eruption patterns, and the parameters of current orthodontic care is critical to a successful outcome. Impacted teeth in children often have common clinical presentations. Surgeons also may encounter patients with certain craniofacial disorders, a history of maxillofacial trauma, and pathology in infancy or early childhood. These distinct situations require a more complex level of evaluation and management. Advanced dentomaxillofacial radiology imaging techniques, such as the cone beam CT scan, have begun to play an important role in helping surgeons care for these patients.

Etiology and incidence

There are many documented causes for the eruption failure of teeth. In many circumstances, however, the cause remains unknown. Eruption failure of teeth can be caused by any number of causes or can be part of a constellation of problems, such as those seen in patients with craniofacial disorders. Common local causes include dense fibrotic gingiva, premature exfoliation or loss of the primary dentition, and mechanical obstruction secondary to pathologic lesions or the presence of supernumerary teeth. Regional causes, such as skeletal facial deformities and true Bolton tooth size discrepancies, also may contribute to mechanical obstruction. Systemic causes include metabolic and endocrine and genetic disorders. Inappropriate downregulation of the pituitary axis (hypopituitarism) and functional problems with the thyroid gland itself (hypothyroidism) can contribute to impacted teeth in childhood. Common genetic disorders that include impacted teeth include cleidocranial dysostosis, certain craniostenoses, and facial clefting, although the disease etiology is multifactorial [1].

Little argument exists regarding the incidence of impacted teeth in children, which has been well documented in several studies [2]. The most frequently impacted tooth normally found in the primary and mixed dentition is the maxillary canine, followed by the mandibular second premolar, the maxillary incisors, and the molars, although this is an uncommon occurrence. Impacted supernumerary teeth are often first diagnosed in childhood and may cause impaction of teeth in the permanent dentition. The most commonly impacted supernumerary teeth in pediatric patients in order of frequency are the mesiodens, supernumerary maxillary incisors, additional or fourth molars, and supernumerary mandibular premolars. The management of third molars, although a frequent problem in adolescence, is more commonly dealt with in the mature or nearly ma-

* Corresponding author.
 E-mail address: paul.tiwana@louisville.edu (P.S. Tiwana).

ture facial skeleton and is not included in the scope of this article.

Impacted maxillary canines

The impacted maxillary canine is the most frequently impacted tooth seen in childhood. The canine tooth is tremendously important in long-term orofacial function and aesthetics. Often in adult patients with preterminal dentition, it is the last tooth extracted within the arches because of its importance and strength. Management of this tooth in pediatric patients takes on a special imperative by surgeons to preserve these fundamental roles. The most likely position of the impacted maxillary canine is palatal rather than buccal by a significant margin. The overall incidence of impacted canine teeth is approximately 2% [3]. The decision to remove the cuspid should be guided by whether significant pathology exists or whether it is orthodontically unfeasible to position the tooth within the arch in a functional relationship.

Of critical importance in the management of the impacted canine are the radiographic techniques involved in its localization within the alveolus. When the tooth is palpable, either buccally or palatally, a surgeon is guided by the physical examination as to which approach is used. When not palpable, the decision requires detailed radiographic evaluation beyond obtaining the standard panoramic radiograph. On a panoramic radiograph, however, the tooth closest to the film is the most well defined. If the canine is clearer than the incisor roots, it is labial or buccal. The most common technique currently in use is the tube shift technique, with radiographic analysis specifically directed at the buccal object rule. In review, as the tube of the x-ray unit shifts away from the object (maxillary canine), if the canine seems to move radiographically in the opposite direction, the tooth is in the labial side of the alveolus. If the tooth seems to move radiographically in the same direction as the x-ray unit tube, the tooth is located in the palatal alveolus. Occasionally, the tooth is located in the central alveolus and does not seem to shift at all. Additional radiographs also may be helpful, such as the lateral cephalogram and specifically the cone beam CT scan, which is discussed later [4].

The approach to the palatally impacted maxillary canine traditionally involves one of two methods [5,6]. If the crown of the tooth is readily palpable, then a "window" approach generally is used, in which a full-thickness mucoperiosteal incision is made with removal of the overlying soft tissue directly over the tooth. This procedure is followed by removal of remaining palatal bone surrounding the crown with either a rotary handpiece or hand instrumentation. The wound is then packed for patient comfort during the healing period. If the surgeon does not readily palpate the crown of the impacted cuspid but has confirmed its presence on the palatal aspect of the alveolus, an envelope incision with a full-thickness palatal flap can be used. The incision on the palatal aspect of the erupted teeth is created full thickness, and the mucoperiosteum subsequently is elevated. Care must be taken to extend the incision far enough anteriorly and posteriorly so as not to create undue tension on the flap and cause a rent or tear.

Infiltration of small amounts of local anesthesia subperiosteally on the palate, after regional block, note only aids in hemostasis but also secondarily provides some hydrodissection as the tissue is bound firmly to the bone. The surgeon accomplishes bone removal around the crown of the impacted cuspid with a surgical handpiece. A small stab incision is made for the wire ligature of the bonded orthodontic appliance to pass through the palatal flap or the incision itself. The surgical management of the labially impacted maxillary canine demands that the surgeon recognize the significance of the surrounding connective tissue, specifically the preservation of a band of fixed gingival tissue to maintain periodontal health. The apically repositioned flap is usually the incision of choice. Vertical incisions are used with a wider base and the tip of the flap being composed of fixed tissue from the alveolar ridge. The flap is dissected superiorly, and in a manner similar to one described previously, bone is removed as necessary from around the crown of the impacted tooth. The tissue is then sutured apically to allow for gradual descent with the tooth during orthodontic traction, which preserves the keratinized tissue band around the labial aspect of the tooth. If the root of the impacted tooth is not fully formed, spontaneous eruption of the tooth can occur if sufficient bone is removed (at least to the gingival one third of the crown). Allowance of 6 to 8 weeks for observation should be sufficient to determine if spontaneous eruption will occur. If the root is fully formed or eruption does not ensue, the initial application of the orthodontic appliance usually rests with the surgeon. Contemporary treatment calls for the placement of an orthodontic button or gold chain. The visible light cure cements have made secure attachment of the devices routine. Hemostasis and a dry field are paramount, however, although some of the newer bonding agents are more adaptable to working in a

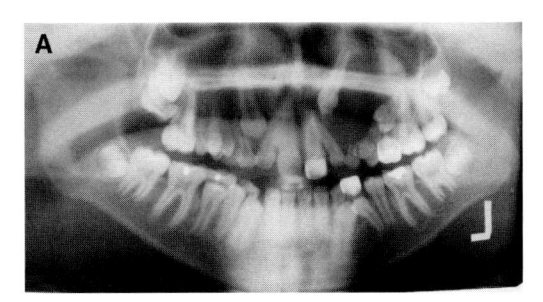

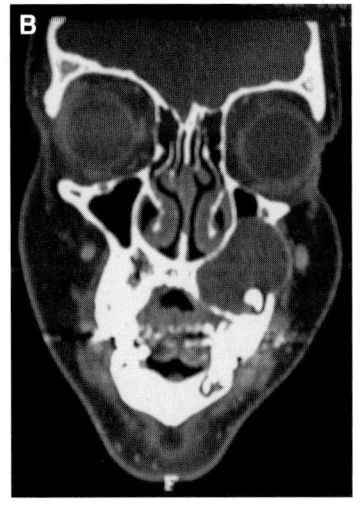

Fig. 1. (*A*) Impacted maxillary cuspid with associated dentigerous cyst. (*B*) Coronal CT scan demonstrates impacted maxillary cuspid and associated dentigerous cyst.

wet environment. The appliance is wire or suture ligated to the archwire to allow for easy access by the orthodontist after initial soft tissue healing (Fig. 1) [7].

Impacted mandibular premolars

Although impacted premolars can be found in the maxilla, they are predominately found in the mandible. Management of the impacted premolar requires assessment of a patient's overall occlusal scheme. If true tooth space exists in the arch or no extractions are planned for relief of malocclusion, then consideration should be given by the surgeon to surgical exposure rather than removal. The most likely position of this impaction is on the lingual aspect of the alveolus or the center of mandible. Care must be exercised three dimensionally by the surgeon to prevent indiscriminate bone removal with possible subsequent injury to the roots of the adjacent teeth or the inferior alveolar nerve.

Exposure is performed through a sulcular incision. The incision is extended enough to permit an adequate operative field and prevent trauma to the flap. The tooth is exposed with a surgical handpiece or hand instrumentation. The follicular remnants are excised, and a button is bonded or, if the root apex remains open, is allowed to erupt spontaneously. In the authors' experience with spontaneous eruption of impacted mandibular premolars, however, the more dense cortical bone makes eruption less likely to occur to satisfaction without the aid of some orthodontic anchorage and traction (Fig. 2).

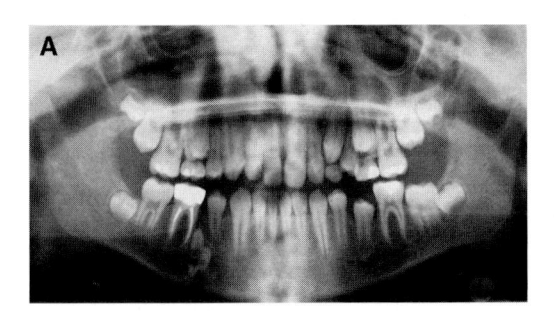

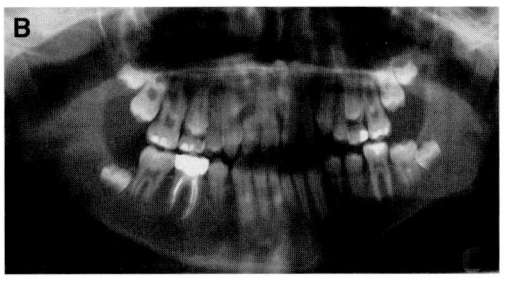

Fig. 2. (*A*) A 12-year-old boy who sustained a mandibular body fracture 5 years earlier as a result of child abuse. The original rigid fixation hardware subsequently was removed. Note screw holes evident through impacted mandibular premolar and supernumerary. (*B*) Postoperative panorex demonstrates removal of impacted mandibular premolar and supernumerary.

Impacted maxillary incisors

Impacted maxillary incisors are the most likely to demonstrate failure of eruption secondary to external factors, such as premature loss of the deciduous incisors, or as a result of history of previous trauma or infection. Whatever the cause, management remains relatively straightforward. If the root of the impacted incisor is fully formed, exposure remains dedicated to bonding and allowing orthodontic traction to move the tooth into the contiguous arch. The immature root should have eruption potential remaining, and it is not unreasonable to expose the tooth and allow for spontaneous eruption to take place over the following 8 weeks.

The incision is made on the crestal aspect of alveolar ridge with reflection of the tissue labially or palatally, depending on the radiographic assessment of location or physical confirmation of tooth location. The crown of the tooth is exposed with removal of the surrounding follicular tissue and bone reduction to below the gingival third of the crown. The tooth can be allowed to erupt spontaneously or be bonded for orthodontic traction.

Impacted molars

Of the impactions discussed, perhaps the unerupted molar has the most serious consequences to the alveolus and orthodontic rehabilitation. It is fortunate that this event remains rare. Management is directed at surgically assisted eruption or repositioning rather than exposure and bonding, which have not been proved to be effective because of anchorage issues. Root development can be used to predict, with relative surety, the outcome. As expected, molars with incomplete root formation have a higher success rate than molars with fully formed roots. Another alternative that has been used successfully involves removal of the impacted molar with subsequent use of the remaining distal molars, which are allowed to move forward and replace the extracted tooth. Skeletal anchorage combined with orthodontics, as discussed later, also may prove to be useful in this clinical problem.

The technique for surgical repositioning of the tooth requires a sulcular incision and removal of the remaining soft tissue and follicle covering the crown, if present. The tooth should be luxated gently into position just slightly below the occlusal plane. Bone should be removed judiciously so as to allow for a positive seat in the alveolus. Consideration also should be given to attaching the tooth to a continuous archwire (if present) to lend additional support (Figs. 3, 4).

Impacted supernumerary teeth

The most commonly found impacted supernumerary tooth in childhood is the mesiodens, followed by supernumerary maxillary incisors. The surgical management of these impactions should take into consideration the eruption status and root development of the adjacent permanent teeth. The mesiodens is frequently located on the palatal aspect of the alveolus, which should be confirmed radiographically before surgical removal is attempted. The surgeon also should ensure that the adjacent permanent central incisors have completed one half to two thirds of their root development, which decreases the likelihood of injury to the permanent dentition. The impacted supernumerary central incisor, in likewise fashion, should be confirmed in its position radiographically using the tube shift technique unless obviously palpable. Allowing for most root development to take place in the adjacent permanent dentition

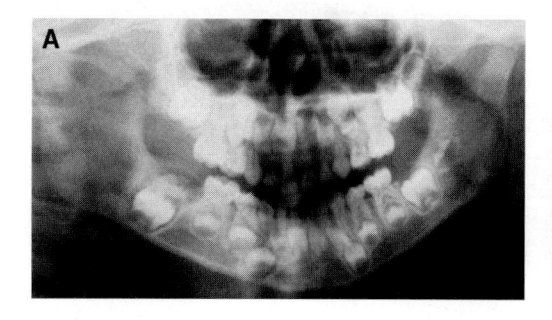

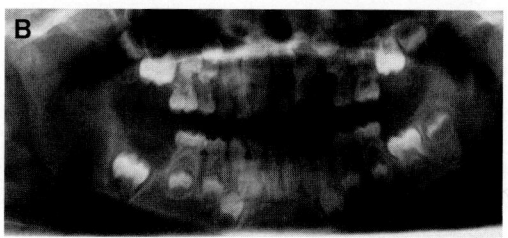

Fig. 3. (*A*) Impending eruption failure of mandibular first molar secondary to the presence of odontoma superiorly. (*B*) Postoperative panorex demonstrates removal of pathologic lesion.

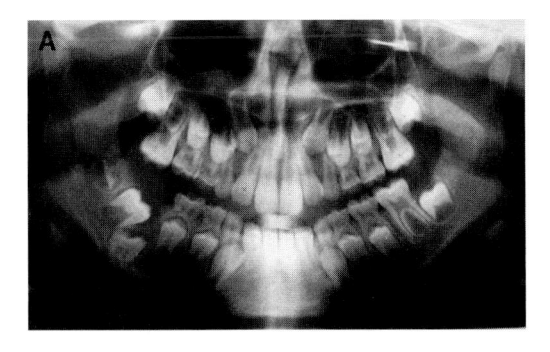

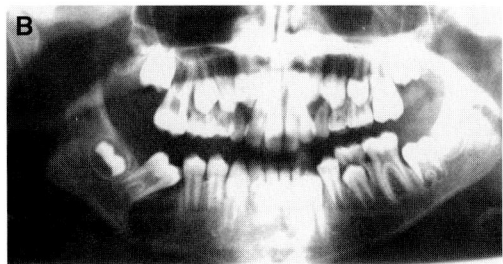

Fig. 4. (*A*) Eruption failure of mandibular first molar. (*B*) Postoperative radiograph demonstrates removal of the impacted mandibular first molar.

decreases the incidence of injury to those teeth. The management of fourth molars is more pertinent to a discussion concerning third molars and is outside the scope of this article. Uncommonly, impacted supernumerary premolars are diagnosed. The removal of these teeth is similar to the management of unerupted premolars. From a timing and growth perspective, however, a surgeon should allow for most root formation to occur in the adjacent permanent teeth to lessen the chance for injury. The supernumerary tooth also should be identifiable radiographically and its position in the alveolus confirmed before attempting removal. In the mandible, the surgeon should be cognizant of the location of the inferior alveolar canal and mental foramen in relation to the impacted supernumerary tooth.

Impacted teeth in the patient with cleft lip and palate

In addition to numerous other clinical challenges, an infant born with cleft lip and palate often presents with impacted and supernumerary teeth later in childhood. The staged reconstructive approach for management of these children frequently calls for bone graft reconstruction of the cleft maxilla [8–10]. This procedure usually is undertaken based on a child's dental age. The surgeon should allow for two-thirds formation of the canine root before graft placement. The cleft maxilla significantly complicates the removal of impacted and supernumerary teeth. Ideally, any attempt at removal of these teeth should be accomplished at the time of bone graft placement. The problematic teeth are usually located in the readily adjacent paracleft regions of the alveolus, and the soft tissue dissection performed during the course of bone graft reconstruction is more than sufficient to provide access for removal of the teeth. Contemporary soft tissue flap design for closure of the cleft maxillary skeletal defect usually consists of the sliding advancement flap or the vestibular (cheek) rotational flap. In either case, any attempt to retrieve an impacted tooth from the cleft site before bone graft reconstruction may compromise the vascular supply to the later elevated soft tissue used in closure of the defect. Scarring from removal of the impacted tooth only serves to increase technical difficulty during bone grafting. From a psychological standpoint, children with facial clefts are understandably "orally defensive," and the number of surgical procedures a child must undergo always should be mitigated by this consideration. Rarely, because of presurgical requirements during the first phase of orthodontic treatment, it may become necessary to remove an impacted tooth before bone graft reconstruction. This situation should be approached with caution because of the potential negative outcome for the reasons stated previously. In this case, the surgeon who removes the tooth should be thoroughly familiar with the planned approach for

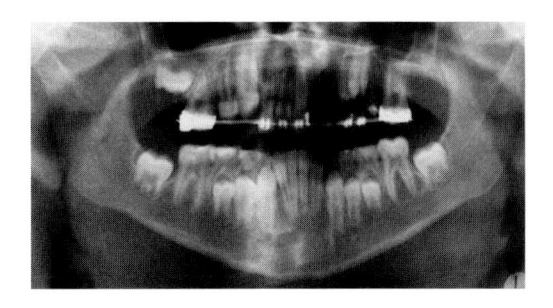

Fig. 5. Child with unilateral cleft lip and palate in phase I orthodontic care before bone grafting. Note impacted supernumerary in cleft site.

elevating the soft tissue flaps during bone grafting. When designing the incision and minimizing the dissection required for tooth removal, every attempt should be made not to compromise future circulation and viability of the tissues surrounding the premaxilla. This is especially true of children born with bilateral cleft lip and palate (Fig. 5) [11].

Advanced imaging techniques

Cone beam CT scanners are based on volumetric tomography, a principle that uses a two-dimensional extended detector and a three-dimensional x-ray beam. This configuration allows for a single rotation of the gantry to generate multiple basis images of the entire region of interest. Cone beam CT systems are well suited for imaging of the craniofacial area; the robotic hardware and acquisition software are controlled by personal computers. They provide good images of highly contrasted structures and are useful for evaluating bone. They are capable of providing submillimeter resolution images, with short scanning times (10–70 sec) and greatly reduced radiation dose compared with conventional CT scans. Because the data are volumetric, images can be generated in any plane with equal resolution. In particular, numerous display modes unique to maxillofacial imaging are available. Although current limitations exist in the application of this technology for soft tissue imaging, it has proved to be an effective clinical tool in the

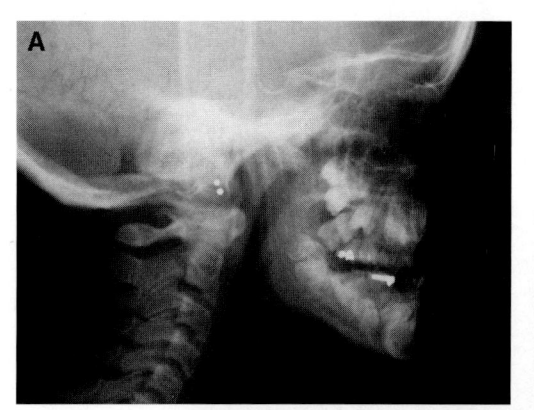

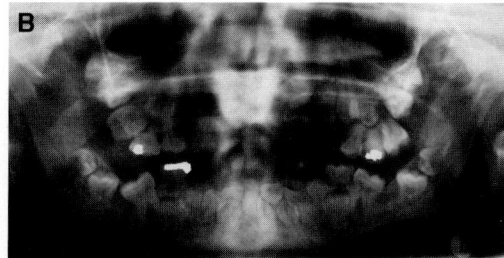

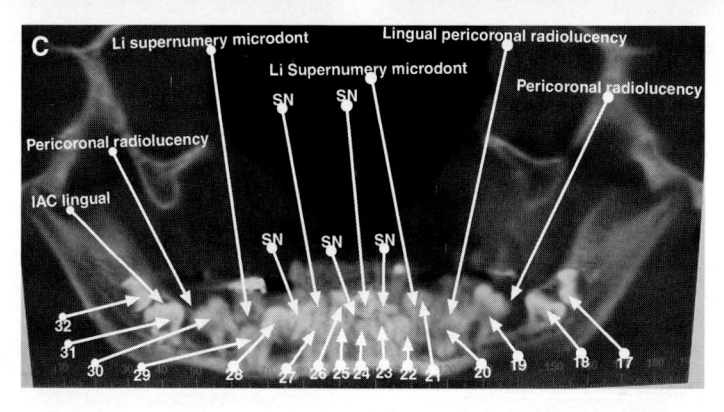

Fig. 6. (*A*) Lateral cephalometric radiograph of a 13-year-old child with cleidocranial dysostosis. (*B*) Panoramic radiograph demonstrates multiple impacted and supernumerary teeth in the same child. (*C*) Cone beam CT panoramic view of same child with overlay of comments by oral and maxillofacial radiologist identifies all permanent teeth and supernumerary teeth. (*D*) Cropped 0.4-mm axial images at the level of the alveolus in the maxilla (*top*) and mandible (*lower*) identifies supernumerary teeth, retained deciduous teeth, and pericoronal pathology. (*E*) Volumetric three-dimensional reconstructions with minor transparency that provide images in right (*A*), left (*B*), AP (*C*), and 30° superior anteroposterior (*D*) projections demonstrate retained deciduous teeth and orientation of supernumerary and unerupted teeth. (*F*) Volumetric three-dimensional reconstructions with minor transparency that provide cropped images in right and left inferior 30° oblique posteroanterior projections demonstrate retained deciduous teeth and orientation of supernumerary and unerupted teeth.

management of difficult or numerous impacted teeth. With this new technology, oral and maxillofacial radiologists have the ability to help surgeons identify teeth correctly, anatomically provide accurate information concerning the relative proximity of structures within the operative field (such as the inferior alveolar nerve), and provide an incredibly detailed roadmap as to the location of the teeth in question within the maxillae. One potential drawback to the use of this emerging technology is cost, and although not prohibitive, it is still a substantial concern. In the authors' opinion, however, this concern is mitigated effectively by the importance of the information provided and its potential to improve operative ease and patient safety.

Impacted teeth in patients with craniofacial disorders

Craniofacial syndromes present with varying degrees of oral and facial malformations. One aspect pertinent to the comprehensive management of this group of patients is a functional and aesthetic dentition. Impacted teeth can present an obstacle to achieving full rehabilitation and as such must be dealt

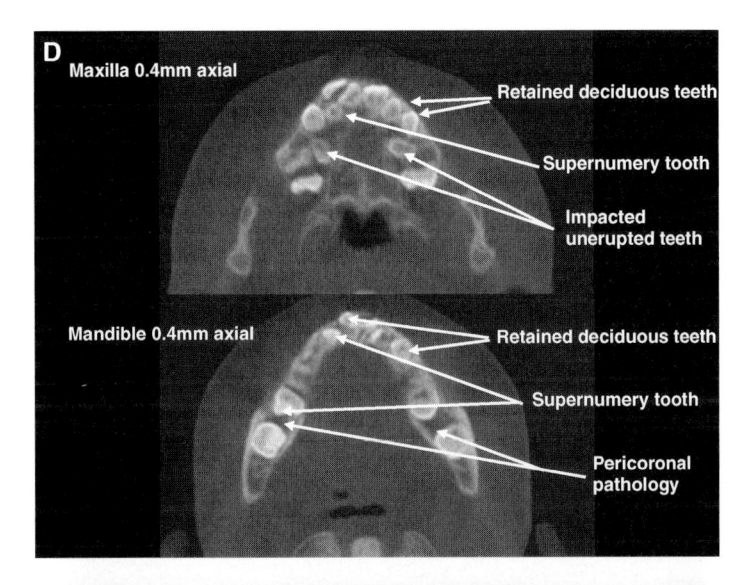

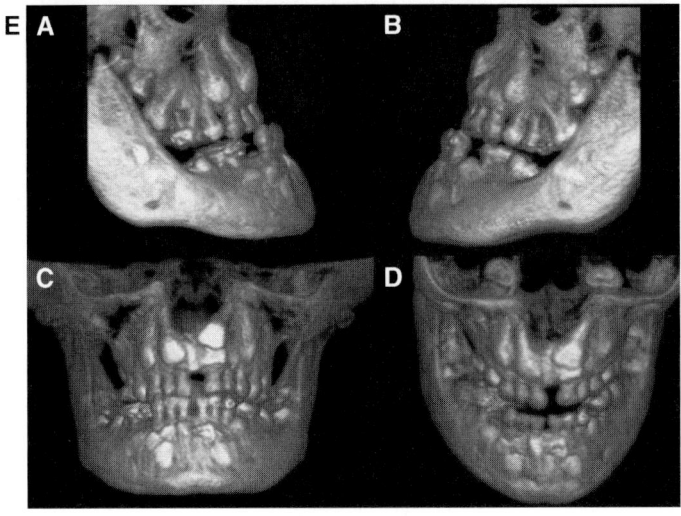

Fig. 6 (*continued*).

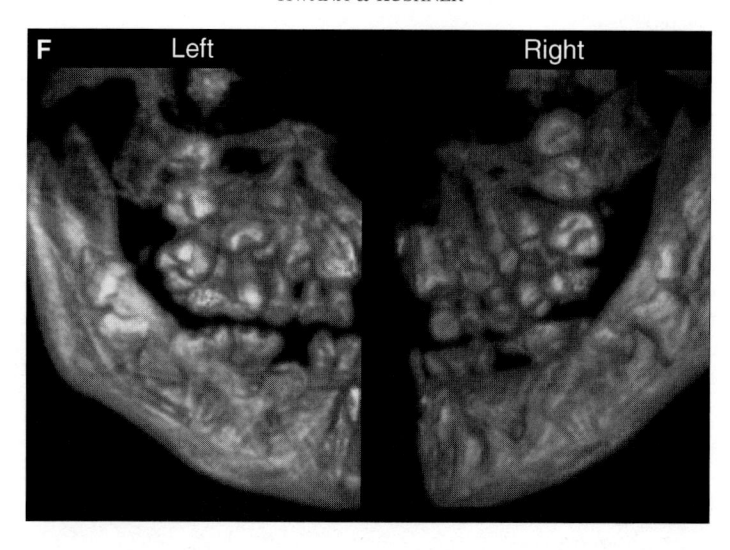

Fig. 6 (*continued*).

with during treatment planning. Although any child with a craniofacial anomaly can have an impacted or supernumerary tooth, there are certain syndromes in which this becomes a pronounced problem. These syndromes include certain craniostenoses and require a mature level of management, taking into consideration the sequential nature of their staged reconstructive efforts. Once incorporated into the treatment plan, however, they usually do not require significantly greater technical management than in nonsyndromic children. The craniofacial syndrome that is most often related when discussing impacted teeth is cleidocranial dysostosis [12,13]. Children with this syndrome present with frontal bossing, absent clavicles, skeletal facial deformity, and multiple impacted teeth. In addition to the other craniofacial concerns, their dental issues often become paramount in management. The treatment planning and technical execution for the removal of supernumerary teeth and assisted eruption of the other teeth in children with this craniofacial anomaly are arguably some of the most challenging procedures in dentoalveolar surgery and orthodontics to accomplish (Fig. 6).

The study of the orthodontically assisted eruption of impacted teeth in children with cleidocranial dysostosis is the study of mechanics. The objective goal of getting the teeth into the arch in a functional position rests with the surgeon and orthodontist to collaborate effectively and create useful anchorage. With this concept in mind, traditional treatment planning should center on getting the first molars (if present) into the arch. Once this stage is complete, attention is directed anteriorly and teeth should be erupted into the arch using the stable first molars as anchorage [14]. Occasionally, interarch elastic can be applied carefully to aid in eruption. The formation of the supernumerary teeth also can be somewhat predictable. Often, supernumerary teeth form in the incisor region from age 5 to 7 years, whereas the posterior supernumerary teeth form several years later. Cone beam CT technology is useful in this group of patients and should be used to aid surgeons and orthodontists in treatment planning. The advent of plate- and screw-type skeletal anchorage has the potential to revolutionize this treatment concept. If applied selectively, anchor screws and plates should make treatment planning substantially more straightforward for these children. Theoretically, it would allow surgeons and orthodontists to select teeth for eruption and assist the process as needed with anchorage placed in areas of maximal mechanical advantage.

Summary

Ankylosis remains one of the major complications associated with impacted teeth in children. Orthodontically assisted eruption of an ankylosed tooth may intrude or displace the adjacent teeth. Where arch length discrepancy is not present, impacted teeth should alert the surgeon to this possibility. Children who undergo orthodontically assisted eruption should be followed closely to ensure that movement of an impacted tooth is occurring. In general, the removal or assisted eruption of impacted teeth in children requires a thoughtful interdisciplinary evaluation between the surgeon and orthodontist/primary dental care provider. Factors that must be considered include operative feasibility, orthodontic management, future growth, and psychosocial considerations. The use of emerging technology, such as cone beam CT and skeletal anchorage, should better equip surgeons to navigate the anatomy three dimensionally and provide assistance in management of difficult cases.

Acknowledgments

The authors wish to express their sincere appreciation to Dr. William C. Scarfe for his outstanding radiographic interpretation and assessment of our patients.

References

[1] Gorlin RJ, Cohen MM, Hennekam RC. Syndromes of the head and neck. 4th edition. Oxford: Oxford University Press; 2001.
[2] Trankmann J. The frequency of retention of permanent teeth. Dtsch Zahnarztl Z 1973;28:415–20.
[3] Bass T. Observation on the misplaced upper canine tooth. Dent Pract Dent Rec 1967;18:25–33.
[4] Jacobs SG. Localization of the unerupted maxillary canine. Am J Orthod Dentofacial Orthop 1999;115: 314–22.
[5] Felsenfeld AL, Aghaloo T. Surgical exposure of impacted teeth. Oral Maxillofac Surg Clin N Am 2002; 14(2):187–99.
[6] Kaban LB, Troulis MJ. Pediatric oral and maxillofacial surgery. Philadelphia: Elsevier; 2004. p. 125–45.
[7] Becker A, Shpack N, Shteyer A. Attachment bonding to impacted teeth at the time of surgical exposure. Eur J Orthod 1996;18:457–63.
[8] Abyholm F, Bergland O, Semb G. Secondary bone grafting of alveolar clefts. Scand J Plast Reconstr Surg 1981;15:127–40.
[9] Boyne PJ, Sands NR. Secondary bone grafting of alveolar and palatal clefts. J Oral Surg 1976;30:80.
[10] Bergland O, Semb G, Abyholm F. Elimination of residual alveolar clefts by secondary bone grafting and subsequent orthodontic treatment. Cleft Palate J 1986;23:175–205.
[11] Fridrich KL. Management of impacted teeth in patients with congenital clefts. Oral Maxillofac Surg Clin N Am 1993;5(1):105–10.
[12] Jenson BL, Kreiborg S. Development of the dentition in cleidocranial dysplasia. J Oral Pathol Med 1990; 19:89.
[13] Jenson BL, Kreiborg S. Dental treatment strategies in cleidocranial dysplasia. Br Dent J 1992;21:242.
[14] Ferraro NF. Pediatric dentoalveolar surgery. Oral Maxillofac Surg Clin N Am 1994;6(1):51–67.

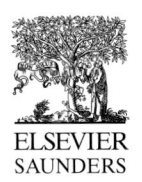

Dental Implants in Children

Jaime S. Brahim, DDS, MS

National Institutes of Health, National Institute of Dental and Craniofacial Research, Building 10, Room 1N 117, MSC 1191, 10 Center Drive, Bethesda, MD 20892, USA

In adult patients, implant success depends on the quality and quantity of bone, treatment planning, sound surgical technique, optimal restorative prostheses, and good long-term oral hygiene. The same factors apply to the placement of implants in children and adolescents, but the unique and critical difference between pediatric and adult patients is that children have ongoing dental and skeletal growth, which may make outcomes less predictable. Only a few reports specifically have discussed the use of endosseous implants in children [1–5]. The last consensus development from The National Institutes of Health on Dental Implants concluded that "children need special consideration given long-term morbidity concerns, requirements of growth, manual dexterity, and coping skills" [6].

Some children and adolescents have anodontia, partial anodontia, congenitally missing teeth, and lost teeth as a result of trauma, and they may benefit from early placement of dental implants. Clinicians should have an understanding of the potential risks involved in placing implants in jaws that are still growing and developing and consider the effect that implants have on craniofacial growth. Implants may act as ankylotic teeth and fail to move together with the surrounding structures, which produces an infraocclusion that leads to difficulties with prosthetics. Young patients may require general anesthesia for the procedure and there may be limited cooperation in maintaining good oral hygiene.

Facial growth

This article does not intend to cover in great detail craniofacial growth, because there are excellent reviews by Cronin and Oesterle [7–9] that describe this process elegantly. The studies of Bjork in the 1960s demonstrated the maxillary and mandibular growth radiographically with the use of skeletal implants [10]. It is essential that clinicians understand the dynamic development of these young patients and the effects of skeletal growth on implants. Osseointegrated implants can be considered analogous to ankylosed teeth that remain stationary in bone.

The amount of growth of a particular person is specific to that individual and is influenced by many factors, including genetics and confounding factors, such as chronic illness. Growth determination is an important factor when planning implant placement in children and adolescents. No reliable indicator is available to determine when growth has ceased, however, although a good quality method is the use of serial cephalometric radiographs taken 6 months apart with superimposed orthodontic tracings. If no changes occur over a period of 1 year, one may assume that the growth is complete.

Maxillary growth

As a general rule, the midface grows in a downward and forward direction relative to the anterior cranial base, with maxillary growth occurring as a result of passive displacement and enlargement. During the early years of growth, passive growth is the predominant factor, whereas growth from the enlargement of the maxilla itself becomes the major factor after 7 years of age. Maxillary growth occurs in the anteroposterior, transverse, and vertical dimensions. The transverse growth of the maxilla is controlled mainly by the midpalatal suture and ends with eruption of the second permanent molars. Anteroposterior maxillary growth occurs at the sutures of the

E-mail address: jbrahim@dir.nidcr.nih.gov

palatine bones and at the maxillary tuberosities and is complete by the onset of puberty, with subsequent growth occurring primarily in the vertical plane. Vertical growth of the maxilla occurs by resorption on the nasal surface and deposition on the palatal and alveolar surfaces. Given this developmental mechanism, vertical maxillary skeletal growth dramatically affects the placement of an implant in this area at an early age.

Mandibular growth

Growth of the mandible is not as closely associated with the cranial base as is the maxilla. The pattern of mandibular growth closely follows that of general body growth, with an increase experienced during puberty. The studies of Bjork using metallic implants showed that the mandible rolls forward, with apposition below the symphysis and resorption below the gonial angle, and tends to rotate with the center of rotation, which is influenced by direction of condylar growth. The transverse growth of the mandible occurs primarily in the posterior mandible, whereas the width in the anterior mandible stabilizes relatively early before the eruption of deciduous teeth.

There is considerable individual variation in facial growth [11]. Predictions from general databases are not necessarily helpful for clinicians who are trying to decide on the timing of placement of dental implants in children.

Table 1
Craniofacial growth

Patient #	Age	Sex	Year follow-up	SN	S PG	Angle(°)
1	10 y, 5 mo	male	0 y	72.0 mm	121.0 mm	78
			1 y	73.0 mm	123.0 mm	78
			2 y	77.0 mm	130.0 mm	78
			3 y	79.0 mm	132.0 mm	80
2	9 y, 8 mo	male	0 y	74.0 mm	117.0 mm	65
			1 y	75.0 mm	117.0 mm	67
			2 y	76.0 mm	119.0 mm	67
			3 y	78.0 mm	121.0 mm	69
3	10 y, 3 mo	male	0 y	69.0 mm	107.0 mm	63
			1 y	70.0 mm	109.0 mm	63
			2 y	73.0 mm	112.0 mm	65
4	12 y, 2 mo	male	0 y	78.0 mm	129.0 mm	84
			1 y	86.0 mm	139.0 mm	87
			2 y	87.0 mm	140.0 mm	88
5	12 y, 7 mo	male	0 y	73.0 mm	124.0 mm	80
			1 y	79.0 mm	135.0 mm	85
			2 y	80.0 mm	137.0 mm	86
6	12 y, 3 mo	male	0 y	71.0 mm	125.0 mm	69
			2 y	73.0 mm	130.0 mm	76
			4 y	74.0 mm	132.0 mm	80
7	12 y, 9 mo	male	0 y	76.0 mm	122.0 mm	43
			1 y	76.0 mm	122.0 mm	43
			2 y	77.0 mm	125.0 mm	45
			3 y	79.0 mm	128.0 mm	46
8	12 y, 8 mo	male	0 y	77.0 mm	134.0 mm	73
			1 y	78.0 mm	136.0 mm	73
			2 y	78.0 mm	138.0 mm	70
			3 y	81.0 mm	145.0 mm	73
9	13 y, 9 mo	female	0 y	76.0 mm	132.0 mm	72
			1 y	77.0 mm	134.0 mm	70
			2 y	78.0 mm	135.0 mm	72
10	14 y, 5 mo	male	0 y	78.5 mm	129.0 mm	81
			1 y	80.0 mm	131.0 mm	84
			3 y	80.0 mm	131.0 mm	85

Implants in children

Animal studies

Odman and colleagues [12] and Thilander and colleagues [13] developed an animal model to determine whether implants placed in a growing child behave as normally erupting or ankylosed teeth during the dynamic phase of growth. The authors selected six growing Pigham pigs; one served as a control and the others received four fixtures each—three in the lower jaw and one in the upper jaw. Two mandibular implants were placed on one side (in the mesial socket of the second deciduous premolar, and deciduous canine), the third implant was placed in the area of the first deciduous premolar on the opposite side, and the fourth implant was placed in the maxilla in the region of the deciduous lateral incisor. All of

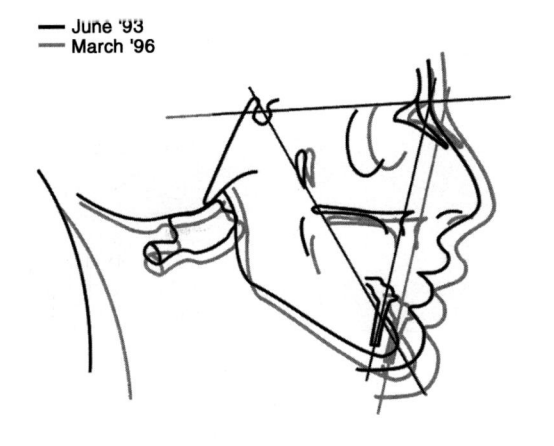

Fig. 1. Cephalometric radiograph showing craniofacial growth.

Table 2
Implant position

Patient #	Age	Sex	Years follow-up	Horizontal measurement	Vertical measurement
1	10 y, 5 mo	male	0 y	3.0 mm	3.0 mm
			1 y	3.0 mm	3.0 mm
			2 y	3.0 mm	3.0 mm
			3 y	3.0 mm	3.0 mm
2	9 y, 8 mo	male	0 y	8.0 mm	3.0 mm
			1 y	8.0 mm	3.0 mm
			2 y	8.0 mm	3.0 mm
			3 y	8.0 mm	3.0 mm
3	10 y, 3 mo	male	0 y	9.0 mm	4.0 mm
			1 y	9.0 mm	4.0 mm
4	12 y, 2 mo	male	0 y	7.0 mm	9.0 mm
			1 y	7.0 mm	9.0 mm
			2 y	7.0 mm	9.0 mm
5	12 y, 7 mo	male	0 y	6.0 mm	5.0 mm
			1 y	6.0 mm	5.0 mm
			2 y	6.0 mm	5.0 mm
6	12 y, 3 mo	male	0 y	10.0 mm	10.0 mm
			2 y	10.0 mm	10.0 mm
			4 y	10.0 mm	10.0 mm
7	12 y, 9 mo	male	0 y	11.0 mm	0.5 mm
			1 y	11.0 mm	0.5 mm
			2 y	11.0 mm	0.5 mm
			3 y	11.0 mm	0.5 mm
8	12 y, 8 mo	male	0 y	8.0 mm	5.0 mm
			1 y	8.0 mm	5.0 mm
			2 y	8.0 mm	5.0 mm
			3 y	8.0 mm	5.0 mm
9	13 y, 9 mo	female	0 y	13.0 mm	7.0 mm
			1 y	13.0 mm	7.0 mm
			2 y	13.0 mm	7.0 mm
10	14 y, 5 mo	male	0 y	8.0 mm	2.0 mm
			1 y	8.0 mm	2.0 mm
			3 y	8.0 mm	2.0 mm

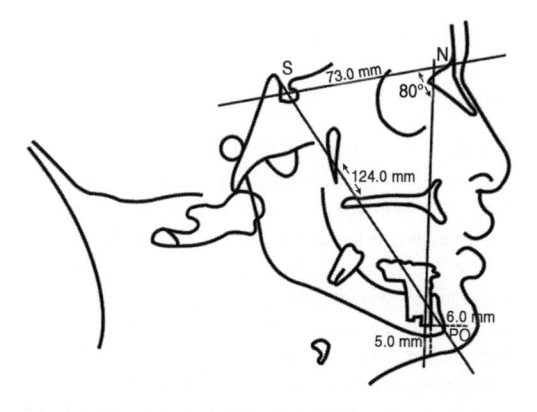

Fig. 2. Cephalometric radiograph showing position of implant.

the fixtures were placed in areas in which dentoalveolar growth was expected. Amalgam markers placed in the buccal cortical layer of the alveolar process adjacent to the implants were used to record growth. In the control pig, only amalgam markers were placed but no implants. The pigs were monitored for 165 days with intraoral and lateral cephalometric radiographs. Six of 20 implants failed to osseointegrate. Implants that integrated in the mandible became displaced to stand lingually in the alveolar process; implants placed in the maxilla

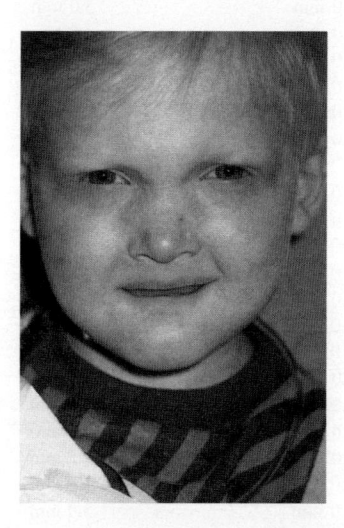

Fig. 3. Three-year-old white male with X-linked hypohydrotic ectoderma dysplasia (Christ-Siemens-Touraine ectodermal dysplasia) had four mandibular and two maxillary IMZ press fit endosseous implants (Interpore International, Irvine, CA). (*From* Guckes A, McCarthy G, Brahim J. Use of endosseous implants in a 3-year-old child with ectodermal dysplasia: case report and 5-year follow-up. Pediatr Dent 1997;19:282–5; with permission.)

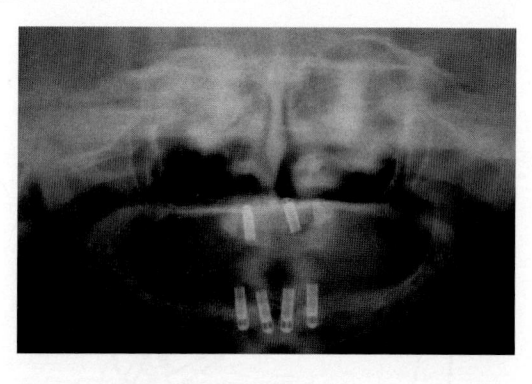

Fig. 4. Panoramic radiograph demonstrates implant placement. Right maxillary implant failed to osseointegrated and was removed. Remaining five implants were osseointegrated. Remaining maxillary implant could not support a prosthesis, and primary closure was achieved without placing an abutment. (*From* Guckes A, McCarthy G, Brahim J. Use of endosseous implants in a 3-year-old child with ectodermal dysplasia: case report and 5-year follow-up. Pediatr Dent 1997;19:282–5; with permission.)

ended up palatally off the alveolar crest. The implants seemed to retard growth of the alveolar process and changed the eruption path of tooth germs located distal to the inserted implants. The results demonstrated that implants placed in the jaws of growing pigs did not behave like normally erupting teeth because the fixtures failed to move together with the adjacent teeth and behaved more like ankylosed teeth.

The authors concluded that it is difficult to correlate their experimental results to the human situation, but based on our knowledge of human maxillary and mandibular growth, osseointegrated implants should not be recommended for use in young children. A possible exception involves chil-

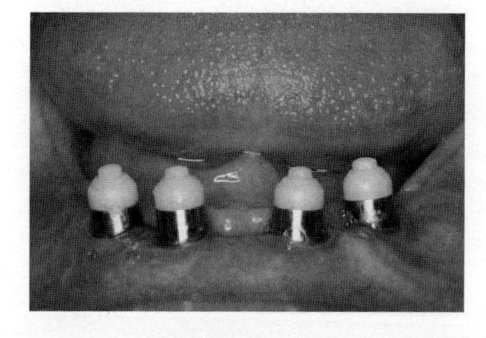

Fig. 5. One month after abutment connection to four mandibular implants. Soft tissue healing was uneventful. (*From* Guckes A, McCarthy G, Brahim J. Use of endosseous implants in a 3-year-old child with ectodermal dysplasia: case report and 5-year follow-up. Pediatr Dent 1997;19:282–5; with permission.)

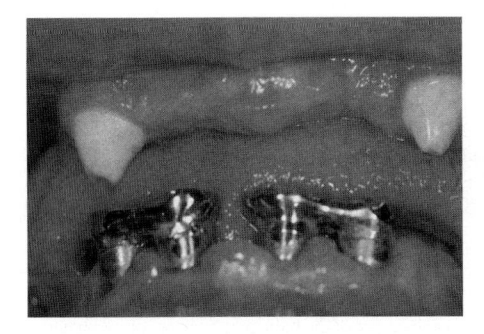

Fig. 6. Patient was fitted with conventional maxillary denture and mandibular overdenture supported by two cast gold bars secured to implants and separated in midline. During 5-year follow-up, prostheses were remade or relined to accommodate eruption of maxillary teeth and facial growth. (*From* Guckes A, McCarthy G, Brahim J. Use of endosseous implants in a 3-year-old child with ectodermal dysplasia: case report and 5-year follow-up. Pediatr Dent 1997;19:282–5; with permission.)

dren in whom growth and development does not follow normal patterns (eg, ectodermal dysplasia).

Endosseous implants in children and adolescents with ectodermal dysplasia

Ectodermal dysplasia is an inherited disorder in which at least two structures derived from the ectoderm are abnormal [14–17]. Oral findings

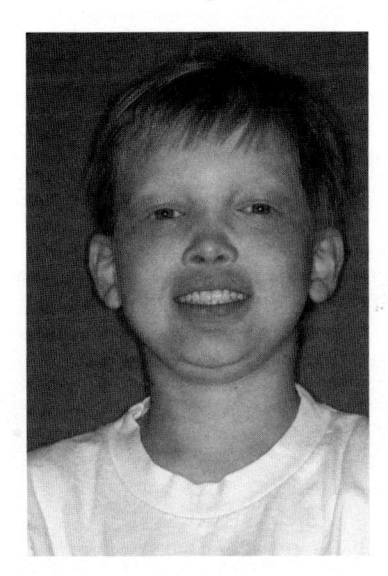

Fig. 7. Patient at age 8 years, 3 months. (*From* Guckes A, McCarthy G, Brahim J. Use of endosseous implants in a 3-year-old child with ectodermal dysplasia: case report and 5-year follow-up. Pediatr Dent 1997;19:282–5; with permission.)

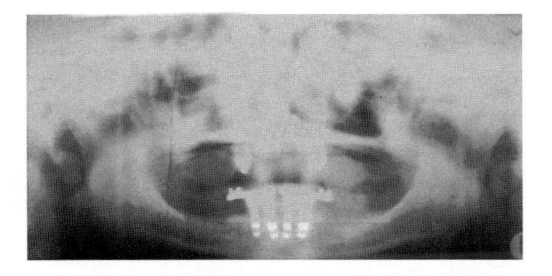

Fig. 8. Panoramic radiographs 5 years after implant placement. Position of implants in anterior mandible remains unchanged. Unloaded maxillary implant did not follow downward and forward growth of maxilla and currently is located in close proximity to floor of nose. (*From* Guckes A, McCarthy G, Brahim J. Use of endosseous implant in a 3-year-old child with ectodermal dysplasia: case report and 5-year follow-up. Pediatr Dent 1997;19:282–5; with permission.)

include multiple tooth abnormalities, such as anodontia, hypodontia, and tapered, malformed, and widely spaced teeth. Abnormal alveolar ridge development also may be present. Other physical signs can involve the sweat glands, scalp, hair, nails, skin pigmentation, and craniofacial structures (eg, cleft lip and palate). Children with ectodermal dysplasia do not have normal patterns of growth, and a risk and benefit analysis must be made to assess the value of implant placement, especially in the anterior mandible, where lateral growth is usually completed by 3 years of age.

The National Institute of Dental and Craniofacial Research conducted a prospective clinical trial that investigated the effects of endosseous dental implants on the mandibles of children with ectoderma dys-

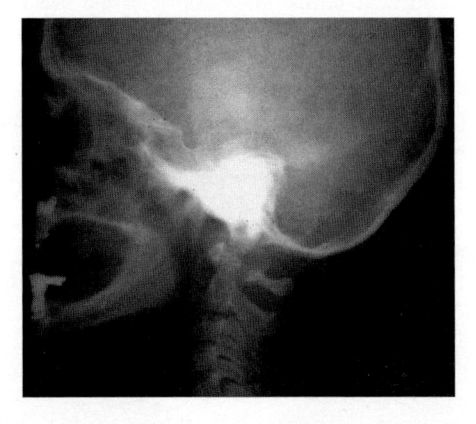

Fig. 9. Cephalometric radiograph of the same patient shown in Fig. 8. (*From* Guckes A, McCarthy G, Brahim J. Use of endosseous implant in a 3-year-old child with ectodermal dysplasia: case report and 5-year follow-up. Pediatr Dent 1997;19:282–5; with permission.)

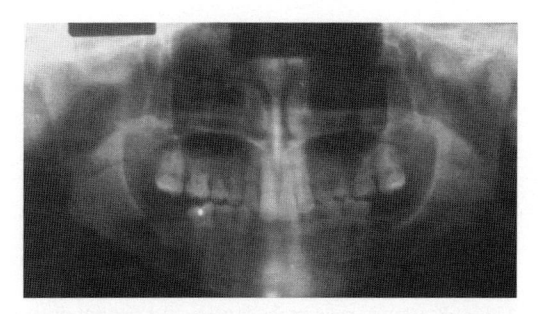

Fig. 10. Panorex of 13-year-old patient with ectodermia dysplasia and multiple missing teeth.

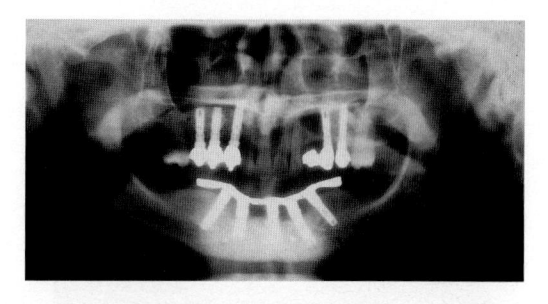

Fig. 12. Panorex of the patient at 18 years old with maxillary implants in place after final craniofacial growth.

plasia [1]. The purpose of this study was to determine if placement of endosseous implants influences growth and development of the craniomandibular complex and to identify the final position of the implant and the ability to fabricate a prosthesis. A total of 23 adolescent (ages 12–17) and 12 preadolescent (ages 7–11) patients were included in the study. The diagnosis of ectodermal dysplasia was established by a geneticist based on clinical examination. A minimum of 16 missing permanent teeth were needed for study inclusion. The craniofacial growth (Table 1) was monitored with lateral cephalometric radiographs by measuring point S to point N and point S to point Pg and then superimposing on point S along the line S N (Fig. 1). The position of implants within the mandible (Table 2) was measured on the cephalometric film by taking the most anterior and inferior image and measuring horizontally to the outer cortical plate of bone at the symphysis. The vertical measurement uses the most anterior corner of the implant that is placed vertically to the outer cortical plate of bone on the lower border of the mandible (Fig. 2).

A total of 255 implants was placed in 23 patients. Twenty-two implants failed, for a success rate of 91.3%. The success rate for the preadolescent group was 88% and 90% for the adolescent group. Given this success rate, the authors concluded that osseointegrated implants in children with ectodermal dysphasia seem to be a feasible treatment option. The mandibles of these patients continued to grow in a normal pattern, and the implants remained in the same position within the bone of the mandible.

Implants in children and adolescents

Indications for implant placement in children include congenital (eg, nonsyndromic hypodontia, cleft lip and palate, ectodermal dysplasia) and acquired (eg, teeth lost by dentoalveolar trauma and tumor resection) absence of teeth (Figs. 3–13). Contraindications to implant placement in the growing patient include adjacent primary teeth, remaining skeletal growth, inadequate quantity or quality of bone, inability to maintain hygiene, and unrealistic expectations of patient or parents.

During childhood, the anterior maxilla is the most traumatized region in the mouth. After tooth loss, 40% to 60% of the bone resorption occurs in the first year, mainly in the facial plate. Traditionally, therapeutic approaches to treat this condition have been removable partial dentures, fixed prostheses, and orthodontic movement of teeth to close spaces, all of which offer only temporary solutions.

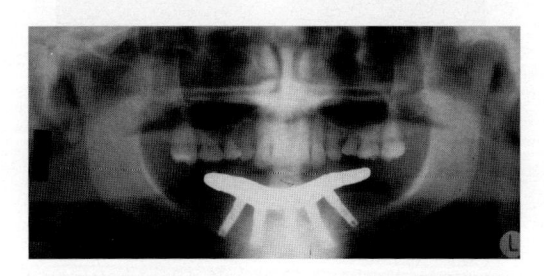

Fig. 11. Panorex of patient after removal of mandibular teeth and placement of five dental implants.

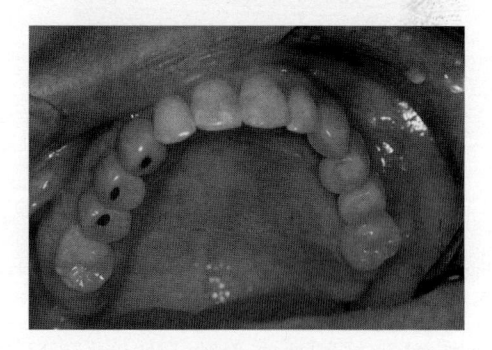

Fig. 13. Final maxillary restoration.

Ledermann and coworkers [11] reported a review of 42 implants placed in 34 patients with a mean age of 15.1 years. They reported a 90% success rate at a follow-up time of 35.5 months. The study reported a positive soft and osseous tissue reaction to the implant. The major complication reported was the ankylotic nature of the dental implant and its failure to respond to the vertical growth of the adjacent teeth and alveolus, which produced an infraocclusion of the implant.

I believe that for unaffected children, the following suggestions should be followed: (1) Extreme caution must be used in placing implants in children because of growth changes of the jaws and the dentition. (2) Whenever possible, implant placement should be delayed until age 15 for girls and 18 for boys. (3) Growing patients treated with dental implants should have adequate follow-up. (4) Further research is needed in the area of implants in growing children.

References

[1] Guckes AD, Brahim JS, McCarthy GR, et al. Using endosseous dental implants for patients with ectodermal dysplasia. J Am Dent Assoc 1991;122:59–62.

[2] Guckes AD, Scurria MS, King TS, et al. Prospective clinical trial of dental implants in persons with ectodermal dysplasia. J Prosthet Dent 2002;88:21.

[3] Kearns G, Sharma A, Perrott D, et al. Placement of endosseous implants in children and adolescents with hereditary ectodermal dysplasia. Oral Surg Oral Med Oral Pathol Oral Radiol Endod 1999;88:5.

[4] Thilander B, Odman J, Gröndahl K, et al. Osseointegrated implants in adolescents: an alternative in replacing missing teeth? Eur J Orthod 1994;16:84.

[5] Westwood RM, Duncan JM. Implants in adolescents: a literature review and case reports. Int J Oral Maxillofac Implants 1996;11:750.

[6] National Institutes of Health. Consensus development conference statement on dental implants. J Dent Educ 1988;52:824.

[7] Cronin Jr RJ, Oesterle LJ. Implant use in growing patients: treatment planning concerns. Dent Clin North Am 1998;42:1.

[8] Cronin Jr RJ, Oesterle LJ, Ranly DM. Mandibular implants and the growing patient. Int J Oral Maxillofac Implants 1994;9:55.

[9] Oesterle LJ, Cronin Jr RJ, Ranly DM. Maxillary implants and the growing patient. Int J Oral Maxillofac Implants 1993;8:377.

[10] Bjork A. Variations in the growth pattern of the human mandible: longitudinal radiographic study by the implant method. JD Res 1963;42:400–11.

[11] Ledermann PD, Hassell TM, Hefti AF. Osseointegrated dental implants as alternative therapy to bridge construction or orthodontics in young patients: seven years of clinical experience. Pediatr Dent 1993;15:327.

[12] Odman J, Grondahl K, Lekholm U, et al. The effect of osseointegrated implants on the dento-alveolar development: a clinical and radiographic study in growing pigs. Eur J Orthod 1991;13:279.

[13] Thilander B, Bodman J, Gröndahl K, et al. Aspects on osseointegrated implants inserted in growing jaws: a biometric and radiographic study in the young pig. Eur J Orthod 1992;14:99.

[14] Freire-Maia N. Ectodermal dysplasias. Hum Hered 1971;21:309.

[15] Lowry RB, Robinson GC, Miller JR. Hereditary ectodermal dysplasia: symptoms, inheritance patterns, differential diagnosis, management. Clin Pediatr (Phila) 1966;5:395.

[16] Guckes AD, McCarthy GR, Brahim J. Use of endosseous implants in a 3-year-old child with ectodermal dysplasia: case report and 5-year follow-up. Pediatr Dent 1997;19:282.

[17] Kere J, Srivastava AK, Montonen O, et al. X-linked anhidrotic (hypohidrotic) ectodermal dysplasia is caused by mutation in a novel transmembrane protein. Nat Genet 1996;13:409.

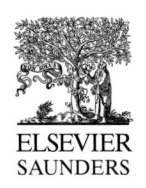

Soft-Tissue Lesions in Children

Dolphine Oda, BDS, MSc

Department of Oral and Maxillofacial Surgery, University of Washington, Box 357134, B-204 Health Sciences Building, Seattle, WA 98195, USA

Fibroma

Fibroma is a mass of collagenous connective tissue that typically presents as an exophytic, dome-shaped, smooth-surfaced, sessile or pedunculated nodule (Fig. 1A) on the buccal mucosa [1]. The most common cause is irritation, especially from chronic chewing of the area. Occasionally, it may represent a true benign neoplasm of fibrous connective tissue origin. Fibroma can affect patients of any age, including children, but it is more common in adults around 30 years of age and has no sex predilection [1]. It occurs anywhere in the oral cavity but most commonly on the buccal mucosa along the plane of the occlusal line, lips, lateral tongue, and gingiva. It can be pink, white, or red (if ulcerated) in color [1-3]. In individuals with dark skin, it can be gray or brown. Sizes range from a few millimeters to several centimeters in diameter, averaging 1 to 2 cm. Unless they are ulcerated, fibromas are usually asymptomatic. Histologically, fibromas are made up of a nodule of connective tissue, usually collagenous (Fig. 1B). The surface epithelium ranges from thin to thick and is usually covered by parakeratin or orthokeratin (Fig. 1B). Conservative surgical removal, whether conventional or laser, and cessation of the chewing habit qualify as appropriate treatment [1,2]. The likelihood of recurrence depends on whether the habit of cheek chewing continues. The differential diagnosis of fibromas of the buccal mucosa and lips should include salivary gland neoplasms.

E-mail address: doda@u.washington.edu

Giant cell fibroma

Giant cell fibroma is not related to peripheral giant cell granuloma. It is a benign nodule of fibrous connective tissue origin believed to be a variant of fibroma but with an unknown etiology; unlike in irritation fibroma, trauma is not implicated [4]. It occurs in patients younger than those with conventional irritation fibroma, usually in the first three decades of life. It is usually smaller than an irritation fibroma, averaging 5 mm in diameter [4,5]. It can be sessile or pedunculated and smooth surfaced (Fig. 2A) or bluntly papillary or lobular; the latter is sometimes clinically mistaken for a papilloma. Giant cell fibroma most commonly occurs on the gingiva, especially the mandibular area, followed by the tongue and palate. Histologically, it is made up of a nodule of delicate connective tissue with stellate fibroblasts, some with multiple nuclei (Fig. 2B) [5]. The surface epithelium is corrugated with slender rete pegs (Fig. 2B). The histology is similar to that of retrocuspid papilla. Treatment ranges from simple surgical excision to laser surgery. The prognosis is good, and the lesion rarely recurs.

Pyogenic granuloma

Pyogenic granuloma constitutes 85% of all reactive gingival swelling, representing a profuse mass of vascular granulation tissue [6]. Local irritants such as excessive plaque, sharp fillings, and dental calculus can induce the lesion. It can occur anywhere in the oral cavity and skin, especially the tongue, lips, fingers, and nail beds [6]. In the mouth, it occurs most commonly in the gingiva (Fig. 3A), especially the

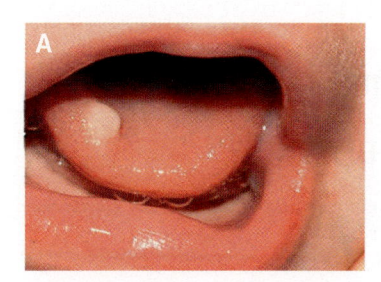

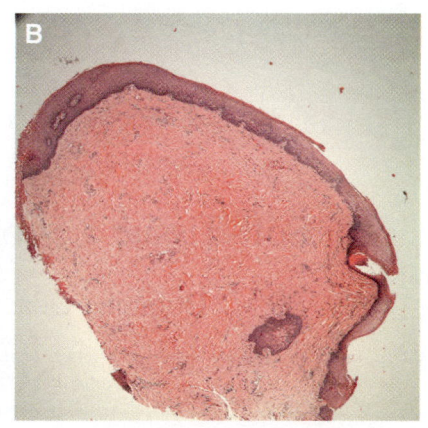

Fig. 1. (A) Fibroma, white dome-shaped and smooth-surfaced nodule on the anterior lateral dorsal surface of the tongue. (B) Fibroma, low-power view demonstrating a mass of collagenous collective tissue.

maxillary buccal and interproximal gingiva [6,7]. Occasionally, it may surround the tooth (Fig. 3B). It is usually highly vascular, fast growing, exophytic, lobular, sessile, and ulcerated (Fig. 3B), or covered by a pseudomembrane. The color changes from red to pink when it starts to heal. It occurs at any age with a slight predilection for young females, affecting 1% of pregnant women. Pyogenic granuloma is usually painless except during eating, when bleeding and pain are described [6]. It can occur from an extraction socket in response to an irritant left in the socket. Histologically, it presents as a mass of loose and vascular granulation tissue, usually with an ulcerated or eroded surface epithelium and many inflammatory cells (Fig. 3B). Various treatment modalities are available, including excision with removal of the local irritant, laser surgery, and intralesional injection with absolute alcohol, steroids, and botulinum toxin [7,8]. Scaling and polishing before surgical removal help shrink the lesion. The prognosis is good, although recurrence is possible, especially during pregnancy.

Peripheral ossifying fibroma

Peripheral ossifying fibroma constitutes 10% of all reactive gingival swelling. It consists of a moderately cellular fibrous connective tissue mass with bony trabeculae or cementumlike hard tissue. It has been reported rarely on edentulous alveolar mucosa. It originates from the periodontal ligament or the periosteum. The lesion is most common in young patients from 1 and 19 years of age and has a predi-

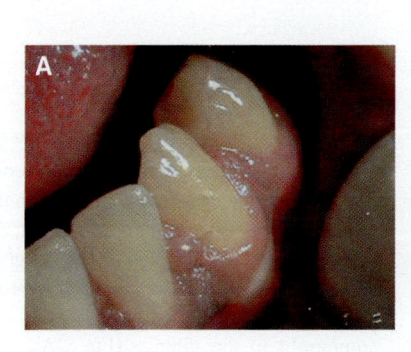

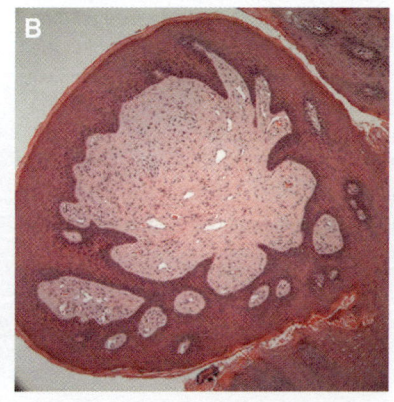

Fig. 2. (A) Giant cell fibroma, exophytic smooth-surfaced pink nodule on the buccal gingiva between the mandibular canine and lateral incisor. (B) Giant cell fibroma, low-power view demonstrating a mass of loose fibrous connective tissue with stellate fibroblasts.

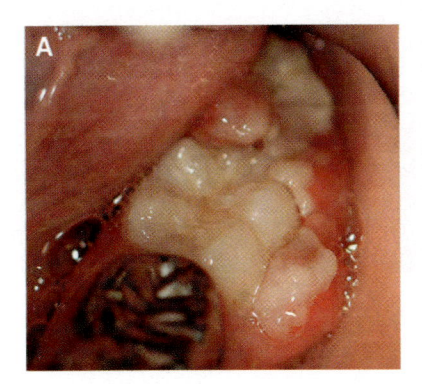

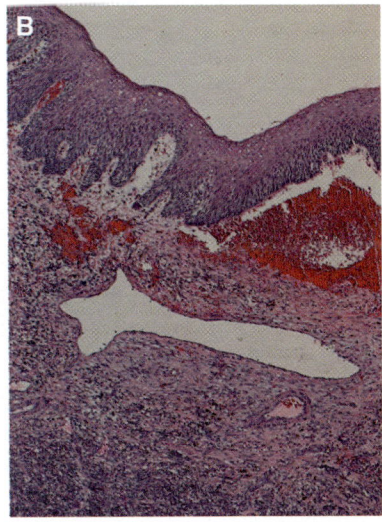

Fig. 3. (A) Pyogenic granuloma, ulcerated and erythematous mass surrounding mandibular molar tooth. (B) Pyogenic granuloma, low-power view demonstrating a mass of vascular granulation tissue.

lection for females over males by a 3:2 ratio [9–11]. It occurs exclusively on the gingiva, especially the anterior gingiva (Fig. 4A), with a slight predilection to the maxilla and rare presentation in primary teeth [11]. It is usually sessile and exophytic and often ulcerated, presenting as well-demarcated sessile nodules that are firm or hard depending on the amount of ossification and calcifications [9–11]. Peripheral ossifying fibroma is usually pink but can be focally red if ulcerated (Fig. 4A). Histologically, peripheral ossifying fibroma is made up of a moderately cellular mass of fibrous connective tissue with calcifications ranging from cementumlike material to calcified bony trabeculae with viable osteocytes (Fig. 4B). The surface epithelium overlying the mass is usually ulcerated. Deep surgical excision to include the periodontal ligament is the preferred treatment, although laser removal has been used effectively. Deep surgery may lead to a gingival defect, which would require gingival grafting, especially if it is located on the anterior buccal gingiva [11]. There is a 16% to 20% recurrence rate [11].

Peripheral giant cell granuloma

Peripheral giant cell granuloma (Fig. 5A) constitutes less than 5% of all reactive gingival swelling

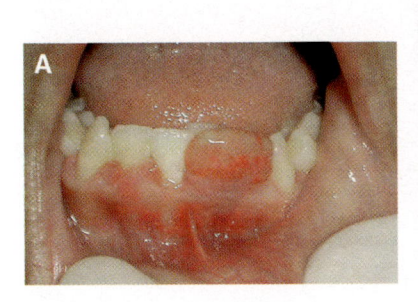

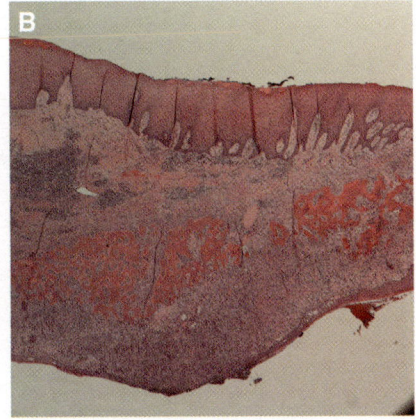

Fig. 4. (A) Peripheral ossifying fibroma, ulcerated exophytic nodule, labial gingiva, anterior mandible. (B) Peripheral ossifying fibroma, nonulcerated moderately cellular mass of fibrous connective tissue with bony trabeculae.

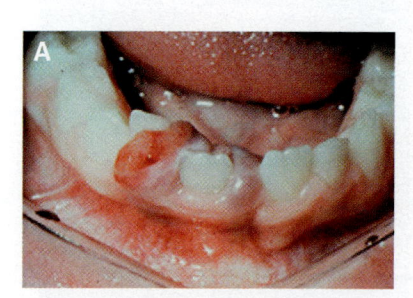

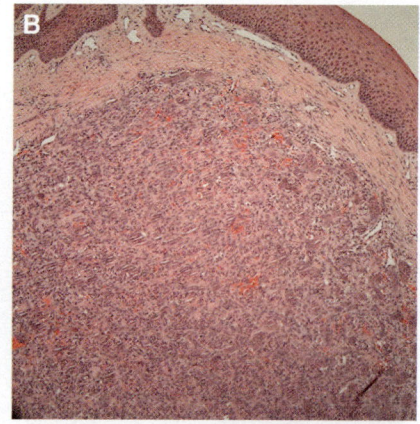

Fig. 5. (*A*) Peripheral giant cell granuloma, colliform mass emanating from the gingiva between the first and second primary molars. (*B*) Peripheral giant cell granuloma, low-power view demonstrating nodule of cellular granulation tissue with many giant cells.

and consists of a hyperplastic mass of vascular granulation tissue with many osteoclastlike multinucleated giant cells (Fig. 5B). It presents as a lobular, purplish-blue exophytic nodule exclusively on the gingiva, both edentulous and dentate, and usually anterior to the molars [12,13]. It originates from the periodontal ligament or the periosteum. It occurs across a wide age range in children and young adults, with females affected more than males by a 2:1 ratio [12–14]. It presents as a sessile or pedunculated and smooth surfaced or lobular lesion. Although usually painless, it can occasionally be ulcerated, painful, and accompanied by bleeding [12–14]. Like pyogenic granuloma, it is usually present on the buccal or lingual gingiva or between teeth but can occasionally surround the teeth [12–14] and act aggressively by displacing teeth much like a sarcoma (Fig. 5A) [12]. It can also resorb the underlying bone in a smooth and concave "saucer-like" manner. Complete excision including curettage of underlying bone is the preferred treatment. The prognosis is good, with a recurrence rate of approximately 10% [14].

Congenital epulis of the newborn

Congenital epulis of the newborn is a rare benign hamartoma of large cells with granular cytoplasm occurring at birth on the anterior alveolar ridge (Fig. 6A). The histogenesis is unknown, and the lesion is not related to the adult granular cell tumor [15]. Immunohistochemistry studies suggest myofibroblastic differentiation or pericytic origin. It oc-

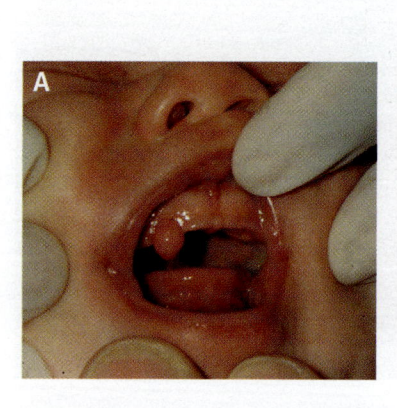

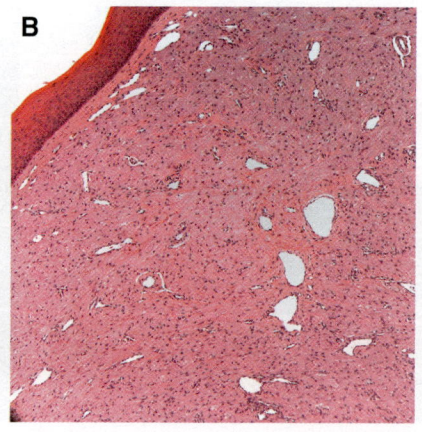

Fig. 6. (*A*) Congenital epulis of the newborn, smooth-surfaced exophytic pink nodule on the anterior maxillary alveolar ridge. (*B*) Congenital epulis of the newborn, low-power view demonstrating sheets of large cells with pale granular cytoplasm.

curs more commonly in females than males, with a 9:1 female-to-male ratio [15], mostly in the anterior alveolar ridge, with a 2:1 ratio of occurrence in the maxilla over the mandible (Fig. 6A). It usually presents as a single pedunculated or sessile, lobular, or smooth-surfaced nodule, typically several centimeters in diameter. It is also described in multiples [16] and in areas other than the alveolar mucosa, such as the tongue; however, such cases are rare. The lesion is sometimes large enough to interfere with feeding and breathing [17]. Histologically, it consists of sheets of large round cells with pale granular cytoplasm and small round-to-oval nuclei (Fig. 6B). The overlying epithelium is usually thin and stretched with no evidence of pseudoepitheliomatous hyperplasia as seen in the granular cell tumor (Fig. 6B). It responds well to conservative surgical removal. It usually stops growing after birth and does not recur even after incomplete resection. Occasionally, smaller lesions have been described to regress spontaneously within a year of birth.

Hereditary gingival fibromatosis

Hereditary gingival fibromatosis is characterized by slow-growing and generalized gingival fibrous connective tissue hyperplasia leading to extensive gingival hyperplasia, occasionally covering the crowns of the maxillary and mandibular teeth. Some of these lesions are hereditary (autosomal dominant or recessive), whereas others are idiopathic in nature. The autosomal dominant type is associated with hypertrichosis, epilepsy, craniofacial deformities, and many other defects [18,19]. The autosomal recessive type presents mostly with gingival hyperplasia and occasionally with facial deformities such as hypertelorism. The gingival hyperplasia is a common presentation in all types; it can be localized, occurring in one quadrant, or diffuse, involving all four quadrants [18,19]. The maxillary gingiva, especially the lingual gingiva, is most commonly affected. Gingival hyperplasia can begin at or before puberty and is associated with erupting teeth, both deciduous and permanent; it may interfere with tooth eruption. The hyperplastic gingiva is made up of dense fibrous connective tissue with little vascularity and dense collagen bundles. Surgical reduction is indicated, especially if the lesion is interfering with function. It has a tendency for slow recurrence taking place over a period of months or years. It is known to disappear when teeth are extracted. The overall prognosis is good.

Melanotic neuroectodermal tumor of infancy

Melanotic neuroectodermal tumor of infancy is a benign lesion of neural crest origin, primarily affecting the maxilla of newborns [20]. The lesion is associated with high urinary levels of vanilmandelic acid, usually diagnostic of a lesion of neural crest origin but not necessarily specific to melanotic neuroectodermal tumor of infancy. This osteolytic lesion is often pigmented with melanin (Fig. 7A). It is a rare lesion mainly affecting infants less than 6 months of age; more than 90% of lesions occur in the first year of life [20–22] with no gender predilection. It most commonly occurs in the anterior maxilla as a swelling with a bluish-black surface. Radiographically, it presents distinctly as an osteolytic le-

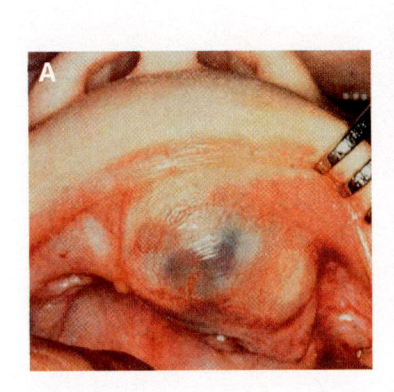

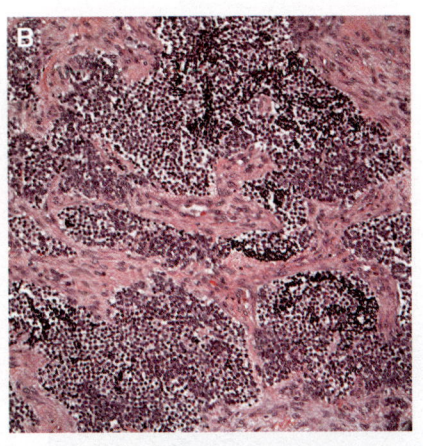

Fig. 7. (A) Melanotic neuroectodermal tumor of infancy, expansile and blue mass, anterior maxilla. (B) Melanotic neuroectodermal tumor of infancy, high-power view demonstrating islands of two cell types: predominant large epithelioid cells and small dark lymphocytic-like cells.

sion with tooth buds floating in space [20]. It has also been described in the mandible, shoulder, scapula, and other areas. The histology is distinct, manifesting in two types of cells arranged in an alveolar pattern. The larger cells contain melanin, whereas the smaller cells are dark blue, simulating lymphocytes (Fig. 7B). It is treated successfully with conservative curettage. Recurrence and transformation are described but are rare.

Hemangioma

Hemangiomas (Fig. 8A) comprise a family of benign developmental vascular anomalies occurring at infancy. They progress through two stages of growth—a rapid growth phase followed by an involution phase [23,24]. Vascular lesions are most common in infants. Lymphangiomas occur at birth and progress with age, whereas hemangiomas mostly occur a few weeks after birth and continue to grow rapidly for the first year. They stop growing and begin to involute within the subsequent few years. Hemangiomas are benign proliferations of blood vessels with many classifications. Capillary and cavernous hemangiomas are the most common types (Fig. 8B). Capillary hemangiomas affect 1% of all newborns in the United States [27]. Half of all hemangiomas occur in the head and neck area, especially the tongue; they are the most common cause of macroglossia [23–26]. They can also occur on the buccal mucosa and lips (Fig. 8A). Hemangiomas have a slight predilection for occurrence in females. The lesion can present as flat or exophytic, smooth surfaced or lobular, and localized or diffuse. Mostly single and localized, they can also present in multiples. Superficial hemangiomas are bright red, whereas deep lesions are purplish-red; they blanche on pressure (Fig. 8A) unless thrombosed. The vast majority will regress and resolve within the first 10 years of age [23]. Treatment of hemangioma depends on its size, its relationship to other anatomic structures, and the rate of blood flow. Observation is important, because many spontaneously involute, especially capillary hemangiomas. If a hemangioma persists, local topical application of injections of corticosteroids has a 75% success rate of involution within 2 weeks to 2 months post injection [25]. Several complications are described with local and systemic use of steroids; interferon alfa-2a has also been used successfully [25]. Surgical procedures include excisional scalpel surgery for small lesions and laser removal for large lesions. Laser use includes the CO_2; argon and other types of lasers have been used with a variable rate of success [24–26]. The prognosis depends on the size and whether the hemangioma is a soft-tissue or bony lesion. It can range from good to extremely poor with gross facial deformity and compromised function.

Sturge-Weber syndrome

Patients with Surge-Weber syndrome present with unilateral port-wine stains on the face. This syndrome also includes hemangiomas involving the lepto-

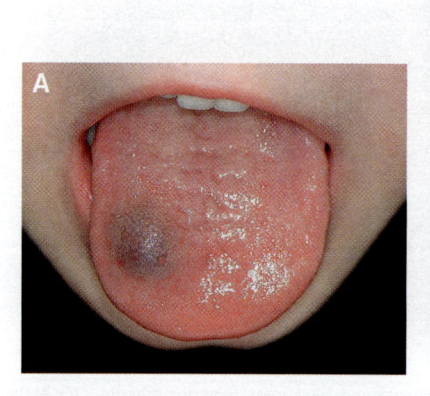

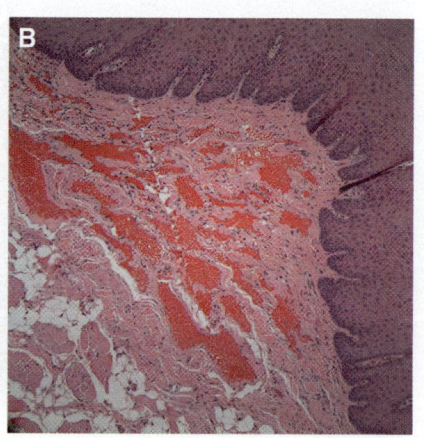

Fig. 8. (*A*) Hemangioma, raised sessile purplish-red mass on the tongue. (*B*) Cavernous hemangioma, low-power view demonstrating multiple large spaces filled with erythrocytes.

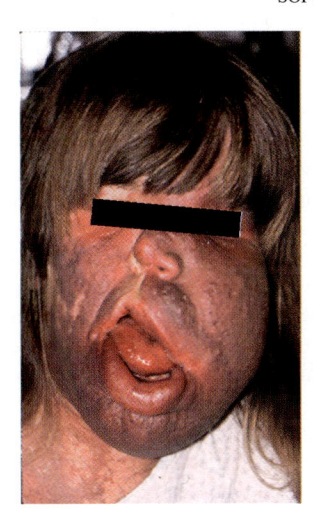

Fig. 9. Sturge-Weber angiomatosis, a rare form involving bilateral face and neck.

meninges [27,28]. The facial hemangiomas are typically unilateral but can be bilateral (Fig. 9) and follow the ophthalmic and maxillary branches of the trigeminal nerve [28]. Most cases are sporadic. The leptomeningeal hemangiomas are more commonly unilateral but can be bilateral. They can develop calcifications with a distinct presentation referred to as "tramline calcifications" [27–29]. The effect of brain hemangiomas, especially when bilateral, includes seizures [29], headaches, learning disorders, and mental retardation. Oral hemangiomas are described on the buccal mucosa and lips and rarely on the gingiva. The syndrome is diagnosed early in life, including at birth. Many of the symptoms appear within the first 2 years of life. Seizures are treated at an early stage. Laser surgery is effective for the cutaneous lesions.

Lymphangioma

Lymphangioma is a benign congenital vascular developmental anomaly of the lymphatic system that commonly occurs in the head and neck area, including the oral cavity. It is best classified as being superficial or deep, with the latter divided into cavernous and cystic types (cystic hygroma). The superficial type is also known as lymphangioma simplex [30,31]. Oral lymphangiomas tend to be of the cavernous type. The head and neck area are the most common location for lymphangiomas, followed by the extremities and buttocks. As many as 50% of lymphangiomas occur at birth and almost 90% develop within the first 2 years of life [30–32]. In the oral cavity, lymphangiomas most commonly affect the tongue. If superficial, they have a cobblestone appearance with clusters of fluid-filled vesicles, some with a dark red color owing to bleeding in the area (Fig. 10A). If it is deep, the lesion will be more diffuse and soft in consistency [30,31]. It may also occur on the lips, resembling an angioedema. It is usually asymptomatic but can be painful if pressed and may drain clear fluid if traumatized. Histologically, lymphangiomas consist of dilated lymphatic vessels present directly beneath the surface epithe-

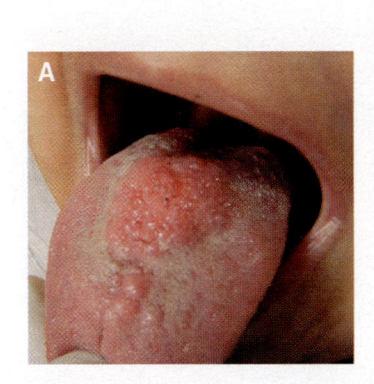

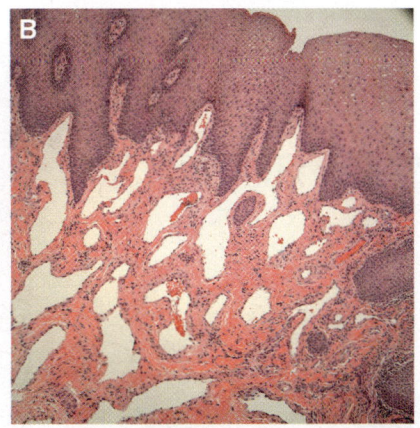

Fig. 10. (A) Lymphangioma, exophytic cobblestone and nodular mass on the middorsal surface of the tongue. (B) Lymphangioma, low-power view demonstrating dilated lymphatic vessels beneath the surface epithelium extending deep into connective tissue.

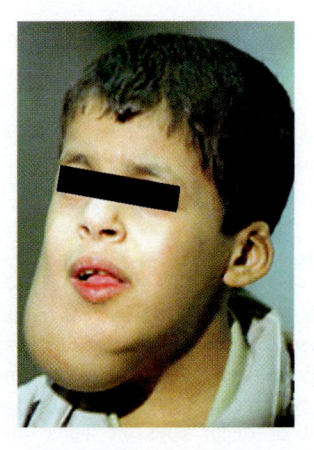

Fig. 11. Cystic hygroma in an 8-year-old-boy from Iraq who was born with this lesion on the right side of his face and treated in 2004 by Swedish Hospital, Seattle, Washington.

lium, some extending into the underlying deep connective tissue (Fig. 10B). Surgery using the scalpel or CO_2 laser is the preferred treatment. Sclerosing agents such as OK-432 and steroids have been used with some success [32]. Local recurrence is common, especially with deep and hard-to-reach lesions. Superficial lesions have better success and less recurrence.

Cystic hygroma

Cystic hygroma is a form of diffuse cavernous lymphangioma present within deep loose connective tissue. It occurs at birth and is most common in the head and neck area (the parotid gland area) (Fig. 11) but has also been described in the axilla and groin [33–35]. It is soft in consistency and tends to grow continuously; therefore, it can reach very large sizes if not treated early in life. It can be life threatening, especially if it interferes with the respiratory system [33–35]. Males and females are affected equally. The posterior triangle is affected, and the lesion may extend into the sternocleidomastoid muscle, as well as anteriorly, crossing the midline. It may extend into the oral cavity to include the posterior tongue and soft palate. The lesion is soft to palpation and can be lobular. It can extend into the axilla, mediastinum, or thorax, causing symptoms such as dyspnea and dysphagia. Infection expedites growth and leads to fibrosis and even bone formation. The latter lesions appear solid on CT scan and other radiographs. Its consistent occurrence at birth, combined with the size, location, and translucent appearance, make the clinical diagnosis of cystic hygroma possible. Like the deep lymphangiomas, cystic hygroma is successfully treated with surgery using the scalpel or CO_2 laser [33,34]. Recurrence is common with deep and hard-to-reach lesions.

Fetal rhabdomyoma

Fetal rhabdomyoma is a benign and rare neoplasm of skeletal muscle origin. It can be misdiagnosed as embryonal rhabdomyosarcoma [36,37]. The head and neck area is the most common location for fetal rhabdomyomas, especially behind the ears and tongue [36]. It occurs predominantly in children, is slow growing, and rarely recurs [36–39]. Histologically, it can be myxoid or cellular and can have mature rhabdomyoblasts without evidence of atypia

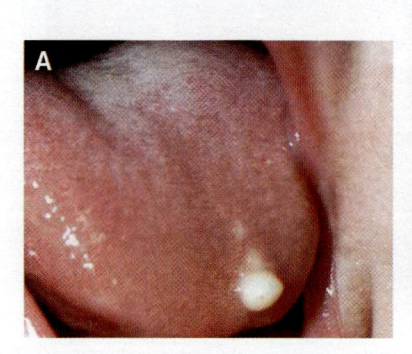

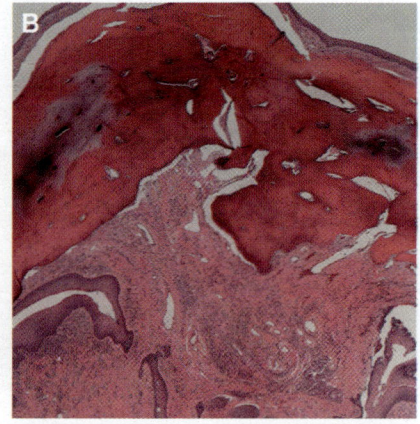

Fig. 12. (*A*) Osseous choristoma, hard exophytic smooth-surfaced white mass on the anterior tip of tongue. (*B*) Osseous choristoma, low-power view demonstrating a mass of lamellar viable bone beneath the surface epithelium.

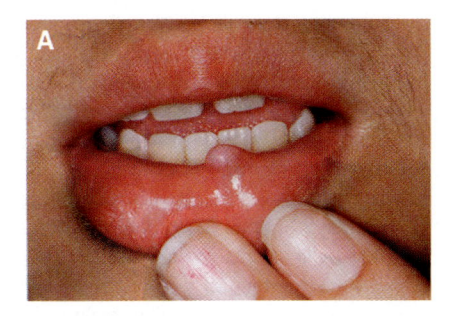

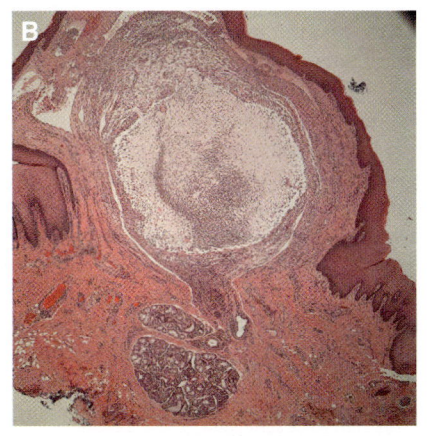

Fig. 13. (A) Mucocele, light blue exophytic nodule on the lower lip. (B) Mucocele, low-power view demonstrating a cystlike structure filled with mucoid material and foamy macrophages present beneath the surface epithelium.

or mitosis [36]. Treatment includes conservative surgical excision.

Choristoma

Osseous and cartilaginous choristomas present as smooth-surfaced nodules on the buccal mucosa or tongue (Fig. 12A) [40]. These lesions are made up of a mass of normal bone or cartilage present in an abnormal area where neither of the two hard tissues typically grow [40–42]. They are benign, self-limiting, and usually less than 1 cm in size. The tongue is a common location for the cartilaginous choristoma [40], whereas the base of the tongue, buccal mucosa, and lips are common locations for the osseous counterpart [42]. The lesions are smooth-surfaced nodules that are hard in consistency. They have no gender predilection and are described mainly in the age range of 12 to 64 years. I have also seen them in infants. Histologically, the nodules are made of normal bone or cartilage covered by intact surface epithelium (Fig. 12B). Conservative surgical excision is the preferred treatment.

Mucocele/ranula

Mucoceles and ranulas are clinical terms describing exophytic, fluid-filled, fluctuant nodules, typically of minor salivary gland origin and present mostly on the lower lip (Fig. 13A) and floor of the mouth (Fig. 14A) [43–45]. More than 90% of these lesions are cystlike structures or pseudocysts

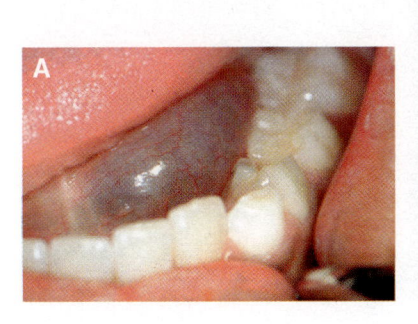

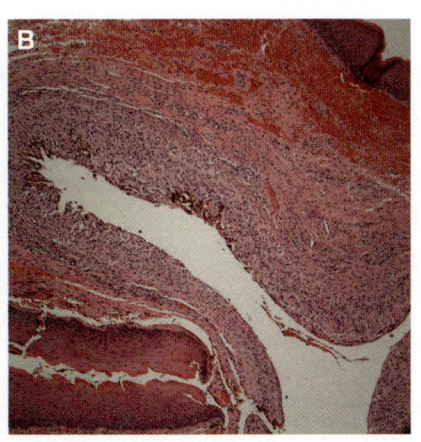

Fig. 14. (A) Ranula, purplish-blue sessile swelling in the floor of the mouth. (B) Ranula, low-power view demonstrating a cystlike structure lined by granulation tissue.

and are mucous extravasation phenomena referred to as mucoceles. Some of the lesions are true cystic structures lined by epithelium and filled with mucus and are called mucus retention cysts or salivary duct cysts; these lesions constitute a small percentage of all mucoceles [43–45]. Ranulas, mucoceles of the floor of the mouth, constitute the other 5% and are divided into those above (the majority) and below the mylohyoid muscle (also known as plunging ranulas or cervical ranulas) [46–48]. Ranulas are of minor or major salivary gland origin and are mostly extravasation in type. The etiology of the extravasation mucoceles is usually sharp trauma cutting through the salivary gland duct and releasing the mucous in the extracellular tissue [43–45]. Histologically, the extravasation-type mucocele consists of a cystlike structure lined by granulation tissue and filled with mucoid material, foamy macrophages, and, at times, small clusters of neutrophils (Figs. 13B and 14B). The mucous retention cysts develop as a result of a duct blockage, which can be caused by trauma, fibrosis, sialolith, or pressure from an overlying tumor [44,45]. Extravasation mucoceles most commonly occur on the lower lip and are extremely rare on the upper lip. They may occur anywhere else in the oral cavity, including the buccal mucosa and floor of mouth (ranulas). The latter can be of minor salivary gland or submandibular or sublingual gland duct origin [46–48]. They are more commonly seen in children and adolescents and present as a swelling with a bluish color if superficial, whereas deep mucoceles tend to take the color of the surrounding mucosa. Mucoceles tend to fluctuate in size. They are usually associated with a history of sharp lip or cheek biting but can also be secondary to surgery in the area, which is especially true for anterior tongue mucoceles.

Surgical excision with associated minor salivary gland removal is the preferred treatment for deep mucoceles; superficial mucoceles can self-heal within 2 to 3 weeks. Superficial mucoceles can also mimic vesiculobullous-type diseases because they look like vesicles [44], especially when presenting in multiples (rare, but described). They can recur if the source of trauma is not eliminated or if they are secondary to surgery. Simple (nonplunging) ranulas are best treated by marsupialization into the floor of mouth [47]. Plunging ranulas require complete excision via an extraoral approach. The technical difficulties associated with complete removal of this thin-walled lesion result in a relatively high recurrence rate.

Mixed tumor (pleomorphic adenoma)

Pleomorphic adenoma is the most common benign neoplasm of the major and minor salivary glands. It originates from the myoepithelial cells and the reserve cells of the intercalated ducts. It accounts for 80% of all benign salivary gland neoplasms, including as many as 77% of parotid, 68% of submandibular, and 43% of minor salivary gland tumors [49]. It is most common in women aged 30 to 50 years but is also described in children (Fig. 15A) [49,50]. One study reports 1% of cases affecting children aged less than 10 years and 5.9% of cases affecting persons aged 10 to 20 years [49]. Pleomor-

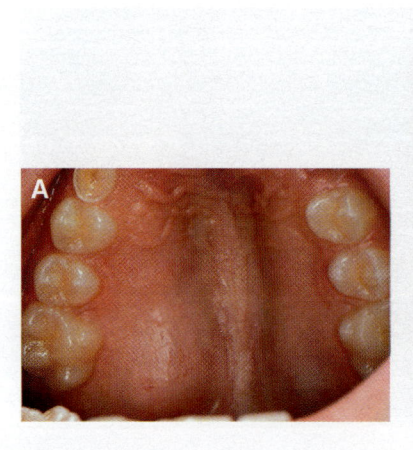

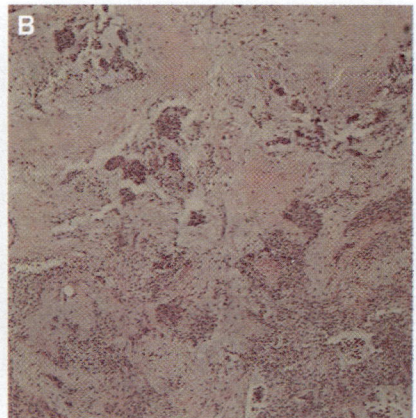

Fig. 15. (*A*) Pleomorphic adenoma, exophytic mass, lateral and posterior hard palate and anterior soft palate. (*B*) Pleomorphic adenoma, medium-power view demonstrating sheets of myoepithelial cells suspended on a myxochondroid background.

phic adenoma presents as a small, painless, slowly enlarging nodule. If left untreated, it can enlarge significantly, sometimes increasing by several pounds in weight [49–52]. It occurs in the oral cavity, especially the palate (Fig. 15A) and lips [49,50]. The palatal mixed tumor is fixed owing to the bone-bound anatomy of the region. The tumor is otherwise movable. The behavior of the tumor in children is similar to that in adults [49]. Histologically, mixed tumor has a wide variety of cellular and pattern manifestations. The main cellular components are epithelial ductlike structures and mesenchymal-like tissue, such as myxochondroid matrix (Fig. 15B). The lesions are generally encapsulated, ranging from predominantly myxoid (36%) to extremely cellular (12%) [52]. The complete histology of mixed tumor is beyond the scope of this article. Complete surgical removal with clean margins is the preferred treatment [49–52]. Palatal lesions respond well to excision in one piece with the periosteum and overlying mucosa. The prognosis is good, but the lesion has a tendency for recurrence (as high as 44%) if not treated thoroughly [49]. The risk of recurrence is less with minor salivary gland involvement (up to 20%). The risk of malignant transformation is about 5% [49].

Multiple endocrine syndrome type 2b

Multiple endocrine syndrome type 2b (MEN2b) frequently presents with multiple small nodules in the anterior oral cavity of children [53]. MEN is a rare group of diseases affecting the endocrine system. Many cases are inherited as autosomal dominant, with the genetic defect (RET) mapped to chromosome 10. Some are the result of a mutation [53]. Three types have been described. Type 2b affects the oral cavity with multiple neuromas, alerting the dentist to identify the more serious components of the syndrome, such as medullary carcinoma of the thyroid and pheochromocytoma of the adrenal glands [53–55]. The dentist can be the first person to identify the multiple oral nodules that are present as early as birth or shortly thereafter. Most are present at childhood. The medullary carcinoma affects 90% of patients and is present between 18 and 25 years of age but has been described in patients as young as 2 years [53]. Pheochromocytoma occurs in the second and third decade, as well as later, and causes profuse sweating, diarrhea, and severe hypertension [53,56]. The multiple neuromas present as nodules of the oral cavity (Fig. 16), eyes, nose, and gastrointestinal tract [57]. The nodules are frequently present

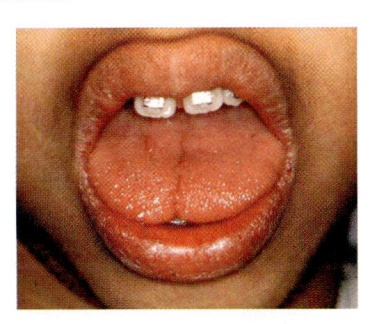

Fig. 16. MEN type 2b, multiple small nodules representing neuromas on the anterior and lateral tongue.

on the tip and anterior dorsal tongue (Fig. 16) and on the lips and bilateral corner of the mouth [53–57]. The latter location is highly characteristic of the disease. Eye and bowel nodules are usually present along with the oral counterpart [57]. In addition, patients may have a marfanoid habitus, a thick lower lip, and an everted upper eyelid [53]. The multiple small neuromas are composed histologically of discrete hyperplastic peripheral nerve bundles surrounded by a fibrotic perineural sheath. High levels of catecholamines and calcitonin are detected if the patients have pheochromocytoma and medullary carcinoma. Preventive removal of the thyroid gland is a life-saving treatment, but other treatments are applied to the various components of the syndrome [53,56,57].

Neurofibromatosis

Neurofibromatosis presents with multiple skin nodules, sometimes involving the oral cavity (Fig. 17A). It is inherited as an autosomal dominant condition with about 25% of cases being the result of a new mutation [58,59]. Neurofibromatosis is a common hereditary condition classified into nine types. Type 1 accounts for 90% of all cases, with the genetic defect localized near the centromere of chromosome 17 [58,59]. Approximately 40% of patients with these lesions manifest the disease at birth and about 60% of patients by the second year of life [58–60]. Cutaneous neurofibromas can occur in large numbers, even thousands, and range in size from small papules to pendulous masses tens of pounds in weight. They occur around puberty. Café au lait spots usually develop first around the first year of life [58–60]. Patients can also have axillary freckling (Crowe's sign), groin freckling, Lisch nodules on the iris, seizures, scoliosis, and many other diseases [58–61]. Although oral lesions are not common, enlarged fun-

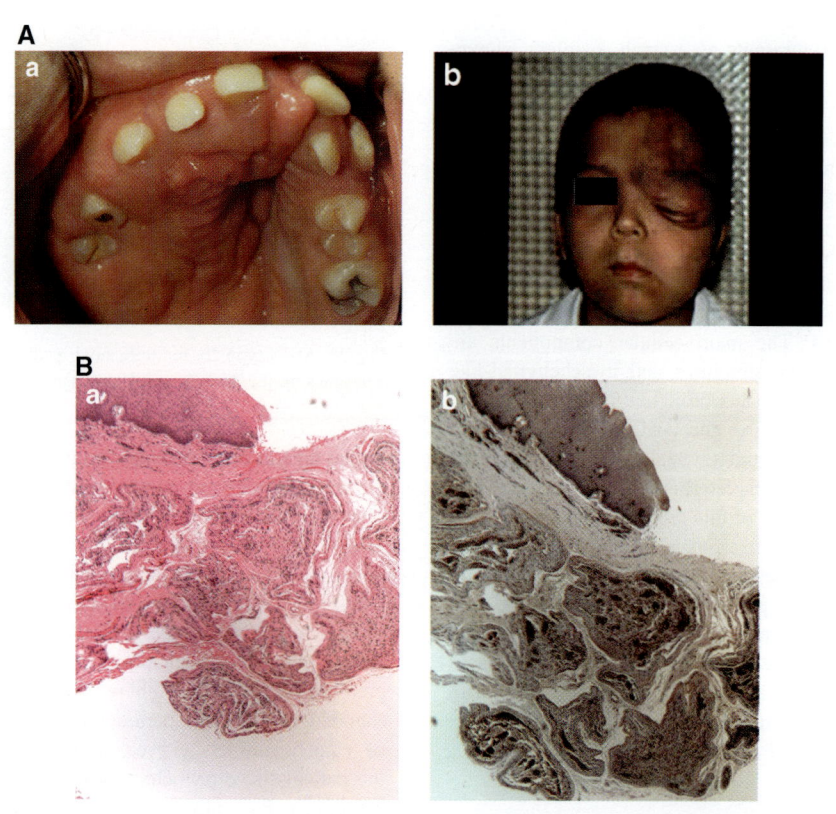

Fig. 17. (*A, a*) Neurofibromatosis, large neurofibroma involving the right side of the palate and maxillary gingiva covering and displacing teeth. (*A, b*) Same patient, pigmented and pendulous neurofibroma covering and displacing the left eye. (*B, a*) Plexiform neurofibroma, low-power view demonstrating lobules of peripheral nerve fibers separated by connective tissue. (*B, b*) Plexiform neurofibroma, low-power view demonstrating lobules of nerve bundles staining positive with S-100 protein.

giform papillae develop in 50% of patients. Multiple oral neurofibromas and jaw neurofibromas may also develop. The latter are most common in the mandible, manifested in a widened inferior alveolar canal and enlarged mandibular foramina [58]. The histology of the cutaneous nodules can be that of typical solitary neurofibromas or plexiform neurofibromas (Fig. 17B) [61]. The latter are pathognomonic for neurofibromatosis type 1. It is difficult to treat hundreds and occasionally thousands of nodules, but conventional and laser surgery are recommended for esthetic and functional reasons. The nodules have a tendency for recurrence.

Verruca vulgaris

Verruca vulgaris, also known as the common wart, is a common papillary epithelial lesion (Fig. 18A,B) of the skin affecting 22% of children [62,63]. Warts are also commonly seen in pediatric transplant patients [64]. They are less common in the oral cavity. They are induced by human papilloma virus (HPV) types 2 and 4 and are transmitted through contact where the virus DNA is incorporated in the host DNA, usually of the basal cell layer of eroded skin or mucosa [62,63,65]. They present as papillary white lesions, commonly in multiples (Fig. 18A). Autoinoculation can occur by the finger and mouth if the child sucks his or her finger [62,63,65]. Thirty percent of common warts will spontaneously disappear in 6 months, two thirds in 2 years, and three quarters in 3 years [62,63]; therefore, treatment should include patient observation for a length of time. Other treatment modalities for cutaneous common warts include liquid nitrogen (the treatment of choice for skin warts) applications, salicylic acid applications, aminolevulinic acid with blue light exposure, 5% imiquimod cream applications, and nonconventional simple duct taping; photodynamic

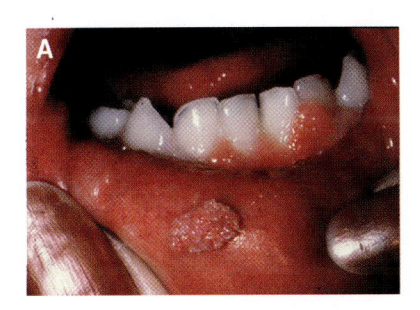

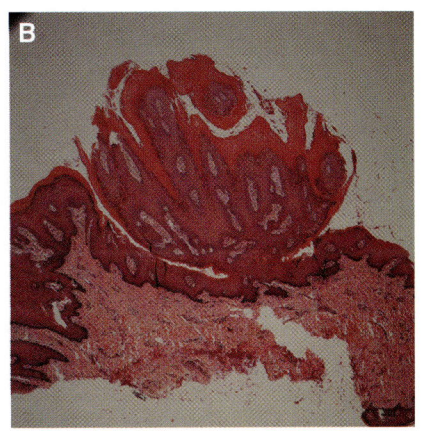

Fig. 18. (*A*) Verruca vulgaris, two papillary lesions (warts) on the mandibular gingiva and lower lip. (*B*) Verruca vulgaris, low-power view demonstrating a pedunculated lesion with epithelial papillary projections covered by alternating parakeratin and orthokeratin and supported by a fibrous connective tissue core.

therapy is used for more resistant warts [62,63,66,67]. For oral warts, conventional and laser surgery are the most effective treatment modalities.

Papilloma

Papilloma is a benign epithelial proliferation that may represent a true neoplasm induced by HPV or may occur as a spontaneous mutation. HPV types 6 and 11 have been described in these lesions. Papilloma occurs at any age, including in children, but most commonly in adults around 30 to 50 years of age. It occurs anywhere in the oral cavity, most commonly in the floor of the mouth, soft palate, and tongue. It presents as a sessile or pedunculated, "cauliflower-like" keratotic lesion around 1 cm in size. Elevated fingerlike projections made up of proliferating epithelial cells are supported by a fibrous connective tissue core. Simple surgical excision is the preferred treatment [65].

Focal epithelial hyperplasia

Focal epithelial hyperplasia, also known as Heck's disease, is common among Native Americans, predominantly the South American Indian population. It is rare in the white and black populations. It is induced by HPV types 13 and 32 and was first described by Archard and coworkers in the Eskimo population of the Greenland area. It has a distinct presentation [65,68], occurring in children living in poor conditions. Multiple small (around 5 mm or slightly larger) slightly elevated, smooth-surfaced and dome-shaped nodules occur that are pink in color, similar to the surrounding mucosa (Fig. 19A) [68,69]. These lesions can be isolated or coalesced, forming a more diffuse and ill-defined elevation of the mucosa. Lip and buccal mucosa are the most common locations (Fig. 19A), but the lesions can also occur on the gingiva, palate, and other areas [68–70]. A similar lesion has been described in AIDS patients; some are also HPV 13 and 32 positive [62]. Histologically, the lesions present as blunt dome-shaped epithelial hyperplasia with mitosoids (the latter are not always present) (Fig. 19B). Treatment includes observation, because the lesions can spontaneously regress. Others respond to laser treatment. Alternative forms of therapy include intralesional injections or topical chemotherapy [70]. The lesions in AIDS patients can be resistant to treatment [62].

Condyloma acuminatum

Condyloma acuminatum is a benign and papillomatous proliferation of the surface epithelium induced by HPV types 6 and 11. Lesions affecting the genitalia are believed to be sexually transmitted, accounting for 20% to 30% of all sexually transmitted diseases. Condyloma acuminatum is more common in the genitalia than in the oral cavity. It presents as a single papillary pinkish to white lesion, or as multiple membranous pink and papillomatous lesions. Cuta-

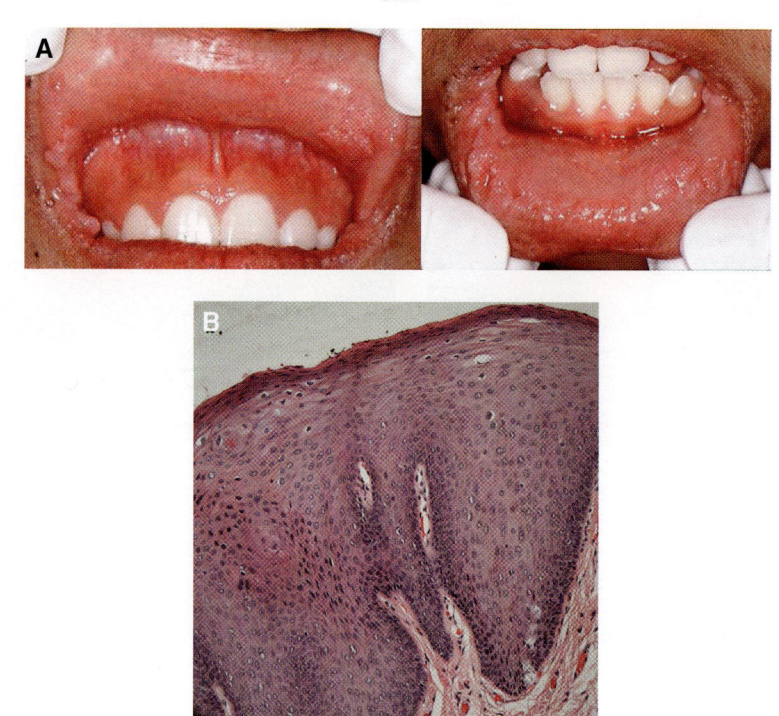

Fig. 19. (A) Focal epithelial hyperplasia, multiple exophytic mucosal nodules on the upper and lower lips. (B) Focal epithelial hyperplasia, medium-power view demonstrating hyperplastic epithelium with blunt papillary arrangement and a few koilocytes with pyknotic nuclei.

neous condylomas are described in children born to mothers with infected genital tracts, as well as in those who spend time with caregivers with hand condylomas or genital condylomas who are not in the habit of washing their hands after use of the bathroom [62,71]. Oral condylomas are not in direct contact with the birth canal during birth; therefore, it is important not to dismiss the possibility of sexual abuse through careful review of the family situation [62]. If sexual abuse is suspected, a physical examination for other signs is advised. Teenagers are also at risk, especially if practicing unprotected sex [62]. Oral condylomas are contracted mostly through oral-genital sex. There are several treatment modalities ranging from chemical cauterization to surgical removal.

Aggressive fibromatosis

Aggressive fibromatosis is sometimes referred to as juvenile or aggressive juvenile fibromatosis. It represents a group of infiltrating fibrous proliferations with a biologic behavior and microscopic appearance that is intermediate between those of benign fibrous lesions and fibrosarcomas [36,72]. The head and neck region, particularly the submandibular area, is a common site of involvement [72]. Intraoral lesions are rare, and 74% of patients are under 10 years of age [36]. No significant sex predilection is apparent. A desmoplastic fibroma is considered the intraosseous counterpart of the soft-tissue fibromatosis [36]. It presents as a firm, painless, poorly demarcated mass that is rapidly or slowly growing (Fig. 20A) [72]. Usually, it involves the tongue or buccal mucosa. The mass is locally aggressive, blends into the surrounding structures, and causes resorption of the underlying bone when it is present on the alveolar ridge (Fig. 20A). The differential diagnosis of fibromatosis includes low-grade fibrosarcoma, myofibromatosis, nodular fasciitis, reactive fibrous hyperplasia, fibrous histiocytoma, and neurofibroma. Histologically, fibromatosis is characterized by a poorly delineated, infiltrating cellular proliferation of mature spindle cells arranged in streaming and interlacing fascicles (Fig. 20B). Infiltration of the adjacent structures is common, but cellular atypia is not present. Treatment consists of wide excision. The reported recurrence rate of 24% for intraoral aggressive fibromatosis is considerably lower than the 50%

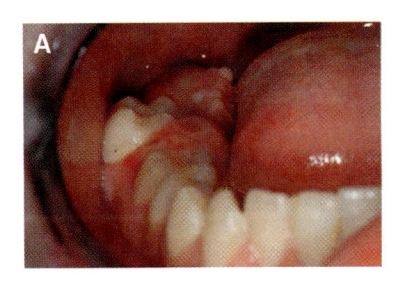

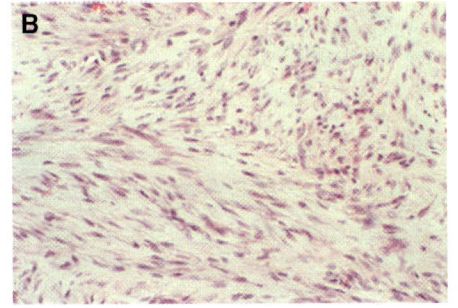

Fig. 20. (*A*) Aggressive fibromatosis, ulcerated and proliferative fibrous connective tissue surrounding and displacing the buccal and lingual right posterior mandibular teeth. (*B*) Aggressive fibromatosis, low-power view demonstrating interlacing fascicles and bundles of fibroblasts with no evidence of atypia.

to 70% rate reported for fibromatosis of the entire head and neck region [36,73,74].

Infantile myofibromatosis

Infantile myofibromatosis is a rare benign soft-tissue lesion with a predilection for the head and neck area, including the oral cavity [75]. The adult counterpart of this lesion is known as myofibroma, although myofibroma can also occur in younger patients [76,77]. The lesion is of myofibroblastic origin, a cell with smooth muscle and fibroblast features. It can be solitary or occur in multiples [75,78], with the latter constituting 25% of the cases of infantile myofibromatosis and affecting visceral organs. It has clinical features similar to those of aggressive fibromatosis but is less aggressive in behavior. Myofibromatosis occurs mainly in infants under 2 years of age and is slightly more common in males; 30% of cases appear congenitally [76]. In the oral cavity, it is more common in the mandible, followed by the tongue and lips, appearing as exophytic and firm swellings, usually asymptomatic [76,77]. Intraosseous lesions, usually in the mandible, range in presentation from well-defined unilocular or multilocular radiolucencies to poorly defined lesions. Histologically, the lesions are a circumscribed mass of spindle-shaped cells arranged in bundles and fascicles with elongated to rounded nuclei and blood vessels with the morphology of hemangiopericytoma [76]. Treatment includes conservative surgical removal; recurrence is rare. Spontaneous regression is described in a large number of infantile myofibro-

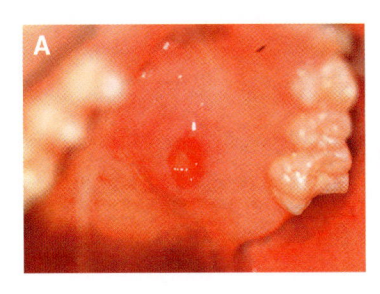

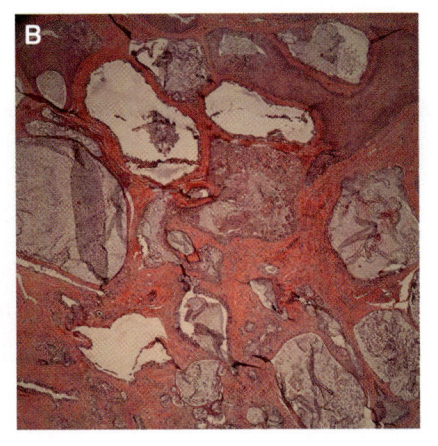

Fig. 21. (*A*) Mucoepidermoid carcinoma, ulcerated swelling in the posterior and lateral hard palate. (*B*) Mucoepidermoid carcinoma, low-power view demonstrating infiltrating but low-grade histology with cystic ductlike structures lined by mucous-producing cells and a few layers of epidermoid cells.

matosis cases. The presence of multiple visceral lesions has a poor prognosis.

Mucoepidermoid carcinoma

This malignant neoplasm of salivary gland origin can present as a smooth-surfaced swelling or a nonhealing ulcer on the palate. It occurs in a wide age range [79,80]. Three histologic types are reported: low, intermediate, and high. The low-grade type is more common in the oral cavity [79]. Mucoepidermoid carcinoma accounts for 10% of all salivary gland neoplasms [79,80]. Although most of the lesions occur in the parotid gland, some occur in minor salivary glands, especially in the palate (Fig. 21A), tongue, buccal mucosa, lips, and retromolar pad areas [79–82]. Mucoepidermoid carcinoma can occur at any age, with a predilection for young people [79]. Armed Forces Institute of Pathology studies demonstrate that 44% of cases occur in patients under 20 years of age, most commonly in the palate [79]. The youngest patient was 9 months old. The low-grade lesions are slow growing and painless and not encapsulated. They sometimes resemble a mucocele, especially those at the retromolar pad area [79,80]. Retromolar pad area mucoceles are rare; therefore, it is best to perform a biopsy early to exclude the possibility of a mucoepidermoid carcinoma masquerading as a mucocele. High-grade lesions tend to be more common in the parotid gland. They present as rapidly growing, painful lesions with facial nerve paralysis and sometimes regional lymph node metastasis. Histologically, mucoepidermoid carcinoma consists of a variety of cell types and architectural patterns which constitute the three histologic gradings. Although low-grade mucoepidermoid carcinoma is characterized by an abundance of mucous-producing cells and ductlike structures with cystic dilation (Fig. 21B), the mere presence of certain types of cells and architecture should not be used to determine the histologic grade. A full discussion of the histology of this lesion is beyond the scope of this article. Complete surgical removal with clean margins is the preferred treatment for the low-grade type. Radiotherapy has also been used successfully, especially when the tumor involves the surgical margins [79–83].

Rhabdomyosarcoma

Rhabdomyosarcoma is a malignant neoplasm of skeletal muscle origin accounting for 4% to 8% of all malignant diseases in children aged less than 15 years. It has been reported that 35% of head and neck rhabdomyosarcomas in children are misdiagnosed [83,84]. The neoplasms primarily occur in the first decade of life with a peak incidence between 2 and 6 years, with the majority of patients aged less than 12 years [83–85], and are slightly more common in males. The orbit is the most common location, followed by the nasal cavity (Fig. 22A), oropharynx, and oral cavity. The oral cavity accounts for 10% to 12% of all head and neck cases [83–85]. The tongue, palate, and cheek are the most common locations in the mouth [83,84]. The clinical appearance ranges from a small cutaneous nodule to an extensive muco-

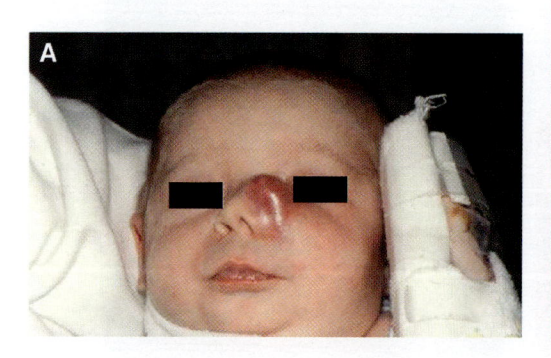

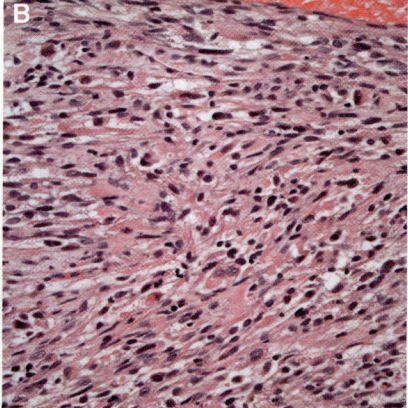

Fig. 22. (A) Rhabdomyosarcoma, exophytic purplish mass of the nasal cavity and left maxillary sinus present at birth. (From Chigurupati R, Alfatooni A, Myall RW, et al. Orofacial rhabdomyosarcoma in neonates and young children: a review of literature and management of four cases. Oral Oncol 2002;38(5):508–15; with permission.) (B) Embryonal rhabdomyosarcoma, medium-power view demonstrating sheets of neoplastic cells including small round cells and rhabdomyoblasts.

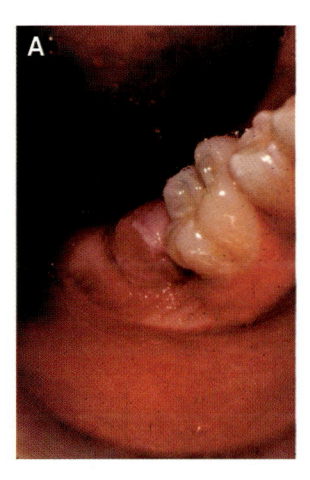

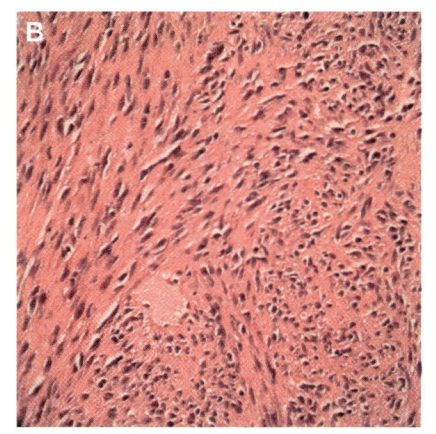

Fig. 23. (*A*) Fibrosarcoma, exophytic pink nodule, posterior maxilla. (*B*) Fibrosarcoma, medium-power view demonstrating bundles of interlacing spindle-shaped cells with hyperchromatic nuclei and herringbone pattern.

sal outgrowth. The lesion may present as a painless or occasionally painful facial swelling. The presenting clinical features are often nondiagnostic and may mimic conditions like infection [83–85]. Trismus, paresthesia, facial palsy, and aural or nasal discharges have been described [83–86]. Histologically, the neoplasms are classified as embryonal (60%) (Fig. 22B) or alveolar (20%) and undifferentiated [83]. The morphologic subtype of the embryonal botryoid accounts for 5% of cases. The tumor is aggressive and, if not diagnosed early, associated with high mortality. With the use of risk-adapted multidrug chemotherapy combined with radiotherapy and surgical excision, the 5-year survival rate has improved from 20% to 70% [83,85,86].

Infantile fibrosarcoma

Infantile fibrosarcoma is a rare malignant neoplasm of fibroblast origin. An adult counterpart exists and is more aggressive, with a 5-year survival rate of 40% compared with the infantile 5-year survival rate of 80%. Like rhabdomyosarcoma, infantile fibrosarcoma can be congenital and usually develops within the first 2 years of life. The neoplasms are slightly more common in males. Only 10% occur in the head and neck area, including the oral cavity. They are more common in the distal portion of the extremities. In the oral cavity, the buccal mucosa, palate, lips, and periosteum of the mandible (Fig. 23A) and maxilla are the most common locations of occurrence. Fibrosarcomas present as fleshly, polypoid, rapidly growing, ulcerated lesions. They can cause asymmetry, tooth displacement, and bone and tooth resorption. Histologically, they consist of bundles of streaming spindle-shaped cells characteristically crossing each other to form a herringbone pattern (Fig. 23B). Treatment includes surgery and chemotherapy. Radiation is used but is not very effective [87,88].

Summary

The soft-tissue lesions discussed herein are among those that occur more commonly in children and are of many different cell origins, including fibroblastic, muscle, nerve, salivary gland, and epithelial. They have been classified in terms of occurrence in single or multiple nodules, behavior, and whether they are benign or malignant. Emphasis is placed on the different treatment modalities when applicable.

Acknowledgments

I would like to thank my colleagues for providing most, if not all, of the clinical photographs used in this article. Professor Robert Myall of the Department of Oral and Maxillofacial Surgery at Oregon Health and Science University was especially generous in his contributions. I would also like to thank Professor Roman Carlos of La Universidad Francisco Marroquin, Department of Pathology; Professor Philip Worthington of the University of Washington, Department of Oral and Maxillofacial Surgery; Professor Mark Egbert of the University of Washington, Department of Oral and Maxillofacial Surgery and Children's Hospital of Seattle; and Professor Helen Rivera of Universidad Central de Venezuela, Department of Oral Pathology, for contributing most of the other clinical photographs. For the microscopic photographs, I would like to acknowledge Dr. Kathleen Patterson and Dr. Raj Kapur from Children's Hospital of Seattle and Professor Thomas Morton Jr. of the University of Washington, Department of Oral Biology for their generous contribution of glass slides. I would like to thank Lysa Rivera of the Department of English, University of Washington, and Arbella Bet-Shlimon of the Center for Middle Eastern and North African Studies, University of Michigan, for their help with typing and editing.

References

[1] Dayan D, Bodner L, Hammel I, et al. Histochemical characterization of collagen fibers in fibrous overgrowth (irritation fibroma) of the oral mucosa: effect of age and duration of lesion. Arch Gerontol Geriatr 1994;18(1):53–7.

[2] Walinski CJ. Irritation fibroma removal: a comparison of two laser wavelengths. Gen Dent 2004;52(3):236–8.

[3] Esmeili T, Lozada-Nur F, Epstein J. Common benign oral soft tissue masses. Dent Clin North Am 2005; 49(1):223–40.

[4] Magnusson BC, Rasmusson LG. The giant cell fibroma: a review of 103 cases with immunohistochemical findings. Acta Odontol Scand 1995;53(5): 293–6.

[5] Bischof M, Nedir R, Lombardi T. Peripheral giant cell granuloma associated with a dental implant. Int J Oral Maxillofac Implants 2004;19(2):295–9.

[6] Fantasia JE, Damm DD. Red nodular lesion of tongue: pyogenic granuloma. Gen Dent 2003;51(2):190–4.

[7] Ichimiya M, Yoshikawa Y, Hamamoto Y, et al. Successful treatment of pyogenic granuloma with injection of absolute ethanol. J Dermatol 2004;31(4):342–4.

[8] Pham J, Yin S, Morgan M, et al. Botulinum toxin: helpful adjunct to early resolution of laryngeal granulomas. J Laryngol Otol 2004;118(10):781–5.

[9] Hanemann JA, Pereira AA, Ribeiro Junior NV, et al. Peripheral ossifying fibroma in a child: report of case. J Clin Pediatr Dent 2003;27(3):283–5.

[10] Walters JD, Will JK, Hatfield RD, et al. Excision and repair of the peripheral ossifying fibroma: a report of 3 cases. J Periodontol 2001;72(7):939–44.

[11] Cuisia ZE, Brannon RB. Peripheral ossifying fibroma—a clinical evaluation of 134 pediatric cases. Pediatr Dent 2001;23(3):245–8.

[12] Flaitz CM. Peripheral giant cell granuloma: a potentially aggressive lesion in children. Pediatr Dent 2000; 22(3):232–3.

[13] Chaparro-Avendano AV, Berini-Aytes L, Gay-Escoda C. Peripheral giant cell granuloma: a report of five cases and review of the literature. Med Oral Pathol Oral Cir Bucal 2005;10(1):48–57.

[14] Neville BW, Damm DD, Allen CM, et al. Peripheral giant cell granuloma. In: Neville BW, Damm DD, Allen CM, et al, editors. Oral and maxillofacial pathology. 2nd edition. Philadelphia: WB Saunders; 2002. p. 449–51.

[15] Olson JL, Marcus JR, Zuker RM. Congenital epulis. J Craniofac Surg 2005;16(1):161–4.

[16] Parmigiani S, Giordano G, Fellegara G, et al. A rare case of multiple congenital epulis. J Matern Fetal Neonatal Med 2004;16(Suppl 2):55–8.

[17] Eppley BL, Sadove AM, Campbell A. Obstructive congenital epulis in a newborn. Ann Plast Surg 1991; 27:152–5.

[18] Katz J, Guelmann M, Barak S. Hereditary gingival fibromatosis with distinct dental, skeletal and developmental abnormalities. Pediatr Dent 2002;24(3): 253–6.

[19] Barros SP, Merzel J, de Araujo VC, et al. Ultrastructural aspects of connective tissue in hereditary gingival fibromatosis. Oral Surg Oral Med Oral Pathol Oral Radiol Endod 2001;92(1):78–82.

[20] Van Middlesworth DG, Fox RC, Freeman MJ. Melanotic neuroectodermal tumor of infancy: a review of histogenesis and report of a case. ASDC J Dent Child 1977;44(2):137–9.

[21] Fletcher C. Melanotic neuroectodermal tumor of infancy: clinicopathological, immunohistochemical and flow cytometry study. Am J Surg Pathol 1995; 17:566–73.

[22] Hoshina Y, Hamamoto Y, Suzuki I, et al. Melanotic neuroectodermal tumor of infancy in the mandible: report of a case. Oral Surg Oral Med Oral Pathol Oral Radiol Endod 2000;89(5):594–9.

[23] Chan YC, Giam YC. Guidelines of care for cutaneous haemangiomas. Ann Acad Med Singapore 2005;34(1): 117–23.

[24] Whang KK, Cho S, Seo SL. Excision of hemangioma and sculpting of the lip using carbon dioxide laser. Dermatol Surg 2004;30(12 Pt 2):1601–2 [author reply, 1602].

[25] Benedetto AV. News in treatment of angiomas. J Eur Acad Dermatol Venereol 2004;18(2):122–3.

[26] Lambrecht JT, Stubinger S, Hodel Y. Treatment of intraoral hemangiomas with the CO2 laser. Schweiz Monatsschr Zahnmed 2004;114(4):348–59.

[27] Taddeucci G, Bonuccelli A, Polacco P. Migraine-like attacks in child with Sturge-Weber syndrome without facial nevus. Pediatr Neurol 2005;32(2):131–3.

[28] Baselga E. Sturge-Weber syndrome. Semin Cutan Med Surg 2004;23(2):87–98.

[29] Jansen FE, van der Worp HB, van Huffelen A, et al. Sturge-Weber syndrome and paroxysmal hemiparesis: epilepsy or ischaemia? Dev Med Child Neurol 2004; 46(11):783–6.

[30] Jian XC. Surgical management of lymphangiomatous or lymphangiohemangiomatous macroglossia. J Oral Maxillofac Surg 2005;63(1):15–9.

[31] Al-Salem AH. Lymphangiomas in infancy and childhood. Saudi Med J 2004;25(4):466–9.

[32] Wheeler JS, Morreau P, Mahadevan M, et al. OK-432 and lymphatic malformations in children: the Starship Children's Hospital experience. ANZ J Surg 2004; 74(10):855–8.

[33] Bryan Y, Chwals W, Ovassapian A. Sedation and fiberoptic intubation of a neonate with a cystic hygroma. Acta Anaesthesiol Scand 2005;49(1):122–3.

[34] Bloom DC, Perkins JA, Manning SC. Management of lymphatic malformations. Curr Opin Otolaryngol Head Neck Surg 2004;12(6):500–4.

[35] Weintraub AS, Holzman IR. Neonatal care of infants with head and neck anomalies. Otolaryngol Clin North Am 2000;33(6):1171–89.

[36] Fletcher CDM. Soft tissue tumors. In: Fletcher CDM, editor. 2nd edition. Diagnostic histopathology of tumors, vol. 2. London: Churchill Livingstone; 2000. p. 1473–540.

[37] Gupta A, Maddalozzo J, Win Htin T, et al. Spindle cell rhabdomyosarcoma of the tongue in an infant: a case report with emphasis on differential diagnosis of childhood spindle cell lesions. Pathol Res Pract 2004; 200(7–8):537–43.

[38] Fernandez JM, Medlich MA, Lopez LH, et al. Fetal intermediate rhabdomyoma of the lip: case report. J Clin Pediatr Dent 2005;29(2):179–80.

[39] O'Callaghan MG, House M, Ebay S, et al. Rhabdomyoma of the head and neck demonstrated by prenatal magnetic resonance imaging. J Comput Assist Tomogr 2005;29(1):130–2.

[40] Toida M, Sugiyama T, Kato Y. Cartilaginous choristoma of the tongue. J Oral Maxillofac Surg 2003; 61(3):393–6.

[41] Kapoor N, Bhalla J, Bharadwaj VK, et al. Cartilaginous choristoma of palatine tonsil—a case report. Indian J Pathol Microbiol 2003;46(4):654–5.

[42] Mintz S, Anavi Y, Barak S, et al. Osseous choristomas of the buccal mucosa. J Mich Dent Assoc 1995;77(3): 30–2, 55.

[43] Kopp WK, St-Hilaire H. Mucosal preservation in the treatment of mucocele with CO2 laser. J Oral Maxillofac Surg 2004;62(12):1559–61.

[44] Silva Jr A, Nikitakis NG, Balciunas BA, et al. Superficial mucocele of the labial mucosa: a case report and review of the literature. Gen Dent 2004;52(5): 424–7.

[45] Taglialatela Scafati C. Mucoceles as a complication of submandibular intubation. J Craniomaxillofac Surg 2004;32(5):335.

[46] Yuca K, Bayram I, Cankaya H, et al. Pediatric intraoral ranulas: an analysis of nine cases. Tohoku J Exp Med 2005;205(2):151–5.

[47] Zhao YF, Jia Y, Chen XM, et al. Clinical review of 580 ranulas. Oral Surg Oral Med Oral Pathol Oral Radiol Endod 2004;98(3):281–7.

[48] Zhao YF, Jia J, Jia Y. Complications associated with surgical management of ranulas. J Oral Maxillofac Surg 2005;63(1):51–4.

[49] Waldrom CA. Mixed tumor (pleomorphic adenoma) and myoepithelioma. In: Ellis GL, Auclair PL, Gnepp DR, editors. Surgical pathology of the salivary glands. Philadelphia: WB Saunders; 1991. p. 165–86.

[50] da Cruz Perez DE, Pires FR, Alves FA, et al. Salivary gland tumors in children and adolescents: a clinicopathological and immunohistochemical study of fifty-three cases. Int J Pediatr Otorhinolaryngol 2004;68(7): 895–902.

[51] Hockstein NG, Samadi DS, Gendron K, et al. Pediatric submandibular triangle masses: a fifteen-year experience. Head Neck 2004;26(8):675–80.

[52] Foote Jr FW, Frazell EL. Tumors of the major salivary glands. In: Foote Jr FW, Frazell EL, editors. Atlas of tumor pathology, section IV, fascicle 11. 1st series. Washington (DC): Armed Forces Institute of Pathology; 1954.

[53] Gorlin RJ, Cohen Jr MM, Hennekam RCM. Multiple endocrine neoplasia, type 2B (multiple mucosal neuroma syndrome). In: Gorlin RJ, Cohen Jr MM, Hennekam RCM, editors. Syndromes of the head and neck. 4th edition. Oxford: Oxford University Press; 2001. p. 461–8.

[54] Kameyama K, Okinaga H, Takami H. Clinical manifestations of familial medullary thyroid carcinoma. Biomed Pharmacother 2004;58(6–7):348–50.

[55] Quayle FJ, Moley JF. Medullary thyroid carcinoma: including MEN 2A and MEN 2B syndromes. J Surg Oncol 2005;89(3):122–9.

[56] Gertner ME, Kebebew E. Multiple endocrine neoplasia type 2. Curr Treat Options Oncol 2004;5(4):315–25.

[57] Prabhu M, Khouzam RN, Insel J. Multiple endocrine neoplasia type 2 syndrome presenting with bowel obstruction caused by intestinal neuroma: case report. South Med J 2004;97(11):1130–2.

[58] Gorlin RJ, Cohen Jr MM, Hennekam RCM. The neurofibromatoses (NF I Recklinghausen type, NF II acoustic type, other types). In: Gorlin RJ, Cohen Jr MM, Hennekam RCM, editors. Syndromes of the head and neck. 4th edition. Oxford: Oxford University Press; 2001. p. 469–76.

[59] Carroll SL, Stonecypher MS. Tumor suppressor mutations and growth factor signaling in the pathogenesis of NF1-associated peripheral nerve sheath tumors. II. The role of dysregulated growth factor signaling. J Neuropathol Exp Neurol 2005;64(1):1–9.

[60] Descheemaeker MJ, Ghesquiere P, Symons H, et al. Behavioural, academic and neuropsychological profile of normally gifted neurofibromatosis type 1 children. J Intellect Disabil Res 2005;49(Pt 1):33–46.

[61] Friedrich RE, Schmelzle R, Hartmann M, et al. Resection of small plexiform neurofibromas in neurofibromatosis type 1 children. World J Surg Oncol 2005; 3(1):1–6.

[62] Silverberg N. Human papillomavirus infections in children. Curr Opin Pediatr 2004;16(4):402–9.

[63] Silverberg N. Warts and molluscum in children. Adv Dermatol 2004;20:23–73.

[64] Fortina AB, Piaserico S, Alaibac M, et al. Skin

disorders in patients transplanted in childhood. Transpl Int 2005;18(3):360–5.
[65] Syrjanen S. Human papillomavirus infections and oral tumors. Med Microbiol Immunol (Berl) 2003;192(3): 123–8.
[66] Schroeter CA, Pleunis J, van Nispen tot Pannerden C, et al. Photodynamic therapy: new treatment for therapy-resistant plantar warts. Dermatol Surg 2005; 31(1):71–5.
[67] Harwood CA, Perrett CM, Brown VL, et al. Imiquimod cream 5% for recalcitrant cutaneous warts in immunosuppressed individuals. Br J Dermatol 2005; 152(1):122–9.
[68] Garcia-Corona C, Vega-Memije E, Mosqueda-Taylor A, et al. Association of HLA-DR4 (DRB1*0404) with human papillomavirus infection in patients with focal epithelial hyperplasia. Arch Dermatol 2004;140(10): 1227–31.
[69] Jayasooriya PR, Abeyratne S, Ranasinghe AW, et al. Focal epithelial hyperplasia (Heck's disease): report of two cases with PCR detection of human papillomavirus DNA. Oral Dis 2004;10(4):240–3.
[70] Akyol A, Anadolu R, Anadolu Y, et al. Multifocal papillomavirus epithelial hyperplasia: successful treatment with CO2 laser therapy combined with interferon alpha-2b. Int J Dermatol 2003;42(9):733–5.
[71] Sinclair R, Yell J. Childhood condyloma acuminatum: association with genital and cutaneous human papillomavirus. Pediatr Dermatol 1994;11(1):85.
[72] Roychoudhury A, Parkash H, Kumar S, et al. Infantile desmoid fibromatosis of the submandibular region. J Oral Maxillofac Surg 2002;60(10):1198–202.
[73] Delloye C, Viejo-Fuertes D, Scalliet P. Treatment of aggressive fibromatosis: a multidisciplinary approach. Acta Orthop Belg 2004;70(3):199–203.
[74] Lackner H, Urban C, Benesch M, et al. Multimodal treatment of children with unresectable or recurrent desmoid tumors: an 11-year longitudinal observational study. J Pediatr Hematol Oncol 2004;26(8):518–22.
[75] Eze N, Pitkin L, Crowley S, et al. Solitary infantile myofibroma compromising the airway. Int J Pediatr Otorhinolaryngol 2004;68(12):1533–7.
[76] Foss RD, Ellis GL. Myofibromas and myofibromatosis of the oral region: a clinicopathologic analysis of 79 cases. Oral Surg Oral Med Oral Pathol Oral Radiol Endod 2000;89(1):57–65.

[77] Lingen MW, Mostofi RS, Solt DB. Myofibromas of the oral cavity. Oral Surg Oral Med Oral Pathol Oral Radiol Endod 1995;80(3):297–302.
[78] Wright C, Corbally MT, Hayes R, et al. Multifocal infantile myofibromatosis and generalized fibromuscular dysplasia in a child: evidence for a common pathologic process? Pediatr Dev Pathol 2004;7(4): 385–90.
[79] Auclair PL, Ellis GL. Mucoepidermoid carcinoma. In: Ellis GL, Auclair PL, Gnepp DR, editors. Surgical pathology of the salivary glands. Philadelphia: WB Saunders; 1991. p. 269–98.
[80] Hicks J, Flaitz C. Mucoepidermoid carcinoma of salivary glands in children and adolescents: assessment of proliferation markers. Oral Oncol 2000;36(5):454–60.
[81] Bentz BG, Hughes CA, Ludemann JP, et al. Masses of the salivary gland region in children. Arch Otolaryngol Head Neck Surg 2000;126(12):1435–9.
[82] Epstein JB, Hollender L, Pruzan SR. Mucoepidermoid carcinoma in a young adult: recognition, diagnosis, and treatment and responsibility. Gen Dent 2004;52(5): 434–9.
[83] Chigurupati R, Alfatooni A, Myall RW, et al. Orofacial rhabdomyosarcoma in neonates and young children: a review of literature and management of four cases. Oral Oncol 2002;38(5):508–15.
[84] Gupta A, Maddalozzo J, Win Htin T, et al. Spindle cell rhabdomyosarcoma of the tongue in an infant: a case report with emphasis on differential diagnosis of childhood spindle cell lesions. Pathol Res Pract 2004; 200(7–8):537–43.
[85] Stevens MC, Rey A, Bouvet N, et al. Treatment of nonmetastatic rhabdomyosarcoma in childhood and adolescence: results of the third study of the International Society of Paediatric Oncology–SIOP malignant mesenchymal tumor 89. J Clin Oncol 2005; 23(12):2618–28.
[86] Punyko JA, Mertens AC, Baker KS, et al. Long-term survival probabilities for childhood rhabdomyosarcoma. Cancer 2005;103(7):1475–83.
[87] Uren A, Toretsky JA. Pediatric malignancies provide unique cancer therapy targets. Curr Opin Pediatr 2005;17(1):14–9.
[88] Grohn ML, Borzi P, Mackay A, et al. Management of extensive congenital fibrosarcoma with preoperative chemotherapy. ANZ J Surg 2004;74(10):919–21.

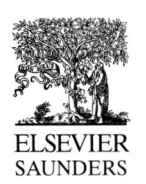

Cysts of the Jaws and Advances in the Diagnosis and Management of Nevoid Basal Cell Carcinoma Syndrome

Jocelyn M. Shand, MBBS, MDSc, FDSRCS, FRACDS(OMS)*,
Andrew A. Heggie, MBBS, MDSc, FFDRCS, FRACDS(OMS)

*Oral and Maxillofacial Surgery Unit, Department of Plastic and Maxillofacial Surgery,
The Royal Children's Hospital of Melbourne, Melbourne, Victoria 3052, Australia*

A cyst is a pathologic cavity filled with fluid or semi-fluid contents that has not been created by the accumulation of pus. Most of the cysts are lined wholly or in part by epithelium [1,2]. Cysts of the jaws are generally described based on the supposed origin of the epithelial lining as either odontogenic or nonodontogenic cysts, and the World Health Organization has classified jaw cysts (Box 1) [3]. The updated World Health Organization classification is anticipated for publication in 2005. Most jaw cysts arise from an odontogenic origin. Any lesion within the spectrum of odontogenic and nonodontogenic cysts may present in children. Examples of lesions found more commonly in pediatric patients include gingival and eruption cysts. A detailed discussion of the histopathologic features is beyond the scope of this article and can be found in specialized texts [1,2].

Aneurysmal bone cyst

The aneurysmal bone cyst is an uncommon lesion in the facial skeleton and is more frequently seen in the long bones, vertebral column, and pelvis. It has been reported that only 2% of aneurysmal bone cyst lesions involve the jaws, and the mandible is affected more often than the maxilla [4–6]. The cause and pathogenesis of the aneurysmal bone cyst remain poorly understood. It may present as a primary lesion or secondarily, where it occurs contiguously with a recognized bone lesion. The aneurysmal bone cyst has been reported in association with various lesions, such as ossifying and cemento-ossifying fibromas, central giant cell granulomas, giant cell lesions, fibrous dysplasia, and osteoblastomas, which have been termed aneurysmal bone cyst "plus" [7,8]. Radiographically their presentation may vary from a unilocular radiolucency to multilocular radiolucencies or manifest as a large multilocular lesion with extensive expansion or "ballooning" (Figs. 1 and 2). Histologically, the aneurysmal bone cyst contains numerous large nonendothelial lined blood-filled spaces, with cellular fibrous tissue and multinucleated giant cells. These lesions are usually managed by curettage of the lesion and bony cavity. Large expansile lesions may necessitate resection and reconstruction.

Calcifying odontogenic cyst

The calcifying odontogenic cyst is usually classified with the spectrum of odontogenic tumors because some lesions are solid. They usually present in patients younger than 40 years of age and most commonly during adolescence. Clinically, the calcifying odontogenic cyst presents as a painless, slow-growing lesion and is usually located in the anterior

* Corresponding author.
E-mail address: jmshand@bigpond.net.au (J.M. Shand).

Box 1. Classification of cysts of the jaws

Epithelial cysts
  Developmental
    Odontogenic cysts
      Gingival cysts of infants
        (Epstein pearls)
      Odontogenic keratocyst
        (primordial cyst)
      Dentigerous (follicular) cyst
      Eruption cyst
      Lateral periodontal cyst
      Gingival cyst of adults
      Glandular odontogenic cyst;
        sialo-odontogenic cyst
    Nonodontogenic cysts
      Nasopalatine duct (incisive
        duct) cyst
      Nasolabial (nasoalveolar) cyst
  Inflammatory
    Radicular cyst
    Apical, lateral
    Residual
    Paradental (inflammatory
      collateral, mandibular infected
      buccal) cyst
Nonneoplastic lesions of bone
  Solitary bone cyst (simple, traumatic, hemorrhagic bone cyst)
  Aneurysmal bone cyst

From Kramer IRM, Pindborg JJ, Shear M. Histologic typing of odontogenic tumours: WHO international classification of tumours. 2nd edition. Berlin: Springer-Verlag; 1992; with permission.

region of the maxilla and mandible. Radiographically it has a variable appearance that ranges from a well-defined unilocular to a multilocular radiolucency, with a varying amount of radio-opacity within the lesion [1,2]. Management of the calcifying odontogenic cyst is by enucleation. The solid variant is potentially more aggressive in behavior compared with the cystic variant, and follow-up is required.

Dentigerous (follicular) cyst

The dentigerous cyst is one of the most commonly encountered jaw cysts. It arises from the dental follicle of a developing or unerupted tooth and either partially or totally encloses the crown. This cyst is more common in male patients and most frequently is associated with teeth that develop impactions, such as third molars and canines. It may be associated with any tooth, however, and can occur at all ages [1,2]. Radiographically, the dentigerous cyst usually appears as a well-defined radiolucency associated with the crown of an unerupted tooth (Fig. 3). The tooth may be displaced because these cysts can attain considerable size before detection and may cause bony expansion. The cyst contains a yellowish fluid; cholesterol crystals also may be present. In the mixed dentition, a variant of the dentigerous cyst has been reported and has been described as an inflammatory follicular cyst, although there is a degree of controversy regarding the terminology and pathogenesis of the lesion [9–12]. The lesion is usually associated with a nonvital deciduous molar tooth and involves the follicle of the permanent successor premolar tooth (Fig. 4). It has been speculated that the periapical inflammation of the deciduous tooth spreads to involve the underlying follicle and that the inflam-

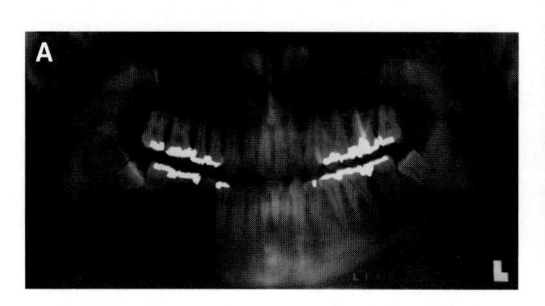

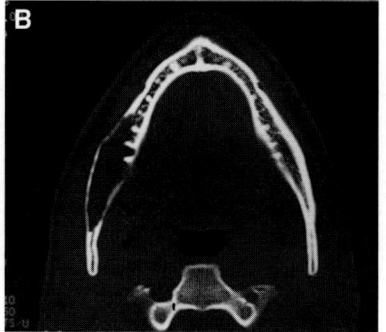

Fig. 1. Aneurysmal bone cyst in a 17-year-old young man. (*A*) Orthopantomogram (OPG) demonstrates a well-defined radiolucent lesion right body and ramus of mandible. (*B*) Axial view, CT scan.

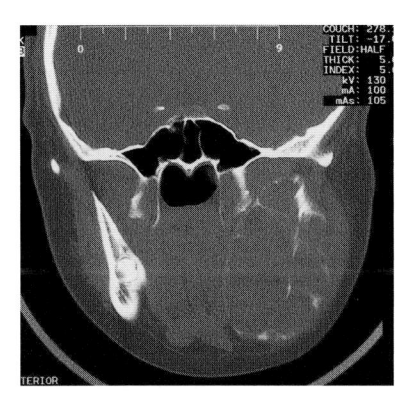

Fig. 2. Aneurysmal bone cyst in a 12-year-old girl. Coronal CT scan demonstrates multilocular lesion left mandible with extensive expansion or ballooning. (Courtesy of Dr. B.J. Costello, Pittsburgh, PA.)

matory response results in the formation of a cyst that involves the premolar, with similar characteristics to a dentigerous cyst. In some cases, irregularities in the enamel of the permanent premolar have been detected [9–12].

Removal of dentigerous cysts is by enucleation with preservation of the inferior alveolar nerve if it is involved in mandibular lesions. In pediatric patients a decision is made on an individual basis for the preservation or removal of the associated tooth. Impacted third molars or teeth that have been displaced a considerable distance are usually removed. If the unerupted permanent tooth (eg, a premolar or canine) has the potential to attain a position within the arch, however, then the enucleation of the cyst with retention of the tooth and monitoring for further root development and eruption may be the treatment of choice. Subsequent failure of eruption of the tooth may necessitate surgical exposure and orthodontic traction.

After removal of large dentigerous cysts the entirety of the lining should be examined histologically as a routine practice. The unicystic ameloblastoma, also described as an "ameloblastoma in situ" or a "microinvasive ameloblastoma," appears radiographically identical to a dentigerous or odontogenic keratocyst (OKC) (Fig. 5). It is speculated that in some lesions the ameloblastomatous change occurs in a pre-existing cyst. The approach to the management of a unicystic ameloblastoma, which is usually diagnosed after enucleation or curettage, is contentious and variable [13–17]. A conservative approach may be undertaken, after enucleation, with routine radiologic review for future recurrence, whereas some authors prefer immediate reoperation with further resection at the margins [13–17].

Eruption cyst

The eruption cyst is a form of dentigerous cyst that occurs during tooth eruption and arises in an extra-alveolar location within the overlying soft tissue of the ridge. It most commonly presents in association with the eruption of deciduous teeth and permanent incisors. As the soft tissues expand, the lesion often appears to have a bluish tinge and is fluctuant [1,2]. In most cases, no treatment is required because the eruption of the tooth results in physiologic marsupialization. In larger cysts with delayed or slow eruption of the tooth, however, surgical exposure and removal of the overlying mucosa may be indicated.

Gingival cyst

Gingival cysts occur most commonly in neonates but may present in adults. In neonates, they appear as multiple firm, white keratinizing nodules along the edentulous ridges and are referred to as Bohn's nodules [1,2]. No surgical management is required because the cysts either involute or rupture and resolve. Gingival cysts in adults occasionally present as gingival swellings, usually in the mandible, and are managed by excision.

Idiopathic bone cavity

This lesion represents an empty cavity in bone with no epithelial lining and is not a true cyst. The idiopathic bone cavity has been reported under various synonyms, including traumatic, solitary or hemorrhagic bone cyst, or extravasation cyst. Most of these lesions occur in the mandible and present most commonly in the second decade. Aspiration of the

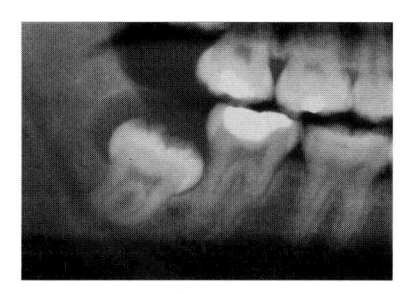

Fig. 3. Dentigerous cyst in a 16-year-old girl. Well-defined coronal radiolucency is associated with impacted third molar.

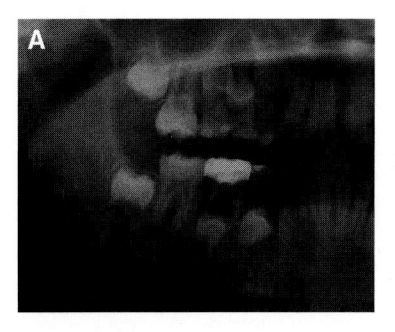

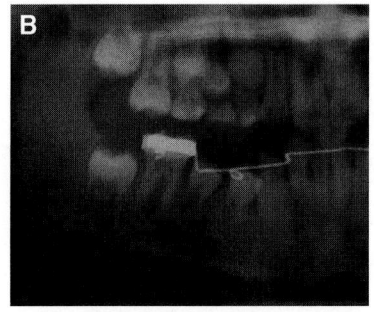

Fig. 4. Inflammatory follicular cyst in a 9-year-old girl. (*A*) Well-defined radiolucent lesion is associated with unerupted first premolar and nonvital deciduous molar. (*B*) Nine months after removal of deciduous molars and curettage of follicular lesion, with the retention of permanent premolar.

lesion often produces blood [1,2]. Radiographically, the idiopathic bone cavity presents as a well-defined radiolucency that is scalloped between the roots of vital teeth (Fig. 6). Management of the lesion involves exploration and curettage of the bony cavity to promote bleeding and subsequent bony regeneration. The surgical exploration is diagnostic to confirm the absence of any content and therapeutic in the production of intralesional hemorrhage.

Lateral periodontal cyst

Lateral periodontal cysts most commonly occur in the canine and premolar regions of the mandible and are uncommon in children. They are usually detected on routine radiographic screening and present as well-defined radiolucencies that are tear drop shaped between the roots of the adjacent vital teeth. The lateral periodontal cyst is believed to develop from

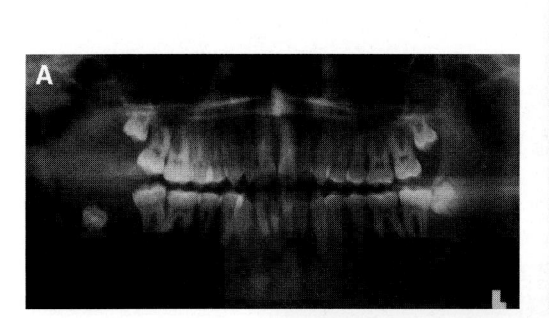

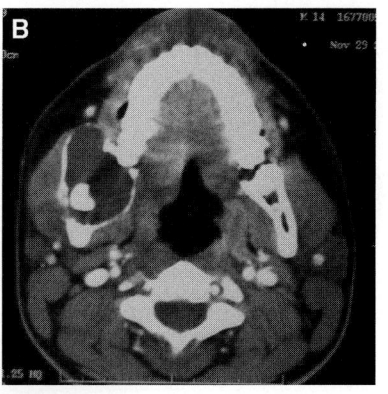

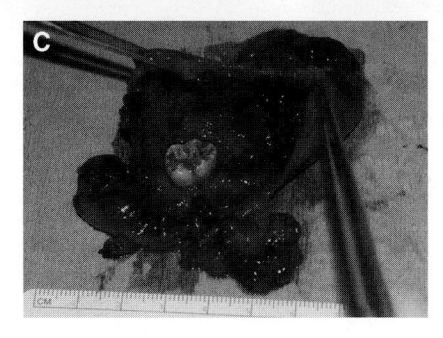

Fig. 5. Unicystic ameloblastoma in a 14-year-old boy. (*A*) Well-defined extensive unilocular radiolucency right body and ramus of mandible, with displaced third molar. Incisional biopsy reported as dentigerous cyst. (*B*) Axial CT scan demonstrates expansive lesion. (*C*) Surgical specimen that histologic examination revealed as a unicystic ameloblastoma.

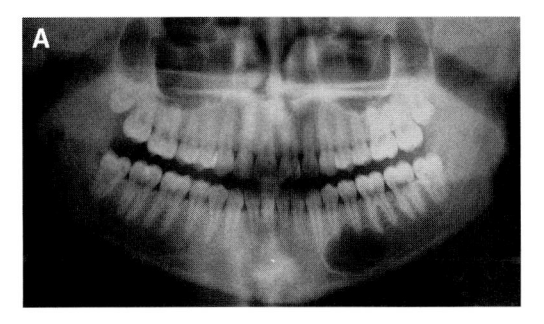

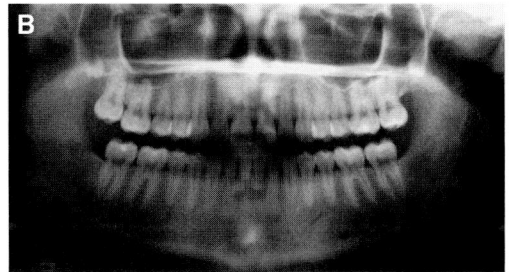

Fig. 6. Idiopathic bone cavity in an 18-year-old girl. (*A*) Preoperative OPG. (*B*) Postoperative OPG after curettage of cavity demonstrates bony healing.

the remnants of the dental lamina. If the lesion is multilocular and resembles a bunch of grapes, then this variant of the cyst is described as a botryoid odontogenic cyst [1,2]. The cyst is managed by enucleation, and recurrence is rare.

Nasopalatine duct cyst

The nasopalatine duct cyst is a developmental lesion that arises from nasopalatine duct remnants. The lesion usually presents in adults and is uncom-

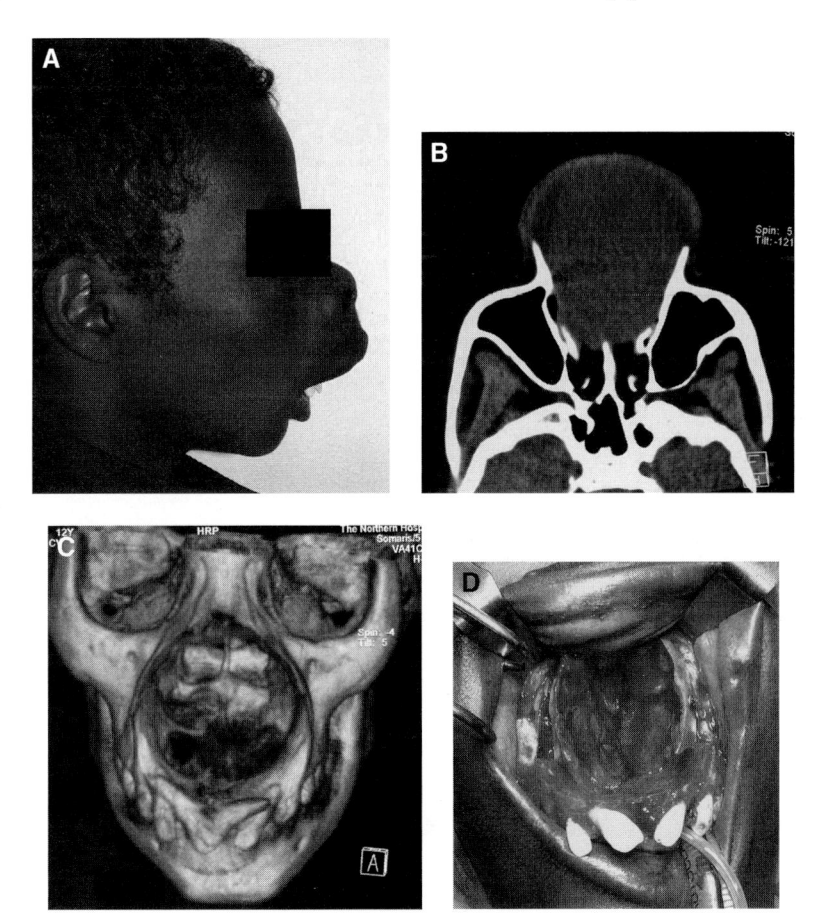

Fig. 7. Nasopalatine duct cyst in a 12-year-old patient. (*A*) Lateral profile view with marked expansion of anterior maxillary and nasal region. (*B*) Axial CT scan demonstrates well-defined expansive lesion. (*C*) Three-dimensional CT reconstruction. (*D*) Intraoperative view after enucleation of lesion via transoral approach.

mon in children. It may present with soft tissue swelling in the anterior palate and occasionally discharges into the oral cavity, which gives rise to a salty taste. Radiographically, the cyst presents as a well-defined radiolucent lesion that is round, ovoid, or heart shaped and usually occurs in the midline of the palate. In small lesions, the cyst must be distinguished from the normal appearance of the incisive canal, and empirically it has been suggested that a radiolucency in this region larger than 6 mm may potentially represent a pathologic entity [1,2]. Untreated, these lesions may expand to marked proportions (Fig. 7). The cyst is managed with enucleation.

Odontogenic keratocyst

The OKC is a common and interesting lesion with behavioral and histopathologic features that differentiate it from all other odontogenic cysts. The cyst occurs in all ages but has a peak occurrence in the second and third decades. Most lesions occur in the mandible, with a predilection for the third molar region. Most cysts present posterior to the premolar region of the mandible and maxilla. The pathogenesis of the OKC has yet to be elucidated fully. Speculatively, it has been proposed that they arise from the remnants of the dental lamina or from the epithelial basal layer of the oral mucosa [18].

The presentation of the OKC demonstrates variability [19,20]. The cysts tend to enlarge in an anteroposterior direction before buccolingual expansion and often attain a significant size before detection. The lesion may be diagnosed after routine radiographic screening or with the investigation of associated symptoms, such as pain or swelling from infection. The radiographic appearance ranges from a solitary small radiolucency or large unilocular and well-defined radiolucency to a multilocular lesion (Fig. 8). There may be displacement of any associated unerupted teeth and the inferior alveolar nerve canal and, occasionally, resorption of adjacent roots. Most OKCs present as solitary lesions; however, multiple primary cysts may present, the most common association being with nevus basal cell carcinoma syndrome (NBCCS) (Gorlin-Goltz syndrome).

The histologic features of the OKC are characteristic. The typical lesion is lined by a regular layer of stratified squamous epithelium, which is between five and ten cells thick and has a palisaded basal cell layer. The cyst wall is usually thin and may be considerably folded. The epithelial layer surface is usually parakeratinized, but areas of orthokeratinization may be present. It has been reported that OKCs with orthokeratinized lining have a lower incidence

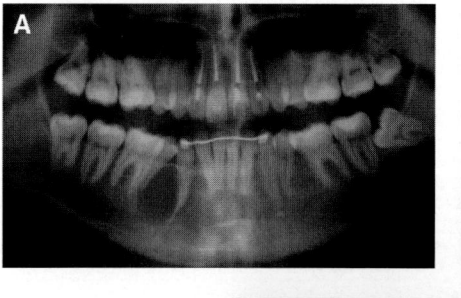

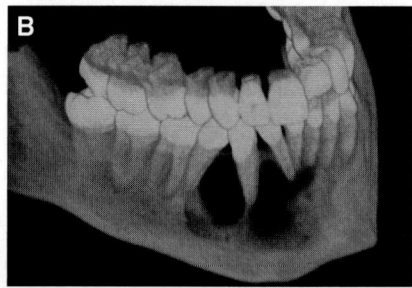

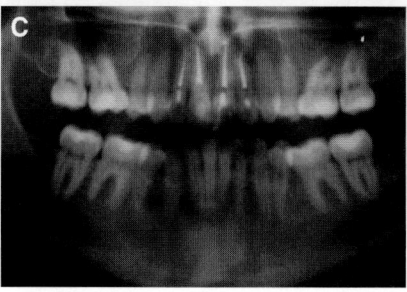

Fig. 8. Odontogenic keratocyst in a 19-year-old man. (A) OPG demonstrates multilocular radiolucent lesion right mandible. (B) Three-dimensional CT scan of lesion. (C) OPG after enucleation of lesion and Carnoy's solution demonstrates bony healing.

of recurrence in comparison to the parakeratinized cysts [21]. The fibrous wall or capsule may contain islands of epithelial cells that are believed to give rise to cyst formation and keratinization and are described as daughter or satellite cysts. A higher incidence of daughter and satellite cysts has been demonstrated in cysts associated with NBCCS. The epithelial cells desquamate into the lumen and the cyst lumen contains variable amounts of keratin. Clinically, the cyst appears to contain a white, cheesy material. The soluble protein level is usually less than 4 g/dL [1,2].

The cystic lesion has the highest recurrence rate of all odontogenic cysts and has been the subject of considerable interest and investigation. The reported recurrence rate varies substantially between studies, and the approach to the management of OKCs has been the subject of discussion and debate [1,2, 17–24]. A range of treatment approaches has been recommended and includes marsupialization, enucleation, enucleation with adjunctive liquid nitrogen therapy or the application of Carnoy's solution, removal with a peripheral ostectomy, and localized or segmental resection [19–24].

Several groups have reported the outcome of marsupialization of OKCs [20,22,24]. This technique involves excision of the overlying mucosa and preparation of an opening into the cyst cavity and, when possible, suturing the mucosal edge to the cyst lining. The patency of the opening is maintained with tubing or an acrylic obturator. Careful patient selection for this technique is required. Pogrel and Jordon [24] reported on the outcome of ten patients managed with marsupialization alone and found that the OKC resolved in all cases. The time for resolution ranged from 7 to 19 months; follow-up ranged from 1.8 to 4.8 years. Nakamura and colleagues [22] reviewed the outcome of 28 primary lesions that were managed by marsupialization followed by curettage and enucleation. The follow-up period was a mean of 6.6 years. In five cases, the lesion resolved with marsupialization alone. A recurrence of the OKC was found in six cases (21%), with the recurrence presenting from 1 to 16 years after surgery. The presence of daughter microcysts in the surrounding fibrous tissue also was demonstrated in 43.5% of cases after the marsupialization procedure. The authors concluded that presurgical marsupialization was effective in minimizing cyst size and that removing the residual cyst and excising the overlying mucosa should be performed to ensure removal of epithelial remnants.

Zhao and colleagues [20] presented the outcome of 255 patients with OKCs who were managed by various surgical techniques. Follow-up ranged from 3 to 29 years, with recurrence detected in 31 cases (12%). The highest recurrence rate was demonstrated in patients who underwent simple enucleation (17%). Patients treated with enucleation and Carnoy's solution had a 6.7% rate of recurrence. No recurrences were detected in the marsupialization/enucleation and resection groups. In a review of 40 patients with a diagnosis of OKC, Morgan and colleagues [25] found a significantly lower rate of recurrence in patients who underwent a peripheral ostectomy than patients who were treated by enucleation.

In a sophisticated, prospective, long-term study, Stoelinga [19] reviewed the outcome of the management of 80 patients who had 82 OKCs over a 25-year period. Of this group, 33 cases (40%) were diagnosed after cyst enucleation and histologic review. The 49 lesions that were preoperatively diagnosed as OKCs were managed by a defined protocol: excision of the overlying mucosa attached to the cyst and application of Carnoy's solution to the bony defect after enucleation. Of the 82 cysts, the parakeratinizing variant predominated and only seven cases exhibited orthokeratinization. The mean follow-up was 11.8 years, with a range of 1 to 25 years. Recurrent lesions were seen in 9 patients (10.9%), and six of the recurrences presented within 5 years. In 6 of the 9 patients, the OKC was diagnosed after simple enucleation and histologic examination. Only 3 of the 9 patients (3%) who experienced recurrence were in the protocol group managed with enucleation and Carnoy's solution. Excision of the overlying mucosa was performed in 44 cases, and histologic examination of the overlying mucosa revealed the presence of microcysts in 23 cases. These clusters of epithelial islands generally were not present elsewhere in the cyst walls.

A promising advance in the diagnosis and management of OKCs is the development of cytokeratin expression profile analysis using immunocytochemistry [26–28]. Research has demonstrated that the epithelial lining of OKCs produces low molecular weight keratin (cytokeratin-10), whereas nonkeratinizing cysts, such as dentigerous cysts, do not. A study by August and collagues [27] demonstrated that of 18 fine-needle aspiration biopsies of cystic jaw lesions, 10 had a strongly positive immunoreaction. The 10 cases were subsequently histologically diagnosed as OKCs and the cytokeratin-10 expression was found to have correlated. The immunocytochemistry technique has been reportedly successful in the analysis of aspiration (cytologic) and tissue (histologic) samples. A recent report by August and colleagues [28] investigated cytokeratin-10 expression in OKCs after decompression and subsequent removal of the residual cyst in 14 biopsy-proven cases. Tissue samples were taken at 3-month intervals after surgical decompression for a mean duration of 8.4 months (range, 6–12 months after operation). At the time of residual cystectomy, which was performed on average at 9 months after decompression, 9 of the 14 cases were cytokeratin-10 negative and no longer had histologic features of an OKC. In 5 cases, histologic features of OKC were present with no evidence of epithelial dedifferentiation and were cytokeratin-10 positive. On average, this group underwent cystectomy at 7 months after decompression.

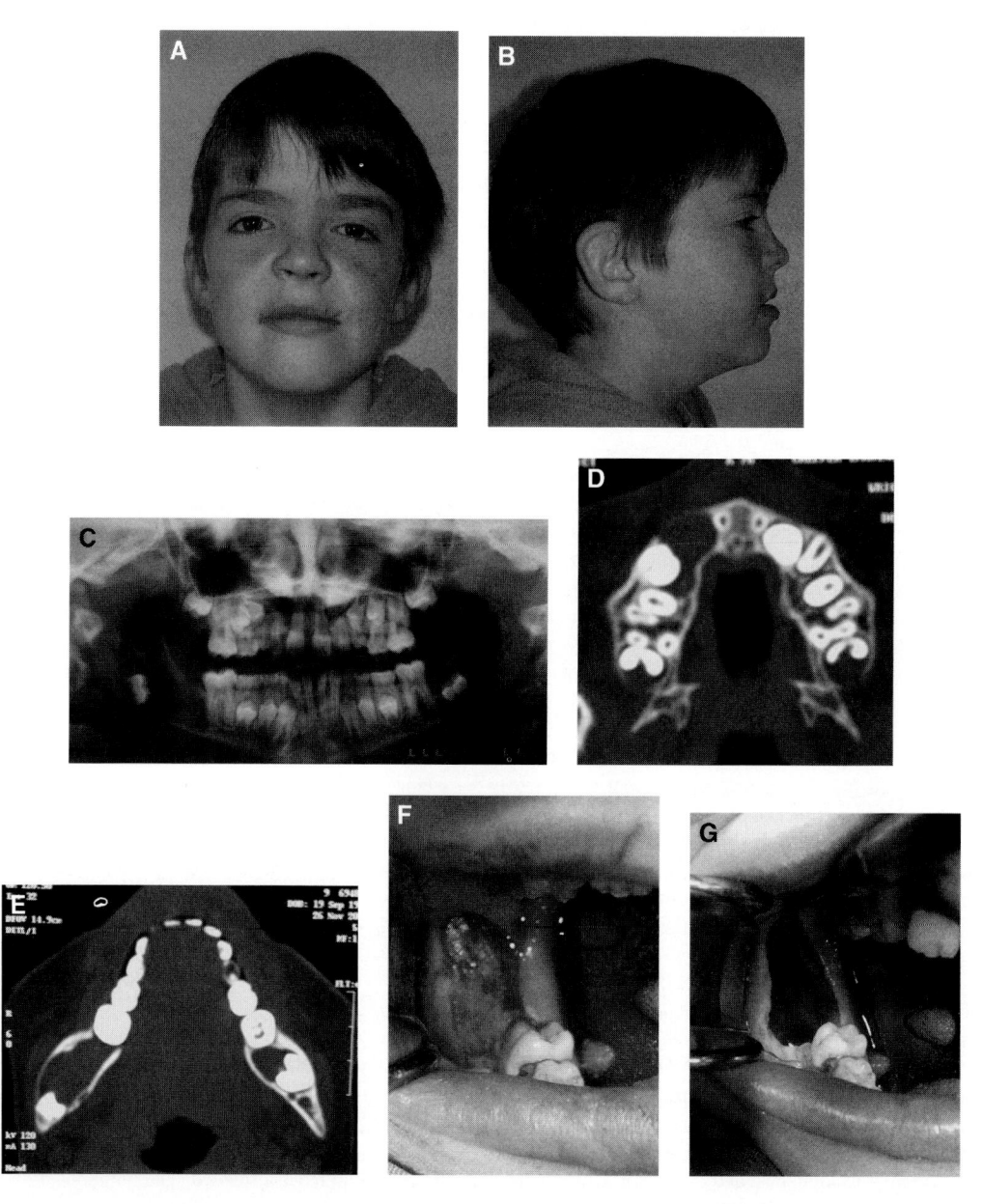

Fig. 9. Nevoid basal cell carcinoma syndrome (Gorlin-Goltz syndrome) in a 9-year-old male. (*A*) Frontal facial view. (*B*) Lateral facial view. (*C*) Preoperative OPG demonstrating well-defined radiolucent lesions right and left mandible, and right maxillary canine region. (*D*) Preoperative axial CT scan of maxilla. (*E*) Preoperative CT scan of mandible demonstrating bilateral lesions and displaced second molars. (*F*) Intraoperative view following exposure of lesion right mandible. (*G*) Bone cavity following enucleation of lesion and Carnoy's solution. (*H*) Surgical specimen. (*I*) 12-month postoperative OPG demonstrating bone healing.

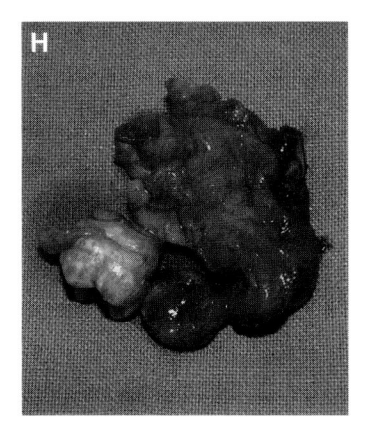

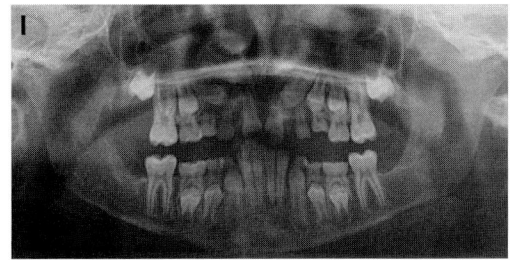

Fig. 9 (*continued*).

The cytokeratin-10 expression analysis has a potential application in the diagnosis and the monitoring of the tissue response after surgical intervention and may prove to be a valuable tool in the management of OKCs.

Paradental cyst

This cyst is inflammatory in origin and has been described as an inflammatory collateral or mandibular infected buccal cyst. It is usually associated with a partially erupted mandibular third molar with a history of pericoronitis and is rarely associated with other teeth. The lesion typically arises on the buccal or distobuccal aspect of a tooth that often has associated developmental enamel defects, ridges, or spurs. Radiographically, it presents as a well-defined unilocular radiolucency associated with the cementoenamel junction or coronal root surface region of the tooth. Paradental cysts have the same histologic features as inflammatory radicular cysts [1,2]. Treatment is the same as for dentigerous cysts, with anticipated resolution and no recurrence.

Radicular cyst

Radicular cysts are associated with nonvital teeth in the deciduous and permanent dentitions. These cysts are the most common lesions in the jaws and arise from epithelial cells—associated with periapical granulomas—that undergo cystic degeneration. As they enlarge, expansion occurs and ultimately perforation of the cortex and development of a discharging sinus may result. Radiographically, they present as a well-defined radiolucency associated with a tooth apex. The histologic appearance and contents of the cyst demonstrate a variable spectrum related in part to the maturity of the lesion [1,2]. The treatment of the radicular cyst involves the management of the nonvital tooth, either by removal or endodontic treatment, and curettage of the lesion at the time of extraction or by subsequent enucleation, apicectomy, and retrograde restoration if required. A radicular cyst may persist after extraction of the associated tooth and the lesion is termed a "residual radicular cyst" or "residual dental cyst."

Nevoid basal cell carcinoma syndrome

Recently in a detailed review, Manfredi and colleagues [29] analyzed the literature and discussed the current understanding of the disorder of NBCCS or Gorlin-Goltz syndrome. Although individual features of this disorder have been described for centuries, with the first evidence reputed to be in historical documents from ancient Egypt, it was not until the late 1890s that a condition with multiple basal nevi was reported [29]. Subsequently, a relationship between basal nevi and jaw cysts and then other anomalies was recognized. The investigations of Gorlin and Goltz [30] led to a definition of the disorder in 1960, however. They characterized the condition as a triad of features: multiple basal cell nevi, jaw keratocysts, and skeletal anomalies and bifid ribs (Fig. 9). A range of other features with variable frequency also is known to be recognized within the spectrum of NBCCS, such as other skin and skeletal anomalies and ocular and endocrine manifestations (Table 1) [29,31,32]. The diagnostic criteria of NBCCS requires the presence of two major or one major and two minor criteria features (Box 2).

Table 1
Some features of nevoid basal cell carcinoma syndrome

	Frequency (%)
Craniofacial anomalies	
Calcification of falx cerebri	35–85
Frontal bossing	25
Macrocephaly	40
Bridged sella turcica	>70
Hypertelorism	40–50
Odontogenic keratocysts	75–85
Cleft lip and palate	4
High arched palate	40
Impacted or ectopic teeth, oligodontia	
Skeletal anomalies	
Rib anomalies; bifid, cervical, fused	60
Kyphosis / scolosis	
Shortened fourth metacarpal	
Polydactyly/syndactyly	
Radiolucencies (pseudocysts) hands/feet	
Skin	
Basal cell carcinoma	50–97
Palmar/plantar pitting	50–90
Neurologic/central nervous system	
Medulloblastoma	3–5
Meningioma	<1
Agenesis of corpus callosum	
Congenital hydrocephalus	
Intellectual disability	
Other anomalies	
Genitourinary tract	
Cardiac	
Ophthamologic	

The genetic background of NBCCS has been a focus of considerable attention and active research worldwide. NBCCS is an autosomal dominant disorder, and the accountable gene has been localized to a microdeletion at chromosome 9q22 [29,33,34]. Recent work has shown that the Patched gene, from the candidate region, is primarily responsible, and its product plays a role in the sonic hedgehog signaling pathway, involving smoothened and GLI-1 [35–38]. Sonic hedgehog signaling seems to be an important regulator of oncogene transformation, and sonic hedgehog, smoothened, and GLI-1 genes have been shown to act as oncogenes. There is increasing evidence that germline mutations in the human Patched gene equivalent are present in NBCCS cases and may result in the development of OKCs and basal cell carcinomas. Deletions of 9q22 have been demonstrated in neoplasms related to NBCCS and in sporadic cases of basal cell carcinoma, OKCs, and medulloblastoma [36,38,39]. In a recent investigation, Ohki and colleagues [35] examined the role of sonic hedgehog signaling in sporadic and NBCCS syndrome associated OKCs. Their findings suggested that abnormality of the Patched gene is essential for the development of OKCs and that the mutations of the Patched gene were distributed in various exons. The results also suggested that the characteristics of sonic hedgehog signaling may differ between NBCCS and sporadic OKCs, however.

In NBCCS, an OKC is frequently the first detected feature of the condition and is usually an incidental finding on radiographic screening during dental or orthodontic care in the first or second decades. OKCs have identical clinical and radiographic features to cysts seen in sporadic cases, except for their propensity to develop multiple cysts. OKCs in

---

Box 2. Diagnostic criteria of nevoid basal cell carcinoma syndrome

Diagnostic criteria

Major
1. More than two basal cell carcinomas or one basal cell carcinoma in a patient younger than 20 years
2. Histologically proven OKCs of the jaw
3. Three or more cutaneous palmar or plantar pits
4. Bifid, fused, or markedly splayed ribs
5. First-degree relative with NBCCS

Minor
1. Macrocephaly
2. One of several orofacial congenital malformations: cleft lip and palate, frontal bossing, hypertelorism, coarse facies
3. Other sketetal anomalies: marked syndactyly, pectus deformity, Sprengel deformity
4. Radiologic abnormalities: bridging of sella turcica, vertebral anomalies, modeling defects or flame-shaped radiolucencies of the hands and feet
5. Ovarian fibroma
6. Medulloblastoma

The diagnosis of NBCCS requires the presence of two major or one major and two minor feature criteria.

NBCCS have a variable but recognized increased rate of recurrence [28]. These rates are difficult to interpret because cases of NBCCS have the potential to develop multiple new cysts that occasionally may be confused with recurrence. In view of the earlier age of presentation in the mixed dentition, multiplicity of lesions, and the potential for recurrence, management of these children into adulthood is challenging and lifelong follow-up is anticipated. Each patient is best given treatment planning on an individual basis, because removal of each affected tooth over a period of time may result in the loss of many teeth. The management of recurrent lesions in pediatric patients must be considered carefully in the context of continued growth, because resection may result in significant long-term deformity. In pediatric patients, an initial approach of cyst enucleation, adjunctive therapy (eg, application of Carnoy's solution), and judicious removal of associated teeth is considered the most prudent approach.

Summary

Cysts are one of the most common pathologic entities that involve the facial skeleton. An understanding of the clinical behavior and pathologic features of each lesion allows for treatment planning that takes into account the developing dentition and the affects of any proposed surgery on the growth of the jaws. Management of the more challenging lesions, such as OKCs, requires that clinicians keep abreast of the emerging studies that will enhance the outcome of treatment.

Acknowledgments

The authors would like to acknowledge the support of the Melbourne Research Unit for Facial Disorders in the preparation of this article.

References

[1] Soames JV, Southam JC. Oral pathology. 3rd edition. Oxford: Oxford University Press; 1998.
[2] Marx RE, Stern D. Oral and maxillofacial pathology: a rationale for diagnosis and treatment. Carol Stream Illinois: Quintessence Publishing; 2003.
[3] Kramer IRM, Pindborg JJ, Shear M. Histological typing of odontogenic tumours: WHO international classification of tumours. 2nd edition. Berlin: Springer-Verlag; 1992.
[4] Motamedi MHK. Destructive aneurysmal bone cyst of the mandibular condyle: report of a case and review of the literature. J Oral Maxillofac Surg 2002;60:1357–61.
[5] Motamedi MHK. Aneurysmal bone cysts of jaws: clinico-pathological features, radiographic evaluation and treatment analysis of 17 cases. J Craniomaxillofac Surg 1998;26:56–62.
[6] Motamedi MHK, Yazdi E. Aneurysmal bone cyst of the jaws: analysis of 11 cases. J Oral Maxillofac Surg 1994;52:471–5.
[7] Chiba I, Teh BG, Iizuka T, et al. Conversion of traumatic bone cyst into central giant cell granuloma: implications for pathogenesis [case report]. J Oral Maxillofac Surg 2002;60:222–5.
[8] Padwa BL, Denhart BC, Kaban LB. Aneurysmal bone cyst "plus": a report of three cases. J Oral Maxillofac Surg 1997;55:1144–52.
[9] Shibata Y, Asaumi J, Yanagi Y, et al. Radiographic examination of dentigerous cysts in the transitional dentition. Dentomaxillofac Radiol 2004;33:17–20.
[10] Aguilo L, Gandia JL. Dentigerous cyst of mandibular second premolar in a five-year old girl, related to a non-vital primary molar removed one year earlier: a case report. J Clin Pediatr Dent 1998;22:155–8.
[11] da Silva TA, de Sa AC, Zardo M, et al. Inflammatory follicular cyst associated with an endodontically treated primary molar: a case report. ASDC J Dent Child 2002;69:271–4.
[12] Benn A, Altini M. Dentigerous cysts of inflammatory origin: a clinicopathologic study. Oral Surg Oral Med Oral Pathol Oral Radiol Endod 1996;81:203–9.
[13] Ackermann GL, Altini M, Shear M. The unicystic ameloblastoma: a clinicopathological study of 57 cases. J Oral Pathol 1988;17:541–6.
[14] Lee PK, Samman N, Ng IO. Unicystic ameloblastoma: use of Carnoy's solution after enucleation. Int J Oral Maxillofac Surg 2004;33:263–7.
[15] Rosenstein T, Pogrel MA, Smith RA, et al. Cystic ameloblastoma: behaviour and treatment of 21 cases. J Oral Maxillofac Surg 2001;59:1311–6.
[16] Olaitan AA, Adekeye EO. Unicystic ameloblastoma of the mandible: a long term follow-up. J Oral Maxillofac Surg 1997;55:345–8.
[17] Stoelinga PJW, Bronkhorst FB. The incidence, multiple presentation and recurrence of aggressive cysts of the jaws. J Craniomaxillofac Surg 1987;15:184–95.
[18] Stoelinga PJW. Studies on the dental lamina as related to its role in the aetiology of cysts and tumours. J Oral Pathol 1976;5:65–73.
[19] Stoelinga PJW. Long-term follow-up on keratocysts treated according to a defined protocol. Int J Oral Maxillofac Surg 2001;30:14–25.
[20] Zhao YF, Wei J-X, Wang S-P. Treatment of odontogenic keratocysts: a follow-up of 255 Chinese patients. Oral Surg Oral Med Oral Pathol Oral Radiol Endod 2002;94:151–6.
[21] Li TJ, Kitano M, Chen XM, et al. Orthokeratinized odontogenic cyst: a clinicopathological and immuno-

cytochemical study of 15 cases. Histopathology 1998;32:242–51.
[22] Nakamura N, Mitsuyasu T, Mitsuyasu Y, et al. Marsupialization for odontogenic keratocysts: long-term follow-up analysis of the effects and changes in growth characteristics. Oral Surg Oral Med Oral Pathol Oral Radiol Endod 2002;94:543–53.
[23] Bataineh AB, Al Qudah MA. Treatment of odontogenic keratocyts. Oral Surg Oral Med Oral Pathol Oral Radiol Endod 1998;86:42–7.
[24] Pogrel MA, Jordan RCK. Marsupialization as a definitive treatment for the odontogenic keratocyst. J Oral Maxillofac Surg 2004;62:651–5.
[25] Morgan TA, Burton CC, Qian F. A retrospective review of the treatment of the odontogenic keratocyst. J Oral Maxillofac Surg 2005;63:635–9.
[26] August M, Faquin WC, Ferraro NF, et al. Fine-needle aspiration biopsy of intraosseous jaw lesions. J Oral Maxillofac Surg 1999;57:1282–6.
[27] August M, Faquin WC, Troulis MJ, et al. Differentiation of odontogenic keratocysts from non-keratinizing cysts by use of fine-needle aspiration biopsy and cytokeratin-10 staining. J Oral Maxillofac Surg 2000;58:935–40.
[28] August M, Faquin WC, Troulis MJ, et al. Dedifferentiation of odontogenic keratocyst epithelium after cyst decompression. J Oral Maxillofac Surg 2003;61:678–83.
[29] Manfredi M, Vescovi P, Bonanini M, et al. Nevoid basal cell carcinoma syndrome: a review of the literature. Int J Oral Maxillofac Surg 2004;33:117–24.
[30] Gorlin RJ, Goltz RW. Multiple naevoid basal cell epithelioma, jaw cysts, bifid rib: a syndrome. N Engl J Med 1960;262:908–11.
[31] Gorlin RJ. Nevoid basal cell carcinoma syndrome. Dermatol Clin 1995;13:113–25.
[32] Ahn SG, Lim YS, Kim DK, et al. Nevoid basal cell carcinoma syndrome: a retrospective analysis of 33 affected Korean individuals. Int J Oral Maxillofac Surg 2004;33:458–62.
[33] Haniffa MA, Leech SN, Lynch SA, et al. NBCCS secondary to an interstitial chromosome 9q deletion. Clin Exp Dermatol 2004;29:542–4.
[34] Boonen SE, Stahl D, Kreiborg S, et al. Delineation of an interstitial 9q22 deletion in basal cell nevus syndrome. Am J Med Genet 2005;132:324–8.
[35] Ohki K, Kumamoto H, Ichinohasama R, et al. PTC gene mutations and expression of SHH, PTC, SMO and GLI-1 in odontogenic keratocysts. Int J Oral Maxillofac Surg 2004;33:584–92.
[36] Gailani MR, Bale SJ, Lefell DJ, et al. Developmental defects in Gorlin syndrome related to a putative tumour suppressor gene on chromosome 9. Cell 1992;69:111–7.
[37] Johnson RL, Rotherman AL, Xie J, et al. Human homolog of patched, a candidate gene for the basal cell nevus syndrome. Science 1996;272:1668–71.
[38] Dahmane N, Lee J, Robins P, et al. Activation of the transcription factor Gli 1 and the Sonic hedgehog signaling pathway in skin tumours. Nature 1997;389:876–81.
[39] Raffel C, Jenkins RB, Frederick L, et al. Sporadic medulloblastomas contain PTCH mutations. Cancer Res 1997;57:842–5.

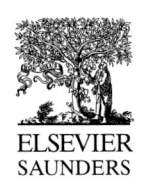

Advances in Diagnosis and Management of Fibro-Osseous Lesions

Maria E. Papadaki, DDS, MD, Maria J. Troulis, DDS, MSc,
Leonard B. Kaban, DMD, MD*

Department of Oral and Maxillofacial Surgery, Massachusetts General Hospital, Harvard School of Dental Medicine, Warren Building 1201, 55 Fruit Street, Boston, MA 02114, USA

Fibro-osseous lesions are benign mesenchymal skeletal tumors in which mineralized tissue, blood vessels and giant cells, in varying proportions, replace normal bone. Included in this group are fibrous dysplasia (FD), cherubism, ossifying fibroma and osteoblastoma, with FD being the most common entity [1]. Although, fibro-osseous lesions have similar histologic and radiographic features, they may exhibit a wide range of biologic behaviors. Because the histologic appearance does not predict the rate of growth or prognosis, treatment is based on the clinical and biologic behavior of the tumor. The purpose of this article is to describe advances in diagnosis and management of fibro-osseous lesions.

Fibrous dysplasia and McCune-Albright syndrome

Background

Fibrous dysplasia (FD) traditionally has been considered a developmental dysplastic disorder of the skeleton in which immature woven bony trabeculae are formed within a stroma of abnormal fibrous connective tissue. It is often a slow-growing lesion that can affect any bone and usually appears in childhood or adolescence, with a median onset at 9.5 years of age. Patients most often present with an asymptomatic swelling of the affected bone. In most cases, growth of the lesion slows down and finally ceases in late teenage years or the early twenties. In young children, however, FD may exhibit a rapid growth pattern with invasion and destruction of adjacent bone, displacement of teeth, and resorption of roots [2].

In 1938, American pathologist Louis Lichtenstein was the first to use the term "fibrous dysplasia" [3]. In 1942, Lichtenstein and Henry Lewis Jaffe described FD as a congenital anomaly caused by a disturbance of the bone-forming mesenchyme. They also noted a relationship among FD, abnormal pigmentation of skin, and premature sexual development [4]. They reported 23 cases of the disease; since then the monostotic form of FD also has been known as Jaffe-Lichtenstein syndrome.

Fuller Albright, an endocrinologist at Massachusetts General Hospital, established the relationship between FD and endocrine disorders. He conducted extensive research in many areas of endocrinology, among them parathyroid disease, bone metabolism, disturbances of sex hormones, and corticosteroid therapy and its side effects. In 1937, Albright and Donovan James McCune, a pediatrician in New York, described in detail a syndrome characterized by "osteitis fibrosa disseminata, areas of pigmentation and endocrine dysfunction with precocious puberty in fe-

---

This work was funded in part by the Massachusetts General Hospital Department of Oral and Maxillofacial Surgery Education and Research Fund, Hanson Foundation, and the AO/ASIF/Synthes Fellowship in Pediatric Oral and Maxillofacial Surgery.

* Corresponding author.
E-mail address: LKaban@Partners.org (L.B. Kaban).

males" [5,6]. This syndrome is currently known as McCune-Albright syndrome, a rare disorder that begins in childhood or early adolescence and is characterized by polyostotic FD of bone, café-au-lait pigmentation of the skin, and endocrine disorders.

In summary, the classic forms of FD are monostotic, polyostotic, and polyostotic FD as part of McCune-Albright syndrome (Fig. 1). Monostotic FD affects only one bone, most commonly the rib, proximal femur, or craniofacial skeleton [7]. In the craniofacial region, the maxilla is affected twice as frequently as the mandible, and the posterior aspects of the jaw are affected more frequently than the anterior aspects [8,9]. Polyostotic FD may affect up to 75% of the skeleton. Eighty percent to 85% of patients who have FD have the monostotic form [8].

Molecular biology

The pathogenesis of FD was discovered only recently. In 1991, mutations of the $G_s\alpha$ gene (GNAS1) were documented in the lesions of patients with McCune-Albright syndrome [10]. In 1995, the same mutations were identified in monostotic FD [11]. GNAS1 encodes the α subunit of G proteins (guanine nucleotide proteins) that act as signal transducers. G proteins consist of three different subunits, α, β, and γ ($G\alpha$, $G\beta$, $G\gamma$), localized to the inner surface of the cell membrane. They are linked with transmembrane receptors (G protein-coupled receptors) of hormones and growth factors. The α subunit is also bound to GDP (inactive G protein) or GTP (active G protein) [12].

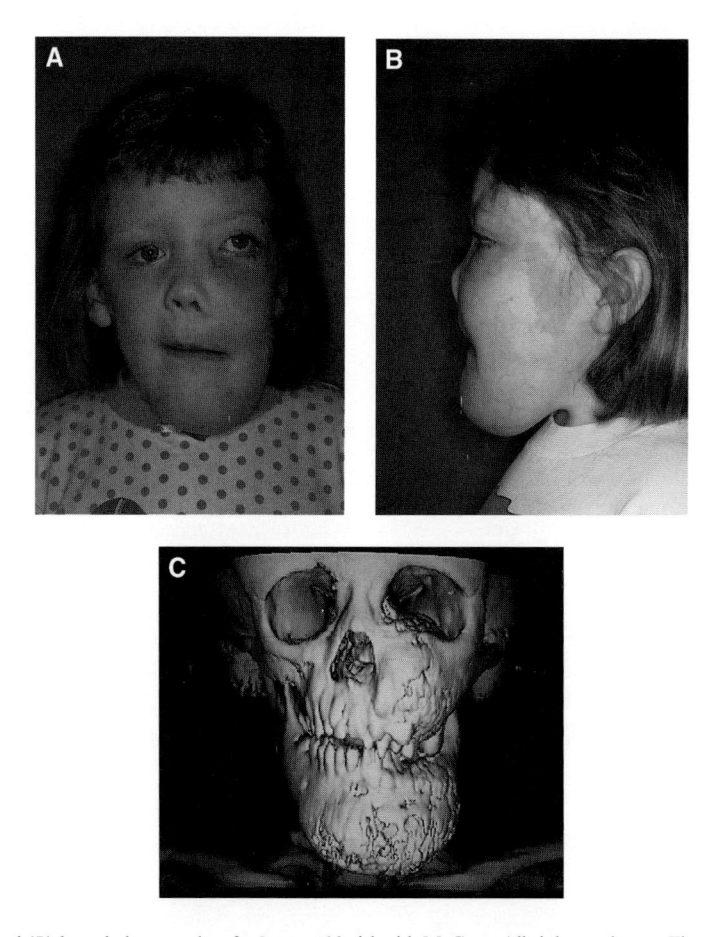

Fig. 1. (*A*) Frontal and (*B*) lateral photographs of a 9-year-old girl with McCune-Albright syndrome. The massive growth of FD in the symphysis region displaced the tongue posteriorly into the oropharynx, which caused airway obstruction that resulted in patient's failure to thrive. She also had nasal airway obstruction caused by obliteration of the left nasal cavity and impaired vision caused by left optic nerve compression. (*C*) Three-dimensional CT image demonstrates the involvement of the mandible, left zygoma, maxilla, and orbit. (*From* Troulis M, William B, Kaban L. Jaw tumors in children. In: Kaban LB, Troulis MJ, editors. Pediatric oral and maxillofacial surgery. Philadelphia: WB Saunders; 2004. p. 224.)

The G protein family includes five types, which are most clearly distinguished by their different α subunits. These types are Gs (stimulatory of adenylyl cyclase), Gi (inhibitory of adenylyl cyclase), Gq (activates phospholipase), and Gt (transducins 1 and 2) [12,13].

The actions of parathyroid, luteinizing, adrenocorticotropic hormones, glucagon, and adrenaline are achieved with mediation of Gs protein [14]. The cascade of events that results in transmission of a signal into the cell through Gs is as follows: (1) binding of the ligand (hormone or growth factor, first messenger) to the receptor (G protein-coupled receptor), (2) dissociation of the α subunit from GβGγ and replacement of the linked to Gα GDP by GTP, (3) activation of the enzyme adenylyl cyclase by binding to the active α subunit, and (4) formation of cAMP (3,5-cyclic adenosine monophosphate) from ATP (catalyzed by adenylyl cyclase). cAMP is the second messenger of the signal that activates intracellular proteins. Eventually, α subunit unbinds from adenylyl cyclase and links again to GβGγ, which is caused by hydrolysis of GTP (linked to Gα) to GDP. G protein is rendered inactive and is ready to act again and repeat the cycle. The gene that encodes α subunit of Gs protein (GNAS1) was mapped in 1991 by Levine and colleagues [15] by in situ hybridization. It was found to be located on 20q13.2.

One of two specific point mutations of GNAS1 is the cause of McCune-Albright syndrome, polyostotic FD, monostotic FD, and pituitary adenoma. These mutations are either C→T, which results in Arg201Cys, or G→A, which results in Arg201His [16–20]. They occur in somatic cells after conception (postzygotic mutations) either during embryonic development or after birth. The extent and form of the disease depend on the stage of development and the location at which the mutation occurs. The earlier during embryogenesis the mutation occurs, the more generalized the FD [21].

In detail, the GNAS1 mutation interferes with hydrolysis of GTP to GDP. $G_s\alpha$ cannot dissociate from adenylyl cyclase and bind to Gβγ. Adenylyl cyclase remains continuously active, which in turn results in continuous high levels of cAMP. Increased cAMP levels result in abnormal osteoblasts, abnormal bone, and increase in sex steroid receptors. These molecular abnormalities result in the pathology of McCune-Albright syndrome, polyostotic FD, monostotic FD, and pituitary adenoma [21]. In 1999, Collins and Shenker [22] reported an additional C→A GNAS1 mutation (Arg201Ser) in FD.

Traditionally, FD has been considered to be a bone disorder. Cohen [23] suggested that FD is a benign neoplasm based on four pieces of evidence: (1) The same activating mutation that causes FD also causes pituitary adenoma, which is a neoplasm [21]. (2) High levels of c-fos proto-oncogene expression were found in cells of FD lesions in eight patients [24]. (3) GNAS1 mutations have been identified in a few neoplasms (thyroid tumors [25], ovarian cysts [26], and Leydig cell tumor [27]). (4) McCune-Albright syndrome is associated with ovarian cysts and neoplasms, such as thyroid tumors, parathyroid adenoma, intramuscular myxoma, and carcinoma of the breast [22].

Diagnosis

For the purpose of communication, treatment, and clinical research, Kaban and colleagues [1] have classified lesions of FD as quiescent, nonaggressive, and aggressive on the basis of clinical behavior and radiographic findings. Quiescent lesions are usually seen in older patients (ie, adolescents and adults) and demonstrate no progressive growth. Teenagers present for evaluation and treatment of an asymptomatic jaw swelling or a facial asymmetry. Plain radiographs and CT scans demonstrate a predominantly radio-opaque expansion of the involved bone. Nonaggressive lesions are often seen in teenagers around the time of the pubertal growth spurt. They are mixed, radiolucent, radio-opaque lesions that demonstrate slow growth. Aggressive lesions usually appear in patients younger than 7 years of age. They are large, rapidly growing tumors often accompanied by tooth displacement, root resorption, cortical thinning, and perforation. There may be impingement on nerves that results in paresthesia and pain [1]. If the orbit or optic canal is affected, changes in visual acuity or blindness can result from optic nerve compression.

Imaging studies, biopsy, and molecular or mutational analysis are currently used in the diagnosis of FD and McCune-Albright syndrome. Laboratory studies to document endocrine disorders (eg, precocious puberty, hyperthyroidism, growth hormone excess, Cushing's syndrome, renal phosphate wasting) are helpful in making the diagnosis of McCune-Albright syndrome. According to Collins and Shenker [22], the definition of McCune-Albright syndrome is FD plus at least one of the endocrinopathies and/or café-au-lait spots.

The appearance of FD on plain radiographs depends on the age of the patient, the chronicity of the lesion, and the activity of the tumor. In quiescent and nonaggressive lesions, the bone is enlarged or expanded and the matrix may be densely radio-opaque or may have a "ground glass" appearance.

The more mature the lesion, the more radiodense it appears on plain radiographs. In patients with aggressive lesions, the bony contour is expanded and there is often cortical thinning, cortical perforation, displaced teeth, and root resorption. FD lesions of the jaws are often poorly defined, whereas in the long bones they are circumscribed with a sclerotic periphery. In the mandible, FD frequently arises below the inferior alveolar canal and displaces it superiorly [8,9].

CT scans display the range of opacification and demonstrate fine details of the pathologic condition, including extent of the lesion, expansion of bone, and local destruction. The characteristic mixed radiolucent and radio-opaque nature of FD and the expansion of bony contour may help distinguish FD from a giant cell tumor, myxoma, or invasive malignant bone tumor. Three-dimensional bone imaging with helical CT provides a superior perspective of the involved bone and overlying soft tissue (Fig. 1). It allows precise preoperative diagnosis and surgical planning [28–30].

MRI of FD demonstrates intermediate signal intensity on T1-weighted images, whereas high signal intensity is present on T2-weighted images, depending on the amount of bone trabeculae and degree of cellularity. MRI offers greater specificity when evaluating neurovascular and ocular involvement. A technetium 99m methylene diphosphonate bone scan is useful to determine if disease is monostotic or polyostotic. Increased uptake of the radioactive isotope is demonstrated in areas of increased blood supply and osteoblastic activity throughout the skeleton.

Biopsy is used to establish the diagnosis, especially in monostotic cases. An open or needle biopsy can be performed (Fig. 2). Histologically, an abnormal collagenous matrix surrounds immature bone or trabeculae that may show regularity in distribution and size. This appearance has been described as that of Chinese letters. Riminucci and colleagues [31] described three histologic patterns of FD. The "Chinese writing" pattern is found in lesions of the extremities, ribs, and vertebrae. The "pagetoid" form, characterized by sclerotic trabecular bone, is observed in cranial bones. The "hypercellular" pattern of FD is observed in the jaws and is characterized by dense, ordered, and often parallel bone trabeculae. Osteoblasts and osteoclasts are scant within the lesions [7]. Clinical growth activity of the tumor may correlate with the number of mast cells and osteoclasts at the periphery of the lesion [2], but standard histologic features do not help a clinician to predict the prognosis.

Serum alkaline phosphatase levels may be elevated depending on the extent of disease and the rate of growth (ie, quiescent, nonaggressive, or aggressive). Serum phosphate levels may be decreased. Thyroid function tests, including tri-iodothyronine, thyroxine, and thyroid-stimulating hormone levels, are performed to exclude hyperthyroidism. Pituitary gonadotropins and gonadosteroids are assessed in the evaluation of precocious puberty [22].

Genetic testing is an additional modality for the diagnosis of FD in selected cases. Mutations of GNAS1 that cause FD or McCune-Albright syndrome are somatic and result in mosaicism. Consequently, lesions and healthy tissues contain various proportions of mutant cells. Mutational analysis, although not routinely used, may be performed in specimen from the lesion or samples from the periphery blood. Karadag and colleagues [32] detected mutations in 49% to 72% of cells from FD specimens. Hannon and colleagues [33] identified

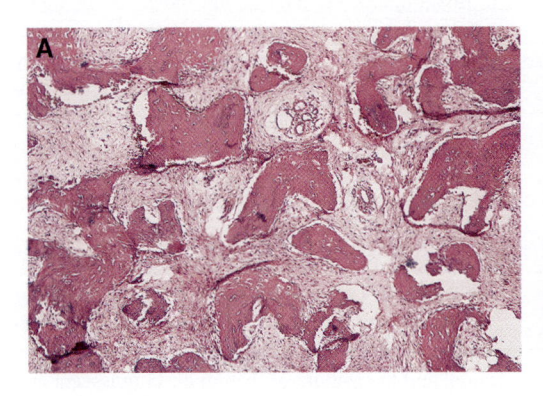

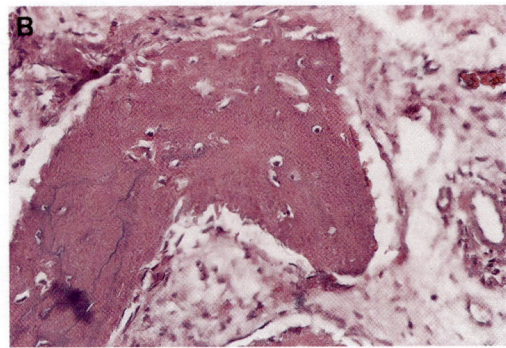

Fig. 2. (*A*) Histology slide of FD (original magnification ×100) shows typical microscopic pattern of the lesion (hematoxylin-eosin). (*B*) Same slide at a magnification of ×400. (*From* Troulis M, William B, Kaban L. Jaw tumors in children. In: Kaban LB, Troulis MJ, editors. Pediatric oral and maxillofacial surgery. Philadelphia: WB Saunders; 2004. p. 224.)

GNAS1 mutations in DNA from periphery blood in five of nine children with monostotic or polyostotic FD. Sequencing of the GNAS1 gene that demonstrates a heterozygous missense mutation on codon 201 confirms the diagnosis of FD. Absence of a GNAS1 mutation does not exclude FD, however, because the sample may not contain mutant cells.

Treatment

Treatment depends on the biologic behavior of the lesion in each patient. Growth of FD lesions is cyclic, with the greatest active change occurring during childhood or coinciding with onset of puberty or pregnancy. The lesion usually becomes quiescent and burns out in late teenage years or in the early twenties. Female patients may experience further growth of FD during pregnancy or with the start of oral contraceptives.

The options for surgical management include either contour excision or en bloc resection with or without bone grafting. Contour excision is performed in patients with quiescent and non-aggressive lesions that have been observed to exhibit no growth for at least 1 year (Fig. 3). Indications for contour resection include aesthetic deformities or functional problems,

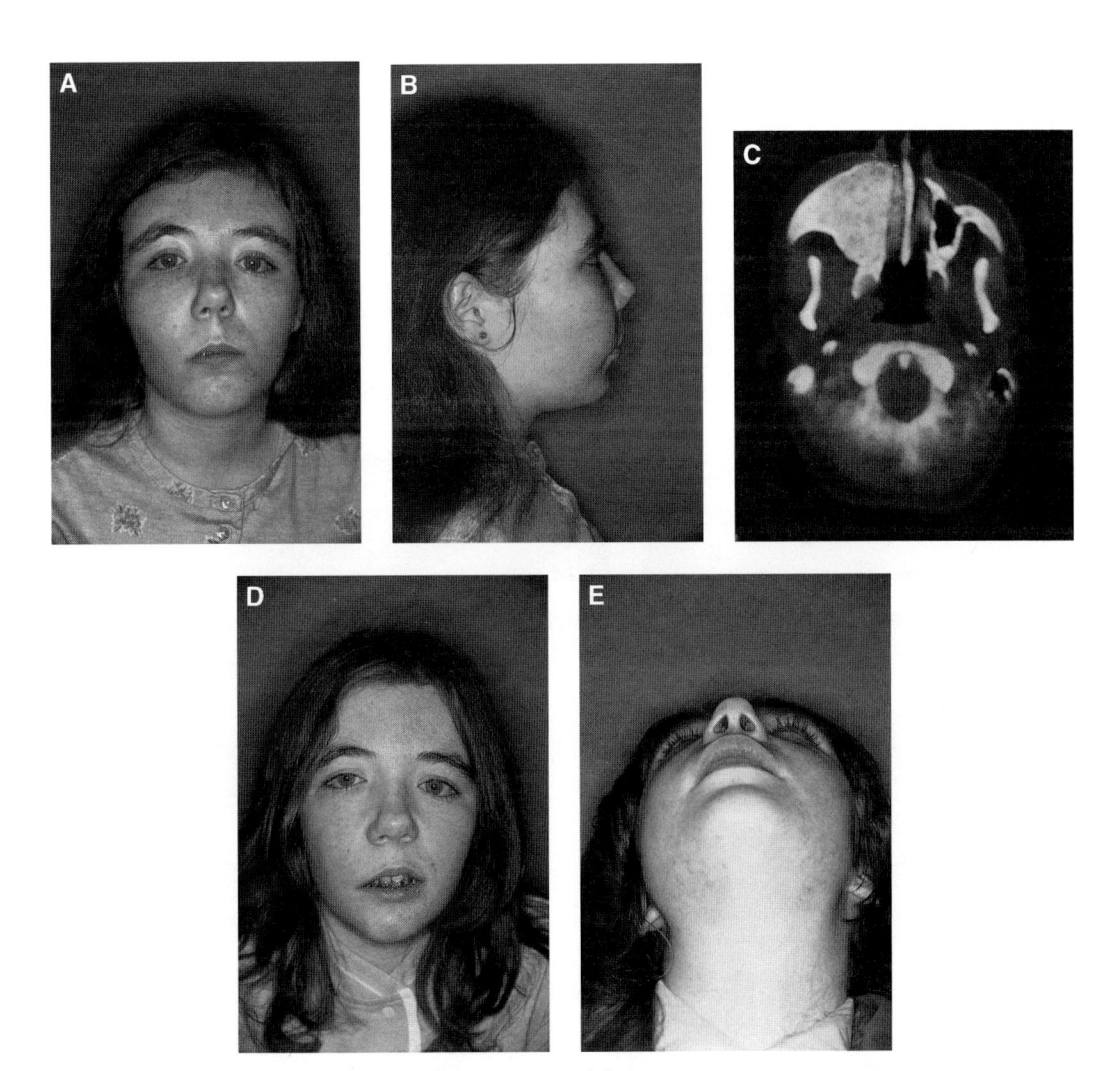

Fig. 3. (*A*) Frontal and (*B*) lateral views of a teenager with FD of the right maxilla, zygoma, and orbit. (*C*) Axial CT image shows the radiopaque lesion occupying the right maxilla. (*D*) Frontal and (*E*) submental photographs 1 year after contour excision of right zygoma and maxilla. (*From* Troulis M, William B, Kaban L. Jaw tumors in children. In: Kaban LB, Troulis MJ, editors. Pediatric oral and maxillofacial surgery. Philadelphia: WB Saunders; 2004. p. 226.)

such as paresthesia, trismus, proptosis, impairment of vision, and pain. Sach and colleagues [34] performed osteotomies of the maxilla and mandible in combination with contour excision in patients with malocclusion secondary to FD. En bloc resection, when possible, is reserved for patients with aggressive lesions that exhibit rapid or extensive growth, cause airway obstruction, or have recurred (Fig. 4). Contour or complete excision should be performed, when indicated, even in the face of continuing growth of the lesion [1]. This option is suggested, despite the risk of recurrence, to prevent serious or life-threatening complications when vital structures, such as nerves or airway, are displaced or compressed (Fig. 5).

The appropriate management of FD around the optic nerve, particularly in patients with normal vision, is controversial. Treatment options include either prophylactic decompression of the optic nerve (unroofing) or observation with regular ophthalmologic examinations in asymptomatic patients. The risks associated with optic nerve decompression include lack of improvement in vision and postoperative blindness. Lee and colleagues [35] studied 38 patients with FD of the sphenoid bone (12 with polyostotic FD and 26 with McCune-Albright syndrome). The patients underwent neuro-ophthalmologic examination and CT of the face and skull. In 38 patients, 67 optic canals were affected by FD. Only 2 patients (2 optic

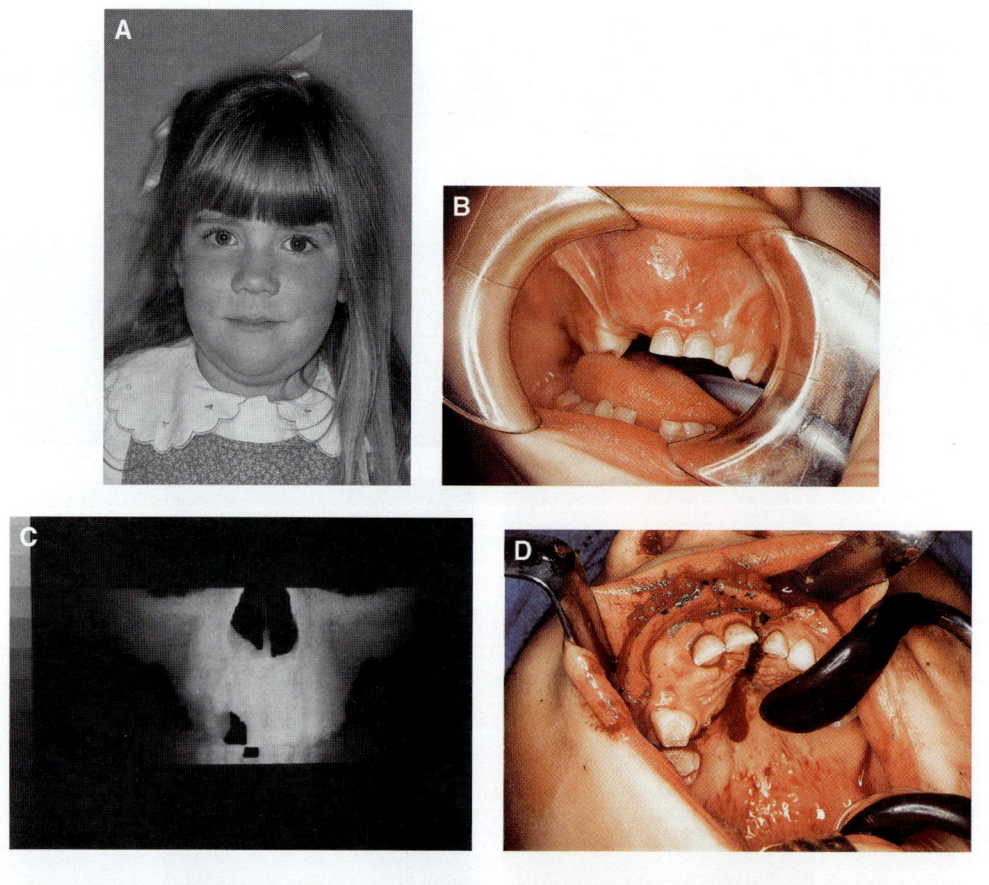

Fig. 4. (*A*) Frontal view of a 3-year-old patient with aggressive FD who presented with rapid onset of swelling in the anterior maxilla. The lesion had been curetted several weeks previously but had recurred. (*B*) Intraoral photograph at time of presentation at the clinic. The anterior maxilla is expanded and the right lateral incisor and canine are missing. They were removed at the first surgery because they were involved with the mass. (*C*) Three-dimensional CT image demonstrates the lesion and its relationship to the floor of the nose. (*D*) En block resection was the treatment of the aggressive lesion. (*E*) Histologic appearance of the lesion. (*F*) Patient 5 years postoperatively after reconstruction of the right maxilla with bone grafting and implants placement (*G*). (*From* Troulis M, William B, Kaban L. Jaw tumors in children. In: Kaban LB, Troulis MJ, editors. Pediatric oral and maxillofacial surgery. Philadelphia: WB Saunders; 2004. p. 225.)

nerves) had abnormal neuro-ophthalmologic findings, however. Narrowing of the affected canal did not always result in visual loss. "Prophylactic decompression of the optic nerve is therefore not necessarily indicated on the basis of the presence of FD on diagnostic images alone" [35].

Currently, bisphosphonates are used in cases of symptomatic polyostotic FD to decrease bone pain. Specifically, intravenous pamidronate administered for 3 days every 3 to 4 months has been proved to relieve pain and decrease bone metabolism in adults with FD [36]. Recently, oral bisphosphonates (alendronate) have been tried and compared with intravenous drugs with good results [37,38]. Plotkin and colleagues [38] first reported on the use of pamidronate treatment in children with polyostotic FD. They treated 18 children for 1.2 to 9.1 years and noticed a decrease in blood levels of bone production markers, such as alkaline phosphatase and urinary collagen type I N-telopeptide. They did not, however, document radiographic evidence of bone fill in lytic lesions or thickening of the cortex surrounding the lesions in any patient. They concluded that pamidronate therapy seems to be safe in children and adolescents with polyostotic FD but that there is no evidence that it has an effect on dysplastic lesions in such patients. Collins and colleagues [39] also found that pamidronate treatment decreased serum alkaline phosphatase but had no effect on the skeletal burden score (clinical severity) in children. Bisphosphonates may be useful for children with maxillofacial FD who experience difficulty with pain control [20]. The drug may slow down bony expansion in some patients.

Recent advances in the understanding of the molecular basis of FD hopefully will lead to effective nonsurgical treatments based on gene therapy in the future.

Cherubism

Background

In 1933, W.A. Jones reported three siblings, aged 6, 5, and 4 years, who developed an unknown bilat-

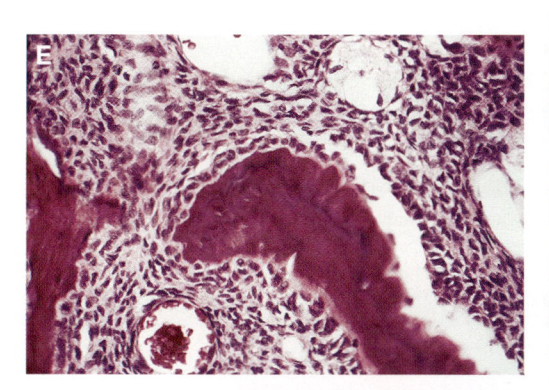

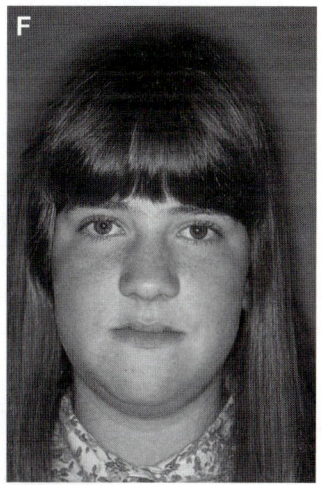

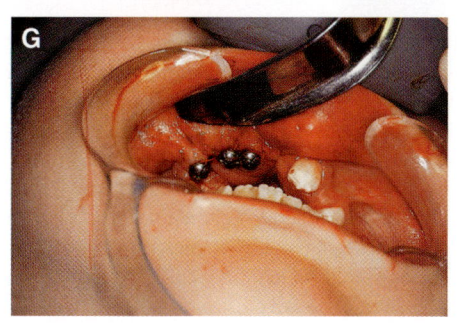

Fig. 4 (*continued*).

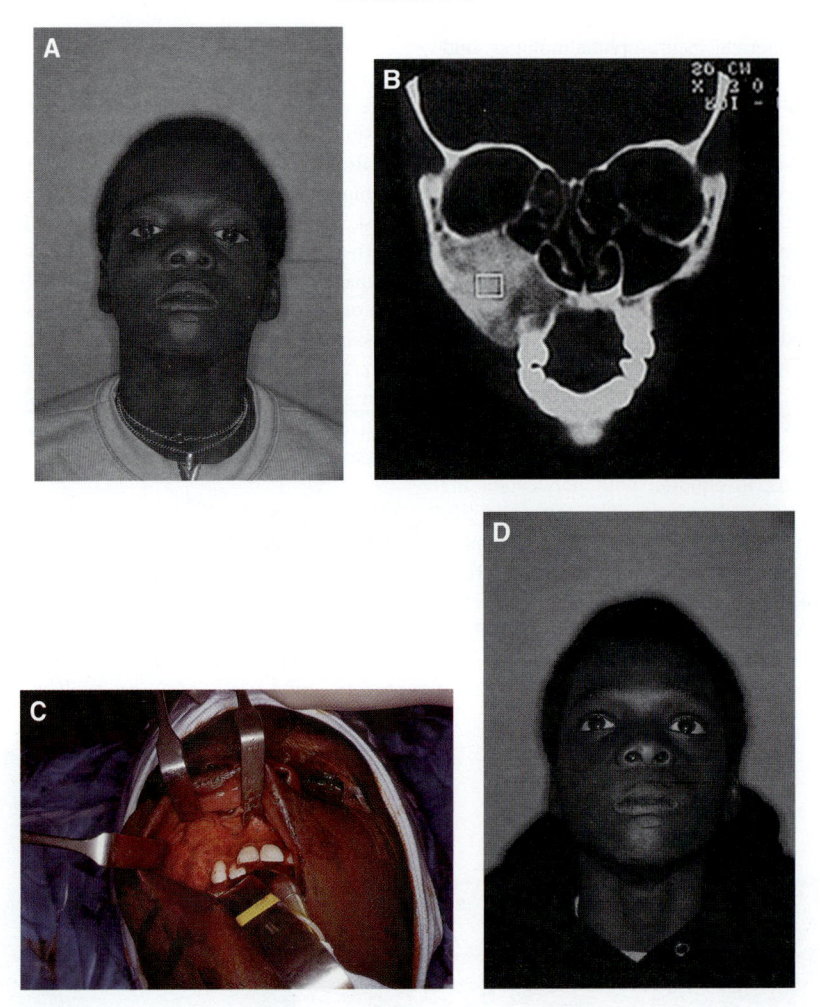

Fig. 5. (A) 10-year-old patient with slowly progressive swelling of the right cheek with paresthesia. (B) CT image shows dense and expanded right maxilla and zygoma with narrowing of the infraorbital foramen. (C) Intraoral photograph during the operation shows the maxilla expansion. Biopsy confirmed FD. The patient underwent contour excision and decompression of the infraorbital nerve. (D) Symmetric face 2 years postoperatively and normal sensory examination. (*From* Troulis M, William B, Kaban L. Jaw tumors in children. In: Kaban LB, Troulis MJ, editors. Pediatric oral and maxillofacial surgery. Philadelphia: WB Saunders; 2004. p. 223.)

eral polycystic disease of both jaws that resulted in fullness of the face. The children presented with "eyes having an upward cast," wide alveolar ridges, and misplaced or absent teeth [40]. Jones believed that these children resembled the cherubs in renaissance art and suggested the name "cherubism" for this disease. Since 1933, almost 215 cases of cherubism have been published [41,42].

Cherubism is a self-limiting, fibro-osseous lesion that primarily affects the jaws of children bilaterally and symmetrically (Fig. 6). The prominence of giant cells in the bone lesions has resulted in reporting them as a form of giant cell tumor [43]. Pierce and colleagues [44] referred to cherubism as "inherited craniofacial FD".

Cherubism is an autosomal dominant disorder with mutations in the gene SH3BP2, mapped on chromosome 4p16.3.3. Point mutations that cause amino acid substitutions have been described. The protein normally produced by this gene affects the cell's responses to incoming signals; these mutations may result in gain of function [45]. Most cases are caused by new dominant mutations. Therefore, the absence of a positive family history does not rule out

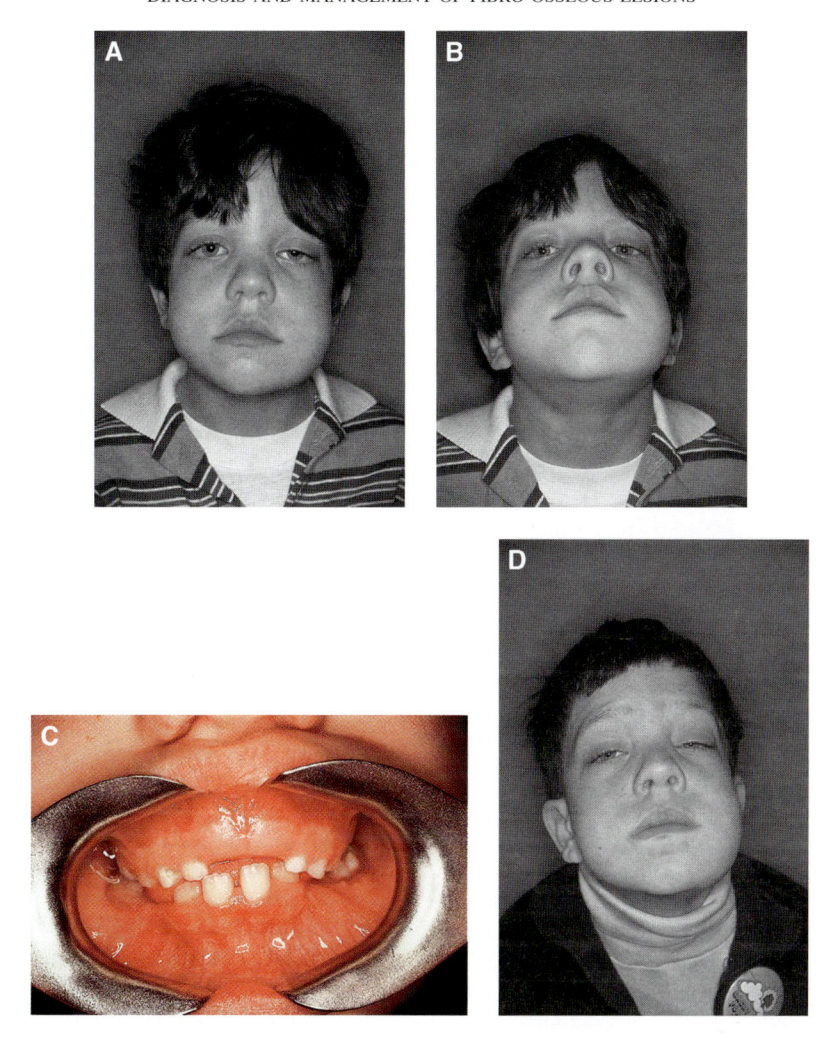

Fig. 6. Frontal (*A*) and submental (*B*) photographs of a 5-year-old patient with the typical cherubic appearance. The face is full with bilateral swelling of the cheeks. (*C*) Intraoral view shows the enlarged maxillary alveolus. (*D*) Patient 7 years later with further growth of the lesions and some increase in the size of the mandible. (*From* Troulis M, William B, Kaban L. Jaw tumors in children. In: Kaban LB, Troulis MJ, editors. Pediatric oral and maxillofacial surgery. Philadelphia: WB Saunders; 2004. p. 229.)

the possibility of cherubism [46,47]. Cherubism may be characterized by incomplete penetrance, with some gene carriers not exhibiting any signs of the disorder. The penetrance is reported 100% in men and 50% to 70% in women [42].

Males are affected twice as often as females. The appearance of affected children is normal at birth, but swelling of the jaws usually appears between 2 and 7 years of age. Cherubism usually has a self-limiting course. Around the age of puberty, the condition begins to regress until age 30, when lesions frequently are not detectable. In a follow-up study of 18 patients with cherubism, Von Wowern [48] found progressive new bone formation in the lesions in patients older than 20 years of age, but by age 41, the bone structure in the affected areas was completely normal. In some patients, cherubism can result in serious complications, such as airway obstruction [49] and extensive orbital involvement with risk of blindness [50,51].

Cases of cherubism associated with other disorders, such as fragile X syndrome, gingival fibromatosis and psychomotor retardation, neurofibromatosis type 1, and craniosynostosis, have been published in the literature [52–55]. In 1989, researchers reported that cherubism also was associated with Noonan syndrome, which is characterized by short stature, hypertelorism, prominent posteriorly angulated ears, congenital heart defect, low normal intelligence or developmental delay, cryptochidism in male patients, and bleeding disorders [56]. Cohen and Gorlin [57], however, proposed a new entity that they named Noonan-like/multiple giant cell lesion syndrome and considered it to be separate from Noonan syndrome and cherubism. They reviewed 15 cases of Noonan-like/multiple giant cell lesion syndrome. After that, 5 more cases of the same disease were published [58–62]. The distinctions between Noonan and Noonan-like/multiple giant cell lesion syndrome are the bleeding problems (secondary to platelet abnormalities and/or coagulation factor deficiencies) in the former and giant cell lesions that are present in the latter [62]. Differentiation between cherubism and Noonan-like/multiple giant cell lesion syndrome is important because the giant cell lesions in the latter syndrome may behave aggressively and produce considerably morbidity if not treated appropriately.

Molecular biology

In 1999, Tiziani and colleagues [63] and Mangion and colleagues [64] identified the locus for the gene for cherubism on chromosome 4p16.3. Tiziani and coworkers genotyped four families affected with cherubism and established the linkage to the same locus in all patients [63]. Mangion and coworkers also localized the cherubism gene to chromosome 4p16.3 in two additional families. They assumed that this gene encodes the production of receptor 3 for fibroblast growth factor, which is associated with various bone disorders, such as achondroplasia [64].

Ueki and others refined the cherubism locus to a 1.5-megabase interval between markers D4S127 and D4S115 by linkage and haplotype analysis of 12 families. The approved name of this gene is SH3-binding protein 2 (SH3BP2). Point mutations that caused amino acid substitutions in the SH3BP2 gene were detected. This adapter binding protein contains three modular peptide recognition domains: an N-terminal pleckstrin homology domain, a 10-amino-acid SH3 binding site, and a C-terminal SH2 domain. All mutations identified so far are in exon 9, and they affect three amino acids within a sequence of six amino acids located 31 to 36 amino acids upstream of the SH2 domain and 205 to 210 amino acids downstream of the SH3-binding domain. Mutations in pro418 (to leu, arg, or his) were the most common and occurred in 8 families. Other mutations resulted in gly420 being replaced by glu or arg and in arg415 being replaced by pro or gln [65]. The accumulation of cosegregating sequence variants in families with cherubism and the absence of these variants in 200 unaffected controls provide compelling evidence that the mutations in SH3BP2 cause cherubism.

Diagnosis

The diagnosis of cherubism is based on bilateral and symmetric swelling of the mandible, maxilla and alveolar ridges, patient age, radiographic findings, and molecular analysis.

The mandible is always involved, whereas involvement of the maxilla varies (Fig. 6). When the latter is involved, the palate may be V-shaped with a high arch. Displaced, impacted, supernumerary, and missing teeth are common findings. Exposure of the sclera below the iris results in an apparent upward gaze that has been attributed to elevation of the eye, retraction of the lower lid, and loss of lower lid support. Orbital involvement in this disease usually appears late in affected individuals. Enlargement of the cervical lymph nodes contributes to the patient's full-faced appearance and is said to be caused by reticuloendothelial hyperplasia with fibrosis [66]. The lymph nodes become enlarged before the patient reaches 6 years of age, decrease in size after the age of 8, and are rarely enlarged after the age of 12 [49].

In 1957, Seward and Hanky [67] suggested a three-tier grading for the disease:

- Grade 1: bilateral lesions confined to the mandible extending up to the coronoid processes
- Grade 2: the same as grade 1, but with lesions in the maxillary tuberosities
- Grade 3: both jaws diffusely affected

In 1998, a modified classification system of cherubism was developed by Kalantar Motamedi [68] to address the location of involvement and the clinical and biologic behavior of the disease:

- Grade I: lesions of mandible without signs of root resorption
- Grade II: mandible and maxilla without root resorption
- Grade III: aggressive lesions of mandible with root resorption
- Grade IV: both jaws involved and root resorption present
- Grade V: rare, massively growing, aggressive and deforming juvenile cases that involve the maxilla and mandible and may include the coronoid process and condyles

Radiographs show bilateral, multilocular, radiolucent areas within the jawbones (Fig. 7). The coronoid processes are commonly involved, whereas the condyles are rarely affected. Although the radiologic characteristics of cherubism are not pathognomonic, the diagnosis is strongly suggested by bilateral symmetric jaw involvement that is limited to the maxilla and mandible. Imaging typically shows expansile remodeling of the involved bones, thinning of the cortices, and multilocular radiolucencies with a coarse trabecular pattern. The teeth may be displaced.

Although histopathologic investigation is not required in most cases to establish the diagnosis, when performed, it reveals multiple osteoclast-like multinucleated giant cells in a moderately loose fibrous stroma. Ovoid- to spindle-shaped cells are also present within the fine fibrillar collagenous stroma, numerous small vessels with large endothelial cells, and perivascular capillary cuffing. Eosinophilic cuffing seems to be specific to cherubism. These deposits are not present in many cases, however, and their absence does not exclude the diagnosis of cherubism [69]. The histologic findings of cherubism are the same as in aggressive and nonaggressive giant cell lesions, myxoma, aneurysmal bone cyst, and hemangioma and other vascular lesions.

For molecular analysis, genomic DNA from a blood sample is used for direct sequencing. A sample of the lesion also is used for DNA analysis [65]. The differential diagnoses for cherubism includes brown tumor of hyperparathyroidism, giant cell lesions, Noonan-like/multiple giant cell lesion syndrome, FD, and aneurysmal bone cyst. Analysis of parathyroid hormone levels, calcium, phosphorous, and alkaline phosphatase rule out hyperparathyroidism, although it is rare in children, except in patients with chronic renal failure (secondary hyperparathyroidism). Cherubism is best differentiated from these other conditions by identifying the gene.

Treatment

Because cherubism is expected to regress spontaneously, operative treatment may not be necessary. Initial management in most cases consists of longitudinal observation and follow-up. When the disease becomes quiescent, the jaw can be recontoured for aesthetic purposes without any risk. Indications for

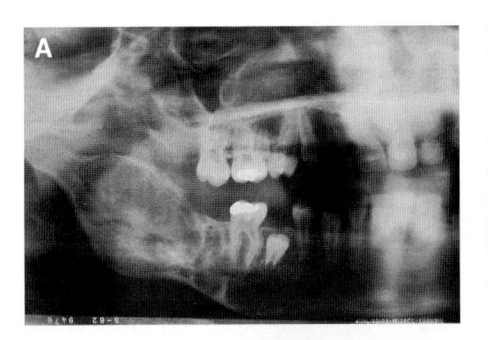

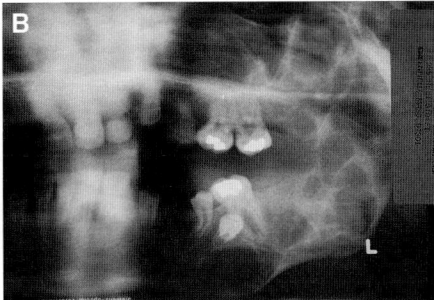

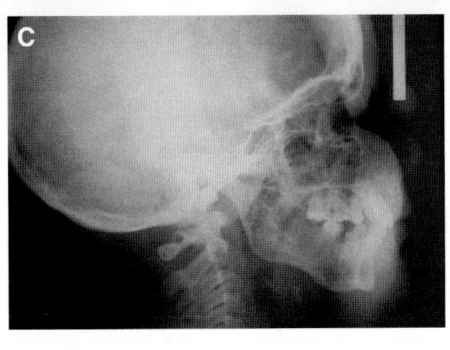

Fig. 7. (*A, B*) Panoramic radiographs of a child with cherubism demonstrate the bilateral multiloculated radiolucent areas in the mandible without involvement of the condyles. Impacted and missing teeth are confirmed. (*C*) Lateral cephalogram shows the multilocular radiolucent areas and the abnormal contour of the jaws. (*From* Troulis M, William B, Kaban L. Jaw tumors in children. In: Kaban LB, Troulis MJ, editors. Pediatric oral and maxillofacial surgery. Philadelphia: WB Saunders; 2004. p. 230.)

surgical intervention (eg, curettage, contouring, or osteotomy) before puberty include severe aesthetic or functional problems, such as airway obstruction. Surgical contouring during the growth phase has been reported to cause rapid regrowth of the tumor [66,70]. Shah and colleagues [71] also reported a case of leiomyosarcoma that arose in the mandible of a 10-year-old child with cherubism after two surgical recontouring procedures. Conversely, favorable results have been published after curettage and recontouring performed during a period of rapid growth of cherubism lesions [72]. Dukart and colleagues [72] found that surgical intervention arrests active growth of remnant cherubic lesions while stimulating bone regeneration. Von Wowern [48] reported 22 patients with cherubism who underwent biopsy with or without autotransplantation of ectopically erupted teeth. Surgical treatment did not provoke progression of the lesions in any of these cases.

The problem of early loss of deciduous teeth and delayed development and eruption of the permanent teeth is difficult, and no satisfactory solution is available. Space maintainers are used while waiting for the permanent teeth to erupt. Surgical exposure of impacted teeth is sometimes necessary [70].

Radiation therapy is contraindicated because of the potential for long-term adverse consequences, such as retardation of jaw growth, osteoradionecrosis, and increased incidence of induced malignancy [70]. In recent years, experimental use of calcitonin in the treatment of cherubism has been described [73].

Juvenile ossifying fibroma

Background

Ossifying fibroma of the jaw is a benign, fibro-osseous lesion first described in 1927 by Montgomery (Fig. 8) [74]. FD and ossifying fibroma are similar, and differentiating between the two may be difficult. They were considered as one entity by most authors until 1948 [75]. In general, ossifying fibroma is a more circumscribed lesion than FD and is usually surrounded by a fibrous capsule [76]. Ossifying fibroma may exhibit a sclerotic margin on plain radiographs and CT [8]. Microscopically, it is characterized by prominent osteoblasts, scant osteoclasts, and relatively prominent stromal cellularity. On the contrary, osteoblasts and osteoclasts are scarce and the stroma presents low to moderate cellularity in FD [7]. Ossifying fibroma is most commonly seen in the third and fourth decades of life. Juvenile ossifying fibroma (JOF), however, is a variant that occurs in children usually younger than age 15. This article focuses on JOF, also known as "aggressive," "active," or "psammomatoid" ossifying fibroma [77].

A lesion with the characteristics of a JOF was first reported by Benjamins in 1938 [78]. This lesion was located in the frontal sinus. The term "juvenile ossifying fibroma" was first used by Johnson in 1952 to describe aggressive forms of ossifying fibroma that occurred in the craniofacial bones of children [79]. Kramer and Pindborg [80] used the same term in the classification of odontogenic tumors in 1992 (World Health Organization). JOF is defined as a fibro-osseous lesion that is characterized by cell-rich fibrous tissue, bands of cellular osteoid trabeculae, and giant cells. It presents in children younger than 15 years of age, behaves aggressively, and tends to recur [81,82].

In most cases, JOF involves the paranasal sinuses, the orbit, the frontoethmoid bones, and the maxilla [83]. Few cases of mandibular JOF have been reported [81,84–87]. JOF sometimes develops in areas of congenitally missing teeth [87]. The reported recurrence rate for JOF ranges from 30% to 58% [88,89]. Local recurrence probably is caused by incomplete removal of tumor, particularly in maxillary/sinus and orbital regions.

Molecular biology

Little has been published on the molecular biology of JOF, probably because of the rarity of the tumor. In 1995, Sawyer and colleagues [90] reported the presence of identical chromosomal breakpoints occurring in three cementifying fibromas (psammomatoid JOFs according to El-Mofty) of the orbit at bands Xq26 and 2q33 [82]. Two of the tumors showed an identical t(X;2)(q26;q33) reciprocal translocation as the sole abnormality. The third tumor revealed an interstitial insertion of bands 2q24.2q33 into Xq26 as the sole abnormality.

Diagnosis

Clinically, JOF may present as an asymptomatic, painless expansion of the affected bone that leads to facial asymmetry. The tumor can grow to a considerable size and may behave as an aggressive lesion that destroys bone. Sometimes JOF exhibits rapid growth. Pain and paresthesia are rarely manifested. Nasal obstruction, epistaxis, exophthalmos, and, rarely, intracranial extension can be associated with

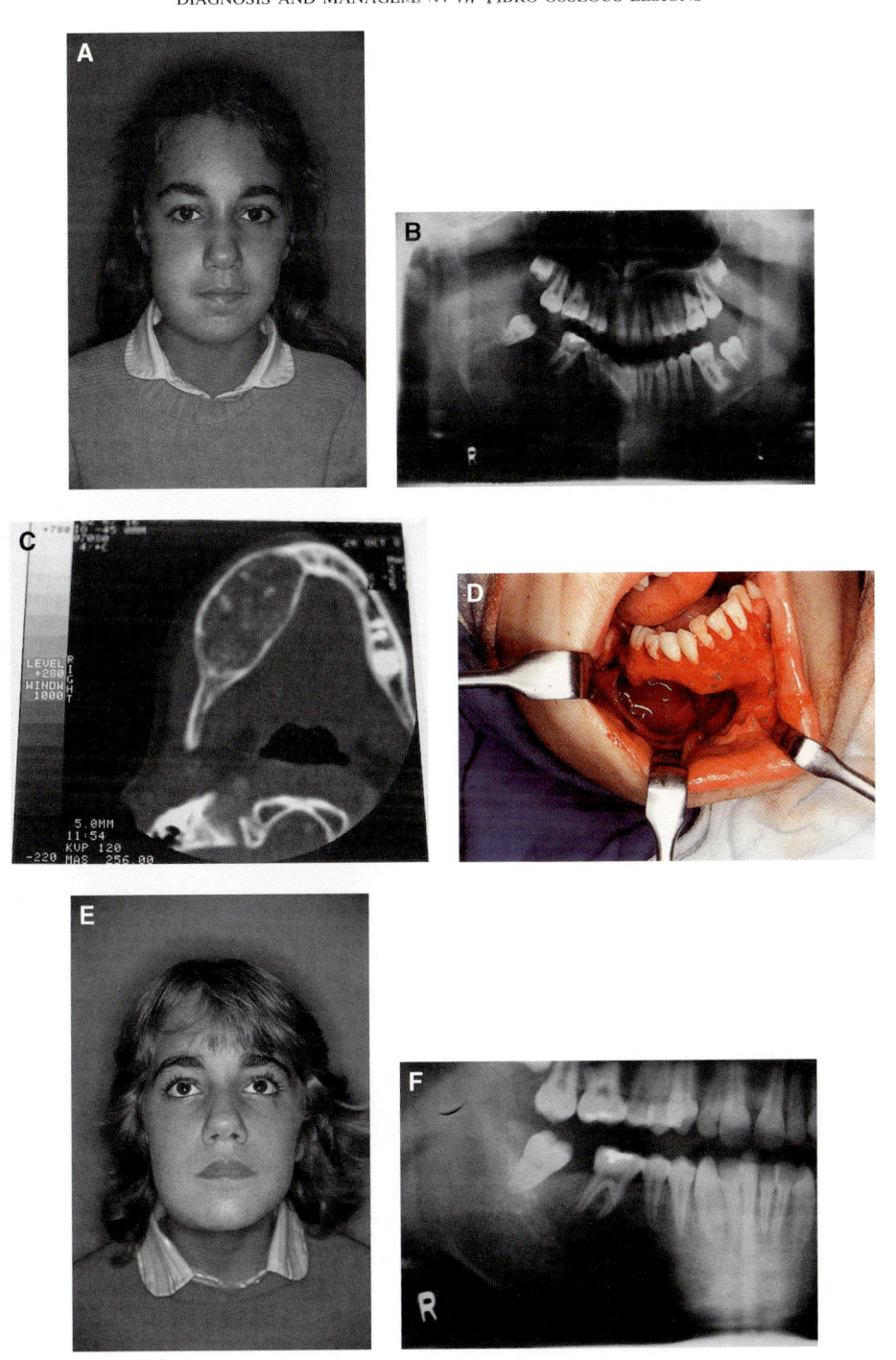

Fig. 8. (*A*) 12-year-old patient with painless right mandibular swelling. (*B*) Panoramic radiograph shows a large radiolucent lesion that extends to the mandibular inferior border and displaces the second molar. (*C*) Axial CT scan demonstrates a solid lesion and expansion of the mandibular cortical plates. (*D*) Intraoperative view of enucleation of the lesion. Histology confirmed ossifying fibroma. (*E*) Frontal view 1 year postoperatively. (*F*) Radiographic demonstration of bone filling. Bone grafting was not needed. (*From* Troulis M, William B, Kaban L. Jaw tumors in children. In: Kaban LB, Troulis MJ, editors. Pediatric oral and maxillofacial surgery. Philadelphia: WB Saunders; 2004. p. 228.)

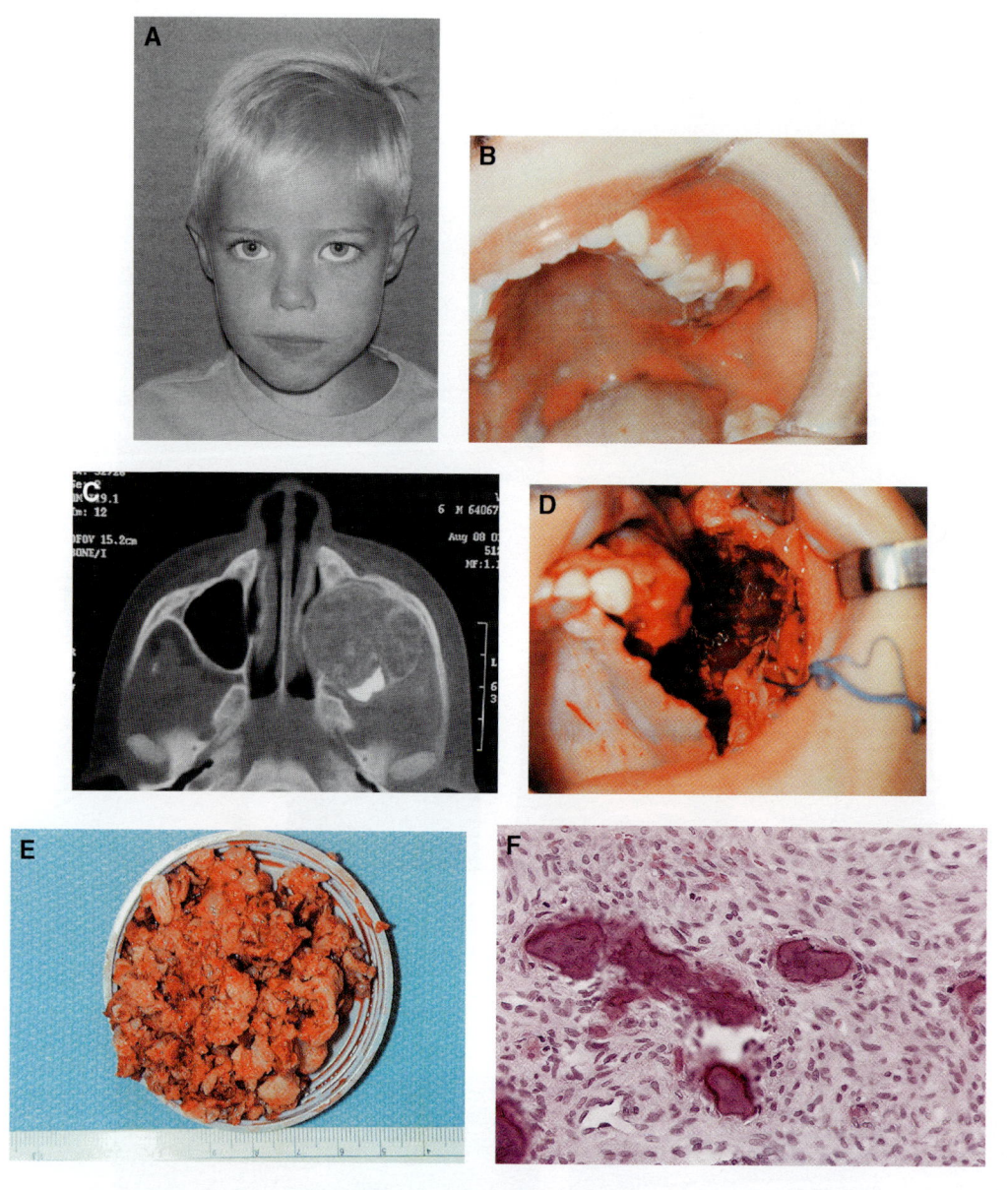

Fig. 9. (*A*) 6-year-old boy with a rapidly expanding lesion of the left maxilla. (*B*) Intraoral view of the maxillary expansion. (*C*) Axial CT image shows a large tumor that involves the left maxilla, occupies the maxillary sinus, and extends into the nasal cavity and the subtemporal space. The tumor that displaces an upper molar, demonstrates thin sclerotic border and calcification areas. Urine basic fibroblast growth factor was normal three times. (*D, E*) Intraoperative views show the thorough curettage. Adjuvant interferon therapy followed for 1 year. (*F*) Histology confirmed juvenile ossifying fibromas. (Courtesy of William Faquin, MD, Boston, MA). Frontal (*G*) and intraoral (*H*) photographs 2 years postoperatively. The child remains tumor free, and urine basic fibroblast growth factor is normal. (*From* Troulis M, William B, Kaban L. Jaw tumors in children. In: Kaban LB, Troulis MJ, editors. Pediatric oral and maxillofacial surgery. Philadelphia: WB Saunders; 2004. p. 227.)

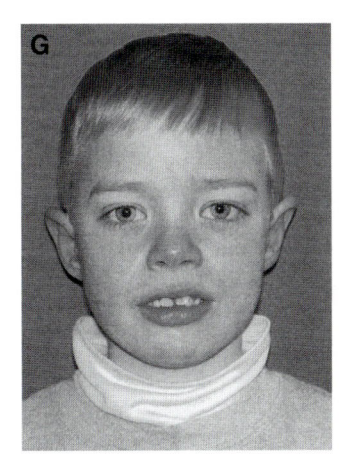

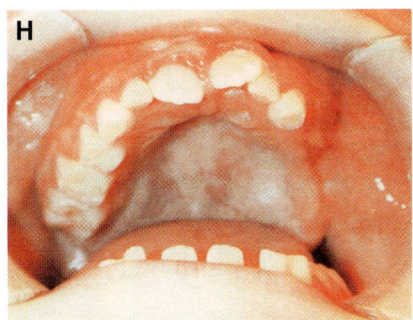

Fig. 9 (*continued*).

lesions that arise in the paranasal sinuses, orbit, and maxilla. Patients' ages range from 2 to 15 years, and a slight male dominance is observed [82].

Radiographically, JOF appears as a unilocular or multilocular radiolucency with defined borders and occasional central opacification. Aggressive lesions may show cortical thinning and perforation. A demarcation line between the neoplasm and the surrounding healthy bone tissue may be present.

CT findings of JOF may include well-defined borders identified by a thin sclerotic shell. Cortical disruption and involvement of adjacent anatomic structures also may be present. The lesion has a predominantly soft tissue consistency with a variable amount of internal calcification or bone. Radiolucent areas also may be noted. CT scan with intravenous contrast may show diffuse enhancement of the lesion. JOF appears to be more invasive and destructive on CT scans when compared with FD and adult or conventional ossifying fibroma [91].

There is an intermediate to low signal intensity on MRI, and the lesion enhances after gadolinium contrast injection. MRI offers great specificity when there is neurovascular and ocular involvement [8]. Accurate diagnosis of JOF is made by correlating the clinical, imaging, and histopathologic findings. Clinical and biologic behavior governs the treatment of this tumor.

Treatment

Nonaggressive forms of JOF are treated by a conservative operation that includes local excision or curettage [92]. Recurrence of JOF also may be managed by local surgical excision [89]. Aggressive JOFs with rapid growth rate, cortical thinning or perforation, tooth displacement, and root resorption may exhibit early recurrence unless treated by en bloc resection, however. The skeletal defect is reconstructed with bone graft once tumor margins are verified [81,93]. Troulis and colleagues [94] suggested a staged protocol for jaw reconstruction after en bloc resection of jaw tumors in children. Stage 1 includes the resection and placement of a rigid internal reconstruction plate. Stage 2 includes skeletal reconstruction with an autogenous bone graft (4–9 months after stage 1). Stage 3 consists of osseointegrated implant placement (5–12 months after stage 2) when possible. Stage 4 consists of prosthetic dental reconstruction (5–7 months after stage 3) [94].

Alternatively, for children with aggressive JOF in the maxilla, orbit, or paranasal sinuses, Kaban and colleagues [95,96] have suggested thorough curettage or enucleation in combination with adjuvant interferon alpha therapy for 1 year (Fig. 9). This protocol is based on the rapid growth, vascularity, and basic fibroblast growth factor (a vascular proliferative marker) production of these tumors in children.

Osteoblastoma

Background

Osteoblastoma occurs most commonly in the vertebrae and long bones (80% of cases), rarely in

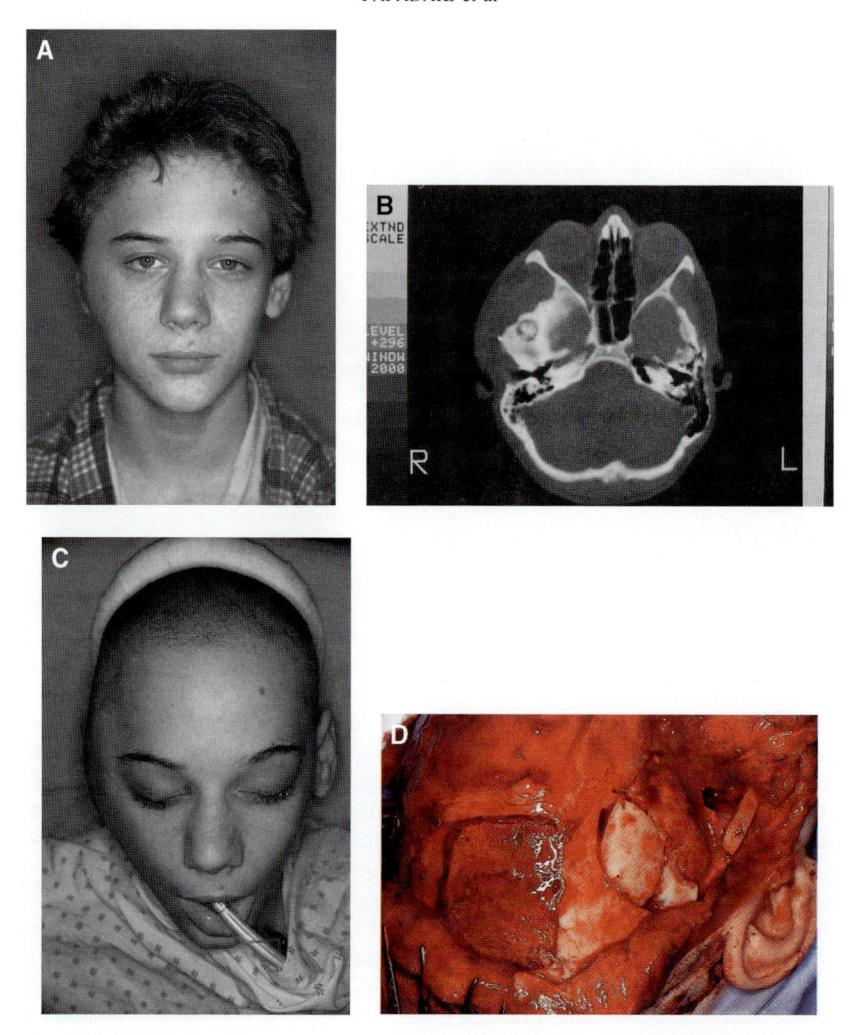

Fig. 10. (*A*) Teenage patient with osteoblastoma of the right temporomandibular joint. He complained of swelling, pain, and decreased motion. The maximal incisal opening was 18 mm. (*B*) Axial CT scan demonstrates the bone lesion involving the right temporomandibular joint and the floor of the middle cranial fossa. (*C*) The patient underwent excision of the tumor via coronal incision. (*D*) Intraoperative view shows reconstructed zygomatic arch, temporal bone, and glenoid fossa with calvarial bone (*arrows*) after tumor removal. (*E*) The patient has a normal range of mandibular motion 1 year postoperatively. (*F*) Frontal photograph shows better facial symmetry. (*From* Troulis M, William B, Kaban L. Jaw tumors in children. In: Kaban LB, Troulis MJ, editors. Pediatric oral and maxillofacial surgery. Philadelphia: WB Saunders; 2004. p. 231.)

the jaws. The tumor affects children and young adults, with an age range of 5 to 22 years [97–100].

Diagnosis

Patients present with swelling and, commonly, with chronic dull pain. The calvarium is the second most common site, and patients may have trismus if the temporal bone (glenoid fossa) and zygomatic arch are involved (Fig. 10). Most cases of jaw osteoblastomas that have been published are located on the condylar process. Radiographically, the osteoblastoma is usually a solitary radiolucent lesion. It may cause root resorption, although this is not common because of the location.

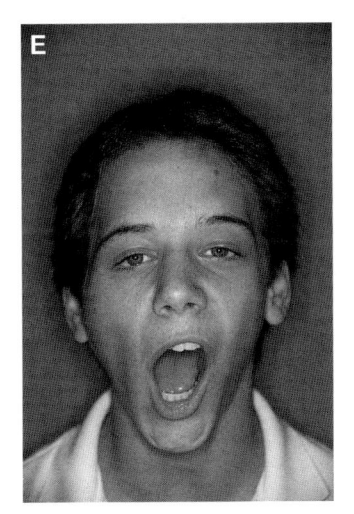

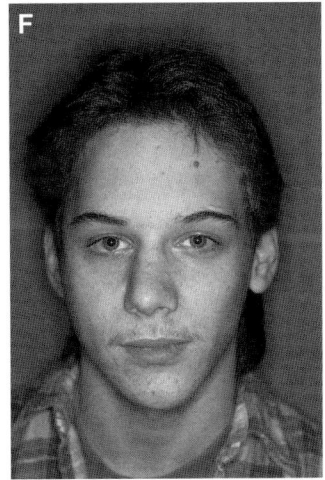

Fig. 10 (*continued*).

Treatment

En bloc resection is the required treatment for osteoblastoma because of the tendency for recurrence [101].

References

[1] Kaban LB. Aggressive jaw tumors in children. Oral Maxillofac Surg Clin North Am 1993;5(2):249–65.
[2] Chuong R, Kaban LB. Diagnosis and treatment of jaw tumors in children. J Oral Maxillofac Surg 1985; 43(5):323–32.
[3] Lichtenstein L. Polyostotic fibrous dysplasia. Arch Surg 1938;36:874–98.
[4] Lichtenstein L, Jaffe HL. Fibrous dysplasia of a bone: condition affecting one, several or many bones, graver cases of which may present abnormal pigmentation of skin, premature sexual development, hyperthyroidism or still other extraskeletal abnormalities. Arch Pathol 1942;33:777–83.
[5] Arbright F, Bulter AM, Hampton AO, Smith P. Syndrome characterized by osteitis fibrosa disseminata, areas of pigmentation and endocrine dysfunction with precocious puberty in females. N Engl J Med 1937;216:727–46.
[6] McCune DJ, Bruch H. Osteodystrophia fibrosa: report of a case in which the condition was combined with precocious puberty, pathologic pigmentation of the skin and hyperthyroidism, with a review of the literature. Am J Dis Child 1937;54:806–48.
[7] Regezi JA. Odontogenic cysts, odontogenic tumors, fibroosseous, and giant cell lesions of the jaws. Mod Pathol 2002;15(3):331–41.
[8] MacDonald-Jankowski DS. Fibro-osseous lesions of the face and jaws. Clin Radiol 2004;59(1):11–25.
[9] Singer SR, Mupparapu M, Rinaggio J. Clinical and radiographic features of chronic monostotic fibrous dysplasia of the mandible. J Can Dent Assoc 2004;70(8):548–52.
[10] Weinstein LS, Shenker A, Gejman PV, et al. Activating mutations of the stimulatory G protein in the McCune-Albright syndrome. N Engl J Med 1991; 325:1688–95.
[11] Shenker A, Chanson P, Weinstein LS, et al. Osteoblastic cells derived from isolated lesions of fibrous dysplasia contain activating somatic mutations of the G(S)-alpha gene. Hum Mol Genet 1995;4:1675–6.
[12] Neer EJ. G proteins: critical control points for transmembrane signals. Protein Sci 1994;3(1):3–14.
[13] Stryer L, Bourne HR. G proteins: a family of signal transducers. Annu Rev Cell Biol 1986;2:391–419.
[14] Pfeuffer T, Helmreich EJ. Structural and functional relationships of guanosine triphosphate binding proteins. Curr Top Cell Regul 1988;29:129–216.
[15] Levine MA, Modi WS, O'Brien SJ. Mapping of the gene encoding the alpha subunit of the stimulatory G protein of adenylyl cyclase (GNAS1) to 20q13.2-q13.3 in human by in situ hybridization. Genomics 1991;11:478–9.
[16] Weinstein LS, Shenker A, Gejman PV, et al. Activating mutations of the stimulatory G protein in the McCune-Albright syndrome. N Engl J Med 1991; 325:1688–95.
[17] Schwindinger WF, Francomano CA, Levine MA. Identification of a mutation in the gene encoding the alpha subunit of the stimulatory G-protein of adenylyl cyclase in McCune-Albright syndrome. Proc Natl Acad Sci U S A 1992;89:5152–6.
[18] Candeliere GA, Roughley PJ, Glorieux FH. Polymer-

ase chain reaction-based technique for the selective enrichment and analysis of mosaic arg201 mutations in G alpha s from patients with fibrous dysplasia of bone. Bone 1997;21:201–6.
[19] Malchoff CD, Reardon G, MacGillivrary DC, et al. An unusual presentation of McCune-Albright syndrome confirmed by an activating mutation of the G(s) alpha-subunit from a bone lesion. J Clin Endocrinol Metab 1994;78:803–6.
[20] Williamson EA, Ince PG, Harrison D, et al. G-protein mutations in human pituitary adrenocorticotrophic hormone-secreting adenomas. Eur J Clin Invest 1991; 25:128–31.
[21] Cohen MM, Howell RE. Etiology of fibrous dysplasia and McCune-Albright syndrome. Int J Oral Maxillofac Surg 1999;28(5):366–71.
[22] Collins MT, Shenker A. McCune-Albright syndrome: new insights. Exp Clin Endocrinol Diabetes 1999;6: 119–25.
[23] Cohen MM. Fibrous dysplasia is a neoplasm. Am J Med Genet 2001;98(4):290–3.
[24] Candeliere GA, Glorieux FH, Prudhomme J, et al. Increased expression of the c-fos proto-oncogene in bone from patients with fibrous dysplasia. N Engl J Med 1995;332:1546–51.
[25] Ballaré E, Mantovani S, Lania A, et al. Activating mutations of the $G_s\alpha$ gene are associated with low levels of $G_s\alpha$ protein in growth hormone-secreting tumors. J Clin Endocrinol Metab 1998;80:1347–51.
[26] Pienkowski C, Lumbroso S, Bieth E, et al. Recurrent ovarian cyst and mutation of the $G_s\alpha$ gene in ovarian cyst fluid cells: what is the link with McCune-Albright syndrome. Acta Paediatr 1997;86:1019–21.
[27] Fragoso MCBV, Latronico AC, Carvalho FM, et al. Activating mutation of the stimulatory G protein as a putative cause of ovarian and testicular human stromal Leydig cell tumors. J Clin Endocrinol Metab 1998;83:2074–8.
[28] Fenlon HM, Breatnach E. 3-D CT aids planning of craniofacial surgery. Diagn Imaging 1995;17(8): 52–7.
[29] Cavalcanti MG, Antunes JL. 3D-CT imaging processing for qualitative and quantitative analysis of maxillofacial cysts and tumors. Pesqui Odontol Bras 2002;16(3):189–94.
[30] Gosain AK, Celik NK, Aydin MA. Fibrous dysplasia of the face: utility of three-dimensional modeling and ex situ malar recontouring. J Craniofac Surg 2004; 15(6):909–15.
[31] Riminucci M, Liu B, Corsi A, et al. The histopathology of fibrous dysplasia of bone in patients with activating mutations of the $Gs\alpha$ gene: site-specific patterns and recurrent histological hallmarks. J Pathol 1999;187(2):249–58.
[32] Karadag A, Riminucci M, Bianco P, et al. A novel technique based on a PNA hybridization probe and FRET principle for quantification of mutant genotype in fibrous dysplasia/McCune-Albright syndrome. Nucleic Acids Res 2004;32(7):e63.

[33] Hannon TS, Noonan K, Steinmetz R, et al. Is McCune-Albright syndrome overlooked in subjects with fibrous dysplasia of bone? J Pediatr 2003; 142(5):532–8.
[34] Sach SA, Kleiman M, Pasternak R. Surgical management of a facial deformity secondary to craniofacial fibrous dysplasia. J Oral Maxillofac Surg 1984;42: 192–7.
[35] Lee JS, FitzGibbon E, Butman JA, et al. Normal vision despite narrowing of the optic canal in fibrous dysplasia. N Engl J Med 2002;347(21):1670–6.
[36] Lane JM, Khan SN, O'Connor WJ, et al. Bisphosphonate therapy in fibrous dysplasia. Clin Orthop 2001; 382:6–12.
[37] Kitagawa Y, Tamai K, Ito H. Oral alendronate treatment for polyostotic fibrous dysplasia: a case report. J Orthop Sci 2004;9(5):521–5.
[38] Plotkin H, Rauch F, Zeitlin L, et al. Effect of pamidronate treatment in children with polyostotic fibrous dysplasia of bone. J Clin Endocrinol Metab 2003;88(10):4569–75.
[39] Collins MT, Kushner H, Reynolds JC, et al. An instrument to measure skeletal burden and predict functional outcome in fibrous dysplasia of bone. J Bone Miner Res 2005;20(2):219–26.
[40] Jones WA. Familial multilocular cystic disease of the jaws. Am J Cancer 1933;17(4):946–50.
[41] Belloc JB, Divaris M, Cancemi GF, et al. Cherubism: apropos of a major case. Rev Stomatol Chir Maxillofac 1993;94(3):152–8.
[42] Ongole R, Pillai RS, Pai KM. Cherubism in siblings: a case report. J Can Dent Assoc 2003;69(3):150–4.
[43] Auclair P, Arendt DM, Hellstein JW. Giant cell lesions of the jaws. Oral Maxillofac Surg Clin North Am 1997;9:655–80.
[44] Pierce AM, Sampson WJ, Wilson DF, et al. Fifteen-year follow-up of a family with inherited craniofacial fibrous dysplasia. J Oral Maxillofac Surg 1996; 54(6):780–8.
[45] Stoler MJ. Molecular genetics and syndrome recognition for the clinician. In: Kaban LB, Troulis MJ, editors. Pediatric oral and maxillofacial surgery. Philadelphia: WB Saunders; 2004. p. 32.
[46] Benetti C, Crippa R, Mazza M, et al. Nonfamilial cherubism: a clinical case report. Minerva Stomatol 1995;44(3):119–26.
[47] Rattan V, Utreja A, Singh BD, et al. Non-familial cherubism: a case report. J Indian Soc Pedod Prev Dent 1997;15(4):118–20.
[48] Von Wowern N. Cherubism: a 36-year long-term follow-up of 2 generations in different families and review of the literature. Oral Surg Oral Med Oral Pathol Oral Radiol Endod 2000;90(6):765–72.
[49] Battaglia A, Merati A, Magit A. Cherubism and upper airway obstruction. Otolaryngol Head Neck Surg 2000;122(4):573–4.
[50] Carroll AL, Sullivan TJ. Orbital involvement in cherubism. Clin Experiment Ophthalmol 2001; 29(1):38–40.

[51] Ahmadi AJ, Pirinjian GE, Sires BS. Optic neuropathy and macular chorioretinal folds caused by orbital cherubism. Arch Ophthalmol 2003;121(4):570–3.

[52] Quan F, Grompe M, Jakobs P, et al. Spontaneous deletion in the FMR1 gene in a patient with fragile X syndrome and cherubism. Hum Mol Genet 1995;4(9): 1681–4.

[53] Yalcin S, Yalcin F, Soydinc M, et al. Gingival fibromatosis combined with cherubism and psychomotor retardation: a rare syndrome. J Periodontol 1999;70(2):201–4.

[54] Ruggieri M, Pavone V, Polizzi A, et al. Unusual form of recurrent giant cell granuloma of the mandible and lower extremities in a patient with neurofibromatosis type 1. Oral Surg Oral Med Oral Pathol Oral Radiol Endod 1999;87(1):67–72.

[55] Stiller M, Urban M, Golder W, et al. Craniosynostosis in cherubism. Am J Med Genet 2000;95(4): 325–31.

[56] Dunlap C, Neville B, Vickers RA, et al. The Noonan syndrome/cherubism association. Oral Surg Oral Med Oral Pathol 1989;67(6):698–705.

[57] Cohen Jr MM, Gorlin RJ. Noonan-like/multiple giant cell lesion syndrome. Am J Med Genet 1991;40(2): 159–66.

[58] Levine B, Skope L, Parker R. Cherubism in a patient with Noonan syndrome: report of a case. J Oral Maxillofac Surg 1991;49(9):1014–8.

[59] Betts NJ, Stewart JC, Fonseca RJ, et al. Multiple central giant cell lesions with a Noonan-like phenotype. Oral Surg Oral Med Oral Pathol 1993;76(5): 601–7.

[60] Addante RR, Breen GH. Cherubism in a patient with Noonan's syndrome. J Oral Maxillofac Surg 1996; 54(2):210–3.

[61] Bertola DR, Kim CA, Pereira AC, et al. Are Noonan syndrome and Noonan-like/multiple giant cell lesion syndrome distinct entities? Am J Med Genet 2001; 98(3):230–4.

[62] Edwards PC, Fox J, Fantasia JE, et al. Bilateral central giant cell granulomas of the mandible in an 8-year-old girl with Noonan syndrome (Noonan-like/multiple giant cell lesion syndrome). Oral Surg Oral Med Oral Pathol Oral Radiol Endod 2005;99(3): 334–40.

[63] Tiziani V, Reichenberger E, Buzzo CL. The gene for cherubism maps to chromosome 4p16. Am J Hum Genet 1999;65(1):158–66.

[64] Mangion J, Rahman N, Edkins S, et al. The gene for cherubism maps to chromosome 4p16.3. Am J Hum Genet 1999;65(1):151–7.

[65] Ueki Y, Tiziani V, Santanna C, et al. Mutations in the gene encoding c-Abl-binding protein SH3BP2 cause cherubism. Nat Genet 2001;28(2):125–6.

[66] Koury ME, Stella JP, Epker BN. Vascular transformation in cherubism. Oral Surg Oral Med Oral Pathol 1993;76(1):20–7.

[67] Seward GR, Hankey GT. Cherubism. J Oral Surg 1957;10(9):952–74.

[68] Kalantar Motamedi MH. Treatment of cherubism with locally aggressive behavior presenting in adulthood: report of four cases and a proposed new grading system. J Oral Maxillofac Surg 1998;56(11): 1336–42.

[69] Lannon DA, Earley MJ. Cherubism and its charlatans. Br J Plast Surg 2001;54(8):708–11.

[70] Kuepper RC, Harrigan WF. Treatment of mandibular cherubism. J Oral Surg 1978;36(8):638–41.

[71] Shah N, Handa KK, Sharma MC. Malignant mesenchymal tumor arising from cherubism: a case report. J Oral Maxillofac Surg 2004;62(6):744–9.

[72] Dukart RC, Kolodny SC, Polte HW, et al. Cherubism: report of case. Oral Surg 1974;32(10):782–5.

[73] Southgate J, Sarma U, Townend JV, et al. Study of the cell biology and biochemistry of cherubism. J Clin Pathol 1998;51(11):831–7.

[74] Montgomery AH. Ossifying fibroma of the jaw. Arch Surg 1927;15:30–44.

[75] Walter JM, Terry BC, Small EW, et al. Aggressive ossifying fibroma of the maxilla: review of the literature and report of case. J Oral Surg 1979;37: 276–86.

[76] Commins DJ, Tolley NS, Milford CA. Fibrous dysplasia and ossifying fibroma of the paranasal sinuses. J Laryngol Otol 1998;112(10):964–8.

[77] Brannon RB, Fowler CB. Benign fibro-osseous lesions: a review of current concepts. Adv Anat Pathol 2001;8(3):126–43.

[78] Benjamins CE. Das osteoid-fibroma mit atypischer verkalkung im sinus frontalis. Acta Otolaryngol 1938; 26:26–43.

[79] Johnson LC. Bone pathology seminar. American Academy of Oral Pathology 1952;18:13–7.

[80] Kramer IR, Pindborg JJ. Histological classification of Odontogenic tumors. In: Kramer IR, Pindborg JJ, Shear M, editors. Histological typing of odontogenic tumours. 2nd edition. Berlin: Springer-Verlag; 1992. p. 28.

[81] Zama M, Gallo S, Santecchia L, et al. Juvenile active ossifying fibroma with massive involvement of the mandible. Plast Reconstr Surg 2004;113(3):970–4.

[82] El-Mofty S. Psammomatoid and trabecular juvenile ossifying fibroma of the craniofacial skeleton: two distinct clinicopathologic entities. Oral Surg Oral Med Oral Pathol Oral Radiol Endod 2002;93(3): 296–304.

[83] Fakadej A, Boynton JR. Juvenile ossifying fibroma of the orbit. Ophthal Plast Reconstr Surg 1996;12(3): 174–7.

[84] Reaume CE, Schmid RW, Wesley RK. Aggressive ossifying fibroma of the mandible. J Oral Maxillofac Surg 1985;43:631–40.

[85] Slootweg PJ, Muller H. Juvenile ossifying fibroma: report of four cases. J Craniomaxillofac Surg 1990; 18:125–31.

[86] Leimola-Virtanen R, Vähätalo K, Syrjänen S. Juvenile active ossifying fibroma of the mandible: a report of 2 cases. J Oral Maxillofac Surg 2001;59:439–44.

[87] Rinaggio J, Land M, Cleveland DB. Juvenile ossifying fibroma of the mandible. J Pediatr Surg 2003; 38(4):648–50.

[88] Johnson LC, Yousefi M, Vinh TN, et al. Juvenile active ossifying fibroma: its nature, dynamics and origin. Acta Otolaryngol Suppl 1991;448:1.

[89] Waldron CA. Fibro-osseous lesions of the jaws. J Oral Maxillofac Surg 1993;51:828.

[90] Sawyer JR, Tryka AF, Bell JM, et al. Nonrandom chromosome breakpoints at Xq26 and 2q33 characterize cemento-ossifying fibromas of the orbit. Cancer 1995;76(10):1853–9.

[91] Khoury NJ, Naffaa LN, Shabb NS, et al. Juvenile ossifying fibroma: CT and MR findings. Eur Radiol 2002;12:109–13.

[92] Slootweg PJ, Panders AK, Nikkels PG. Psammomatoid ossifying fibroma of the paranasal sinuses: an extragnathic variant of cemento-ossifying fibroma. Report of three cases. J Craniomaxillofac Surg 1993; 21(7):294–7.

[93] Troulis M, William B, Kaban L. Jaw tumors in children. In: Kaban LB, Troulis MJ, editors. Pediatric oral and maxillofacial surgery. Philadelphia: WB Saunders; 2004. p. 225.

[94] Troulis MJ, Williams WB, Kaban LB. Staged protocol for resection, skeletal reconstruction, and oral rehabilitation of children with jaw tumors. J Oral Maxillofac Surg 2004;62(3):335–43.

[95] Kaban LB, Troulis MJ, Ebb D, et al. Antiangiogenic therapy with interferon alpha for giant cell lesions of the jaws. J Oral Maxillofac Surg 2002;60(10): 1103–11.

[96] Troulis M, William B, Kaban L. Jaw tumors in children. In: Kaban LB, Troulis MJ, editors. Pediatric oral and maxillofacial surgery. Philadelphia: WB Saunders; 2004. p. 235.

[97] Lewin ML. Nonmalignant maxillofacial tumors in children. Plast Reconstr Surg 1966;38:186.

[98] Farman AG, Nortje CJ, Grotepass F. Periosteal benign osteoblastoma of the mandible: report of a case and review of the literature pertaining to benign osteoblastic neoplasms of the jaws. Br J Oral Surg 1976;14:12.

[99] Ozturk M, Ozec I, Aker H, et al. Osteoblastoma of the mandible with root resorption: a case report. Quintessence Int 2003;34(2):135–8.

[100] Nowparast B, Mesgarzadeh A, Lassemi I. Benign osteoblastoma of the mandible: a clinical-pathologic review and report of a case. Int J Oral Surg 1979;8(5): 386–90.

[101] Remagen W, Prein J. Benign osteoblastoma. Oral Surg Oral Med Oral Pathol 1975;39(2):279–83.

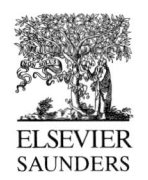

Oral Surgical Aspects of Child Abuse and Neglect

Naomi F. Sugar, MD[a],*, Kenneth W. Feldman, MD[b]

[a]*Department of Pediatrics, Division of General Pediatrics, University of Washington School of Medicine, Harborview Medical Center, 325 Ninth Avenue, Seattle, WA 98105, USA*
[b]*Department of Pediatrics, Division of General Pediatrics, University of Washington School of Medicine, Children's Hospital and Regional Medical Center, 4800 Sandypoint Way NE, Seattle, WA 98105, USA*

A 2-year-old boy presented for evaluation of facial bleeding and bruising. The mother's boyfriend had been roughhousing with him and his older sister. The mother reported that "somehow he flung him, but he did not make it to the bed." The child landed on thinly carpeted and padded concrete. He briefly lost unconsciousness and bled from his nose and mouth. He had bilateral nasal bleeding, blood around his upper central incisors, and a contused, lacerated lower lip. He had a 3-mm midline jaw shift to the left and he resisted jaw movement. Cranial CT showed no brain injury, but his right jaw was broken. The oral surgeon had a consultation and sutured the boy's lip. His skeletal survey confirmed the right jaw fracture; it exited just behind the second molar. An additional fracture was noted below the left condyle.

The first steps in managing child abuse effectively are to suspect that abuse might be the cause of clinical findings and to initiate an effective evaluation. An oral surgeon may be the first to recognize that abuse is a possible cause of injury or may be called as a consultant in a case in which other injuries already have alerted medical providers to suspect inflicted injury. The oral surgeon must consider and respond to suspicious injuries, despite conflicting emotions of abhorrence that a child could be maltreated and concern regarding not harming or displeasing the child's caretaker. The pieces of this diagnostic puzzle require collaboration. The oral surgeon must be able to work with the primary physician, medical consultants, social workers, and community agencies, such as child protective services and law enforcement. The oral surgeon must initiate an evaluation and understand how to seek additional diagnostic and social resources.

Initial evaluation

Central to the evaluation of abuse is whether a child's injuries are congruent with the history. The history may be incomplete or falsified to conceal the caretaker's role. There may be no history of trauma, history of a minor event, or a partial admission, or injuries may be attributed to other small children who are incapable of causing significant trauma. History that changes substantially or is contradicted by other caregivers may indicate falsification.

Even if history is explicit and consistent, it may be inadequate to explain injuries. The scenario should be compared with the child's cognitive, behavioral, and motor skills. Children may be too young to have motor skills leading to an accident, or they may be old enough to have sufficient cognitive and motor skills to avoid injury. The clinically assessed age of injury should be compared with the reported time of injury. As a corollary, multiple vintages of injury raise concern for repeated abuse. Recognizable pat-

* Corresponding author.
E-mail address: nsugar@u.washington.edu (N.F. Sugar).

terns, particularly of skin trauma, may be specific for abuse. When one sees a concerning injury, a child should be examined fully for others. In addition to performing a complete intraoral examination, the oral surgeon should examine the face, neck, ears, nose, and scalp carefully. An examination of the skin of the entire body, including the buttocks and genitalia, and palpation and ranging of bones and joints are required. A young child often must have skeletal and brain imaging and a dilated retinal examination. The oral surgeon must collaborate with medical colleagues to complete these evaluations.

Finally, consideration should be given to a caretaker's response to the child's illness or injury. Was there an unexplained delay in care? Did the caretaker provide unreasonable care at home, such as putting a nonresponsive child in a cold bath, before calling for aid?

Epidemiology

Child abuse is, unfortunately, a common problem. During 2002, protective services agencies in the United States investigated reports of abuse and neglect on 4.38% of children [1]. Twenty-seven percent (1.23% of children) of these reports were substantiated. "Substantiation" is a high threshold, which underestimates the actual level of abuse. Neglect was most common and led to 60.5% of the reports. Physical abuse accounted for 18.9%, emotional abuse accounted for 6.5%, and other issues, such as abandonment, drug exposure during pregnancy, and threats of harm to the child, accounted for 18.9%. Sexual abuse accounted for 9.9% of substantiations. These numbers refer to the most significant form of abuse; children often had multiple types of abuse.

Abuse is primarily an intrafamilial issue; 84.8% of cases involved at least one parent. Mothers were perpetrators in 63.7% and fathers in 38.1% of cases, and many cases involved both parents. Medical and dental personnel made only 7.8% of the abuse reports.

Craniofacial and oral injuries are commonly noted in children with abusive injuries. Of 371 abused, hospitalized children, 92% had soft tissue injuries, 28% of which occurred in the head and face [2]. Infants (40%) and toddlers (38%) had even more frequent head and face injuries. Craniofacial trauma was noted in 49% of 260 hospitalized abused children, but only 14 children had intraoral trauma [3]. Of 1248 patients evaluated for all types of abuse, 37.5% had injuries to the face, head, mouth, or neck [4]. The 511 physical abuse cases were analyzed separately; 75.5% had injuries to these structures. Intraoral injuries, including lip and palate lacerations, tooth and jaw fractures, and frenulum and tongue lacerations, were present in 2%. Three hundred abused children from South Africa sustained a similar frequency of head and face trauma (69%) [5]. Seven percent had oral injuries. Physicians without specialized training in oral medicine performed these studies. The frequency of oral and dental injuries might well be higher with the institution of more skilled oral examination.

Missed injuries

A 5-week-old infant had irritability and possible dehydration. Seven previous pregnancies by five different fathers resulted in miscarriages. Three miscarriages were attributed to being "beaten up badly" by prior partners. The baby was a difficult feeder and growth was poor despite frequent pediatric and public health nurse intervention. At 2 weeks of age, he had unexplained oral bleeding, which was not investigated. From the age of 3 weeks, recurrent vomiting led to multiple formula changes. He was noted to have a large head size and bulging fontanel. At evaluation, his upper lip frenulum had a healed disruption (Fig. 1). His strength was normal, but tone increased. He was nutritionally wasted. His weight was less than fifth percentile, length was twenty-fifth percentile, and head size was ninety-seventh percentile for age. Cranial ultrasound demonstrated extra-axial fluid. An MRI showed bilateral chronic subdural effusions and right frontal cystic encephalomalacia. Cerebral ventricular size was increased. Retinal ex-

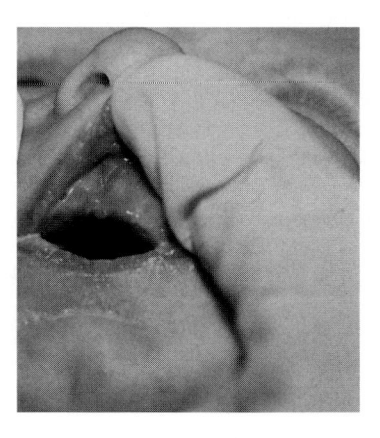

Fig. 1. A 5-week-old infant evaluated for inflicted head injury had a healed disruption of his upper lip frenulum.

amination was normal, but multiple rib fractures in various stages of healing confirmed abuse. He required subdural shunting.

His father admitted that a week before admission he had vigorously shaken the baby while grasping him around the chest. This confession did not account for the multiple injuries of different ages. The father subsequently pled guilty to assault. By 2 years of age, the child's head size had normalized. He was walking and talking but had mild left hand weakness. His MRI showed persistent ventriculomegaly and bifrontal scarring. Although this child is performing well, it remains likely that he will have persistent deficits [6]. Had his oral bleeding been investigated, he might have been spared brain injury.

Missed or inadequately managed child abuse puts a child and siblings at risk of further maltreatment. In Wales, 49 of 69 physically abused infants younger than age 1 year were returned home after investigation [7]. During the subsequent 3 years, 15 (31%) of these children sustained further abuse (8) or neglect (7). Eleven of 63 siblings (17%) also were abused during follow-up.

Skin injuries

Among inflicted injuries, skin trauma is common. Bruises are more likely than abrasions or lacerations to be caused by abuse [2,8]. Bruises are the consequence of normal childhood activity, but their incidence is age and development determined [9]. Less than 0.5% of children younger than age 6 months have any bruises. Until children are "cruising," only 2.2% have a single bruise. Skin injuries, such as scratches or abrasions, were found in 11.4% of infants younger than age 8 months, but only 1.2% had bruises [10]. Activities of younger infants do not create sufficient energy to cause bruising. Bruises at this age deserve a critical look at the history, and if the history is suspect, evaluation for inflicted injury and easy bruising is necessary. Sixty percent of children aged 2 to 3 years have at least one bruise. Bruises in toddlers and preschoolers tend to overlie bony prominences and are determined by a child's normal activity. Of children younger than 36 months with bruises, 73% of the children's bruises were on their knees and shins, and 13% had forehead bruises. Of 973 normal children, however, none had buttock bruises and only 7 had cheek or face injuries [9].

Bruises that form a recognizable shape or pattern usually reflect the shape of the injuring object; a positive imprint may be seen or the shape of the object is outlined by confluent petechiae, which create a negative image. These injuries often could not be acquired by normal accidents. Some patterned bruises are determined by the anatomy of the body, which determines how tissue strains are focused. If a child's ear is boxed, a patterned cheek handprint results. The top of the helix also may have a line of confluent petechiae where it is crimped against the head [11]. Although bruise color evolves over time, clinicians vary in their estimate of bruise color, and color changes over time are only poorly predictable [12]. The only reliable age determination has been the lack of yellowing until 18 to 24 hours after injury [13,14]. Similarly, hemosiderin is not present in microscopic bruise samples until 3 days after injury [15].

Oral injuries

Twin A was taken to an emergency department at age 6 weeks after spitting up blood after bottle feeding. She had multiple bruises of varying color, including fingerprints on her right ribs. Simultaneously, Twin B, still at home with his mother, spit up bright red blood. At the emergency department he had multiple bruises. His facial bruises were of a U-shaped parallel pattern, which indicated fingerprint impacts (Fig. 2). The frenulum of his upper lip was torn. His fontanelle was bulging and he had fresh intraoral blood. A discoid collection of blood overlay Twin B's right frontal cortex, which suggested epidural hemorrhage. He had multifocal subarachnoid hemorrhages. Both twins had low normal hematocrits and normal coagulation studies. Skeletal surveys and retinal examinations were normal. Twin A had a 2-cm sharply incised, penetrating palatal laceration (Fig. 3), which was surgically repaired. The injury appeared to be a sharp stab wound.

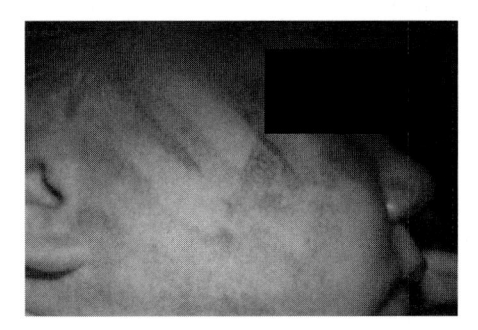

Fig. 2. A 6-week-old infant (Twin B) had a facial slap mark and confluent petechiae outlining pale finger imprints. He also had intracranial bleeding.

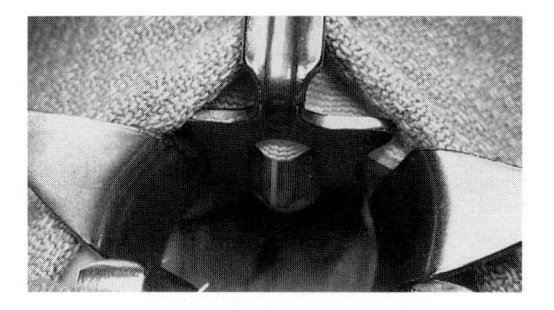

Fig. 3. Twin A sustained a stab wound and soft palate perforation.

Injuries to the mouth of a young infant raise high concerns for abuse. A common inflicted craniofacial injury is laceration of the upper labial frenulum [16]. Like bruising, although this becomes a normal accidental finding in ambulatory children, it is an infrequent accidental injury in infants. It is believed to result when a bottle is jammed into the fussy, difficult-to-feed infant's mouth. This injury may be viewed by parents and professionals as a trivial injury that will resolve without intervention, and they may not even consider how it was caused.

Tooth luxations and avulsions may come to the attention of health care personnel directly or by referral. They are common findings in ambulatory, active children. A thorough injury history should be taken. If a child is able to communicate, a separate history should be obtained from him or her. Associated physical findings, such as abrasions from falls on concrete, may confirm accident scenarios. Alternatively, the lack thereof may place the history in question. If concern about the veracity of the history remains, a complete physical examination for other trauma should be arranged.

Bite marks

Dentists may be called to evaluate abuse in children with bite marks. Because bites by peers are common events, the first question is whether it is a child's bite. In a child's bite, the primary maxillary canines should be less than 3 cm apart [17]. The secondary maxillary central incisors are wider, side-to-side, than the laterals; the primaries are of similar width. Because individual bite patterns are unique, good photographs should be taken to compare with the bite width patterns in a child's environment. The photos should be taken at a true right angle to the plane of the bite to avoid angular distortion. A size scale should be in the plane of the bite, and the photo should document the date and the victim's identity. If a bite mark is evaluated before washing, the surface should be swabbed with a water-moistened cotton swab that is then air dried and bagged in paper. This sample should be transferred to the crime laboratory using "chain-of-evidence" procedures. If saliva is recovered from the wound, the assailant may be identified by blood type and DNA.

Burns

Burns result from either unintentional injury or abuse. Most inflicted burns result from direct contact with hot solids or smoldering objects or from hot liquids. Inflicted contact burns may reflect the pattern of the injuring object, such as the tip of a burning cigarette, the tube of a curling iron, or the grid of an electric hair dryer (Fig. 4). These heat sources also cause accidental burns, but accidental burn injury tends to be smeared out because of the unrestrained child's efforts to escape the burning object. Inflicted injuries are more likely to be directly and clearly imprinted. Accidental burns are usually single and do not appear on body areas normally protected by clothing, and the children lack other trauma.

Inflicted scald burns may be caused by intentionally thrown or poured hot liquids or forced feeding of hot foods. All such injuries result in spattering, which causes irregular lesions of variable burn depth. They may be difficult to differentiate from accidental hot liquid spills. Viscous liquids and liquids hotter than 150°F have enough heat content to cause satellite splash marks. Immersion in basins of hot liquids causes burns demarcated by the waterline contours of the body. Because of restraint, water lines are often sharp and without splash marks, and burn depth tends to be uniform. Often the history suggests that the

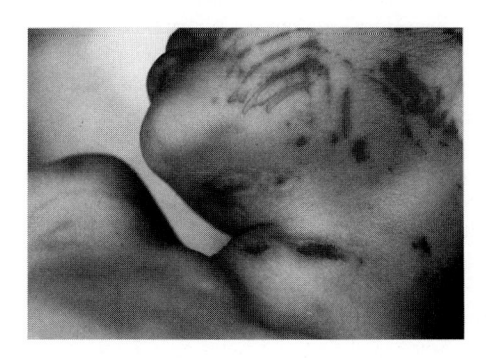

Fig. 4. Cheek burn from a directly imprinted electric hair dryer. The child died of inflicted head injury and 50% body:surface area immersion burn.

burned child did not experience pain before or after injury. The 109° to 113°F pain threshold is well below that required to burn [18]. A thorough scene investigation and consideration of the child's normal behavior and development may differentiate inflicted injury.

In addition to thermal burns, other mechanisms may cause burn-like oral region lesions. Gags cause pressure necrosis of the skin at the corners of the mouth, and they often tail downward. Children may be force fed caustic substances or pepper to "teach them a lesson" [19]. Oropharyngeal and esophageal injury occurs with the caustic agents. Powdered pepper is more hazardous than liquid pepper because it is more likely to be aspirated, with subsequent asphyxia caused by airway edema.

Head injuries

A 17-month-old boy was admitted after a respiratory arrest at home. A week earlier, he developed vomiting and wheezing, which were diagnosed as pneumonia. While at home with his father, he fell backward over a couch arm and landed on his head. Immediately, he became unconsciousness, with gasping respiration. His father performed cardiopulmonary resuscitation until emergency medical services arrived. They found him unresponsive with an arrhythmia. After intubation, he seemed to "wake" briefly and look around before he lapsed into deep coma. Pupils were asymmetric—with the left greater than the right—but reactive.

He had bruising of the forehead, cheek, back, and abdomen. His upper lip was bruised and swollen at the vermilion border, and his upper frenulum was torn deeply. His lower lip was avulsed from his gums. CT scan demonstrated global brain hypodensity, brain swelling, scant high convexity extra-axial blood, and a thin layer of interhemispheric blood. He had extensive bilateral retinal hemorrhages. At autopsy he had bilateral hemispheric and scant spinal subdural hemorrhages, three contusions on the undersurface of the scalp, a posterior right eighth rib fracture, right adrenal hemorrhage, and a small hemopericardium. Bilateral retinal and optic nerve sheath hemorrhages were noted. An older iron-stained subdural membrane also was present. The father later claimed the fall was not from the couch but from a height of 6 feet to a carpeted floor. He also claimed that he had provided cardiopulmonary resuscitation after an aspiration event a week before, which preceded the "pneumonia."

Multifocal trauma is not compatible with a single fall. Extensive retinal bleeding accompanied by optic nerve sheath hemorrhage is rare, except in cases of abuse [20]. The child's severe brain injury is unlike that seen with normal falls, and the rib fracture is not explained by a fall. He sustained severe orofacial trauma with inflicted head injury, which was at least the second trauma episode.

Apparently minor inflicted cranial skin injuries are a common accompaniment of inflicted head injury [21,22]. The most common cause of seriously inflicted intracranial trauma is severe whiplash acceleration head injury, with or without associated cranial impact [23]. Clinical experience and perpetrator confessions strongly suggest that this injury is often the result of caregivers shaking infants and young children [24]. In cases with confessed shaking alone, skull fractures are less common than cases with confessed shaking plus impact or with impact alone. Infants and toddlers are the most frequent victims.

Although many head injured children present with dramatic symptoms, such as apnea, seizures, and coma, some have more subtle symptoms, such as irritability, sleepiness, or vomiting. A distressingly frequent 31% of all children with inflicted head injuries are seen by a medical provider and the diagnosis is missed on the initial evaluation [21]. Thirty-seven percent of these children with a missed diagnosis of inflicted head injury have craniofacial skin injury at that initial visit. The significance of bruising in a preambulatory child may be missed or ignored. Investigation is delayed, which causes greater morbidity. Twenty-eight percent of children sustained further injury and 41% experienced complications because of the missed diagnosis.

Retinal hemorrhage is common with inflicted head injury but occurs rarely with accidental head injury [20]. In fatal cases, there is often accompanying optic nerve sheath bleeding. The pathophysiology of retinal hemorrhage is not defined fully. One leading causal theory is that the bleeding results from whiplash forces on the eye, which distract the vitreous from the retina. Any child with suspected inflicted head injury should be referred for ophthalmologic examination.

Abdominal injuries

Although an oral surgeon is less likely to encounter a child with inflicted visceral injury, intra-abdominal trauma follows brain injury as the most common cause of physical abuse–related fatality. The victims of this abuse are older. Toddler negativism and toilet training accidents are the most common triggers. Blunt impacts to the abdomen with a punch or kick rupture solid organs or bowel. Caretakers usually delay care to try to avoid detection, until the child is in extremis. The mortality rate from hemorrhagic or septic shock is approximately 50% [25,26]. Children usually lack abdominal wall bruising but often have inflicted bruises elsewhere.

Fractures

A 2.5-year-old boy was brought to an outside emergency department with a complaint that he had not been using his right arm since riding his tricycle down the front porch the day before. He had a comminuted fracture of the distal humerus and was referred for definitive care. Although the referring emergency department was only 6 miles away, the family had not arrived until 7 hours later.

When police brought the boy for care, he was noted to be missing three upper incisors. The family reported that he had knocked them out himself by striking the steering wheel of a nonmoving pickup truck. The force of this scenario was incompatible with his dental luxations. He had yellowing bruising and swelling of the right arm from the wrist to the shoulder, which suggested that the injury was older than the proffered history. He had multiple other unexplained bruises: two left scapula fractures, three left lateral rib fractures, a chip fracture of the distal right radius, a pubic ramus fracture, and a right metatarsal fracture (Fig. 5). Periosteal new bone, which indicates subperiosteal bleeding, was present over the right radius, left ulna, right femur, and right tibia. All fractures, except the presenting right humerus injury, were clinically occult. His multiple vintages of unexplained injuries and his parents' failure to show for definitive fracture care strongly indicated abuse.

Fractures are common in abused infants and toddlers. The younger the child, the more frequently fractures are found and the more frequently those fractures are clinically occult [27]. Any young child with signs of physical abuse should have a skeletal survey done [28]. Children younger than 2 to 3 years old are most likely to have occult fractures [27]. In older children, skeletal imaging can be limited to sites of physical signs or symptoms or areas of historical injury or impairment. Fresh fractures are often invisible on plain radiographs. In a young child, if the child's disposition safety plan depends on identifying additional fractures, a nuclear medicine bone scan also should be conducted. It can identify subtle, acute fractures better than the skeletal survey [29]. The nuclear scan is less sensitive to the classic metaphyseal fracture (Fig. 6) of child abuse, however [30]. If a child can be protected from further injury, a follow-up skeletal survey 1.5 to 2 weeks after injury may add more information than the nuclear study [31].

Although bony trauma is the most common cause of abnormal periosteal reaction, other causes, which are infrequent in modern society, warrant attention. Infants and toddlers may develop an inflammatory periostitis, known as Caffey's disease. The most frequently affected bones are the jaw (Fig. 7), clavicle, and tibia. They may have systemic symptoms and elevated acute phase reactants. Other causes of peri-

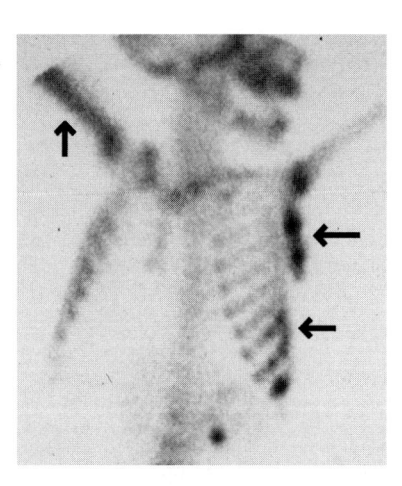

Fig. 5. A 2.5 year-old boy presented for care for a comminuted distal right humerus fracture. Nuclear scan showed the presenting injury, plus two left scapula and three left rib fractures.

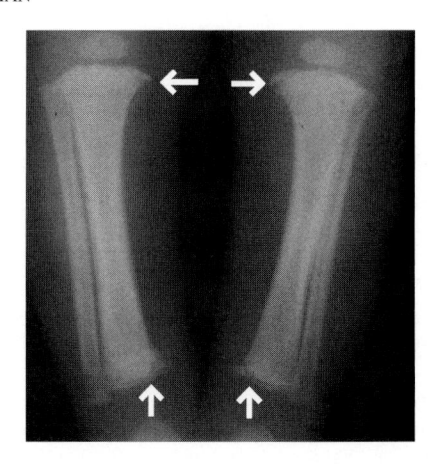

Fig. 6. The classic metaphyseal lesion of child abuse results from ligamentous traction on the ends of the long bones.

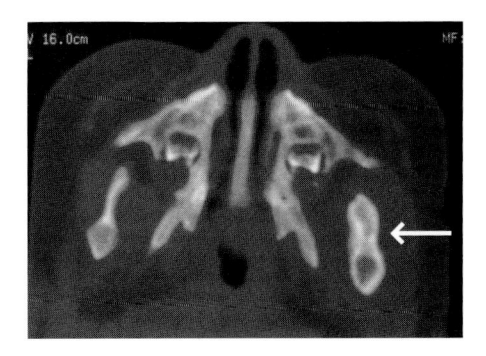

Fig. 7. An infant with Caffey's disease, an idiopathic inflammatory periostitis, has typical left jaw thickening from periosteal reaction.

osteal reaction include congenital syphilis and prostaglandin treatment for ductus-dependent cardiac abnormalities. The periosteal reactions of syphilis are usually accompanied by a moth-eaten appearance in the metaphyses. Subperiosteal hemorrhage and calcification and oral bleeding can occur with vitamin C deficiency, although they occur infrequently with current infant nutrition. Vitamin K deficiency and congenital coagulopathies can cause easy bleeding. Copper deficiency can cause metaphyseal abnormalities, which somewhat resemble classic metaphyseal fracture. Children with the various forms of osteogenesis imperfecta may have dentinogenesis imperfecta (Fig. 8), blue-gray sclerae, and gracile, poorly mineralized bones that are unusually fragile.

Sexual abuse

Sexual abuse is rarely implicated as a cause of oral injury. Forced oral intercourse may result in soft or hard palate petechiae or contusions, but this finding is nonspecific, transient, and rarely documented.

Sexually transmitted infections can present as pharyngeal infection. Sexually transmitted infections can infect mucosal surfaces in a neonate born to an infected mother. Chlamydial infection of the oropharynx is asymptomatic, and in the absence of treatment, it can persist for several years [32]. Pharyngeal gonorrhea is clinically indistinguishable from viral or bacterial pharyngitis. It is uncommonly detected in child sexual abuse [33]. Testing of specimens from oral sites by commercial nucleic amplification tests is not validated; diagnosis should be made by conventional culture. Syphilitic chancres are rarely encountered in children but do indicate sexual contact. Diagnosis of any of these infections should prompt consultation with a specialist in child abuse or infectious disease.

Herpes gingivostomatitis is a common infection of young children. It may be caused by herpes simplex type I or II. In most cases, innocent transmission from family members (who may be asymptomatic) or from infected secretions from playmates is most likely.

Oral condyloma is one manifestation of human papillomavirus (HPV) infection. Although genital HPV in adults is a sexually transmitted disease, several modes of transmission are considered possible in children: prenatally via infected amniotic fluid, perinatally, and through benign household contact, autoinoculation, sexual abuse, and possibly fomite transmission [34]. Although vertical HPV transmission from mother to neonate long has been postulated as a mechanism of infection for young children, recent studies indicate poor concordance of viral DNA between mothers and neonates [35]. Two recent studies showed a high rate of oral HPV positivity in preschool-aged children (45%–50%) but found that the infections were often transient [36,37].

When an oral wart-like lesion is noted in a child, biopsy for diagnosis and viral DNA analysis should be performed, because non–HPV-related lesions may mimic oral condylomata [38]. Insufficient scientific evidence exists at this point to reach a clear conclusion regarding the significance of oral or genital HPV infection in children. Regional medical experts in child sexual abuse may provide valuable consultation.

Behavioral signs

In addition to the craniofacial injuries likely to be seen by an oral surgeon, caretaker and child behaviors in the office can be a sensitive—but less

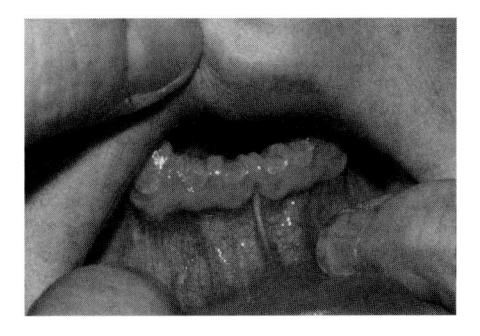

Fig. 8. Dentinogenesis imperfecta in a child with osteogenesis imperfecta.

specific—warning sign of abuse. Rosenberg found that 28% of children under age 2 years who were observed to have abnormal bruising, burns, or bites on emergency department evaluation, and 19% of unkempt children, were abused [39]. If children had these unusual skin injuries in combination with being unkempt, 42% were abused. Thirty percent of unkempt children who had parents with abnormal parenting behavior were abused. The altered caretaker behaviors included intoxications, hostile or aggressive attitudes, rough, demeaning, or belittling interactions with the child, and lack of bonding with the child. These numbers compare with the baseline rate of child abuse in that emergency department of 2.5%.

Domestic violence or significant family dysfunction should alert one to heightened risks for child abuse and neglect. In unselected community samples, the rate of co-occurrence of abuse and domestic violence averaged 6% (range, 5%–21%) [40]. In clinical samples of battered women or abused children, however, the rate averaged 40% (range, 20%–100%). Although the mediating influences are unclear, not only the abusive spouse but also the victim of domestic violence has an increased likelihood of inflicting abuse [41]. Rates of co-occurrence of child abuse with domestic violence in neglected children are increased in the face of single-parent households, parental substance abuse, maternal depression, or mental illness. Children also may react to the domestic violence milieu by adopting problematic behavioral disorders [42], which in turn may put them at risk of violence. Children who grow up with one type of adverse childhood experience, such as abuse, neglect, domestic violence or parental discord, caretaker substance abuse, or mental illness or household criminality, are more likely to have additional adverse experiences [43].

Caretakers who grew up in an abusive environment are less likely to make safe choices in partners and are more likely to have emotional disorders that impair their adult coping skills [44]. Anxiety, depression, posttraumatic stress, and caretaker somatic symptoms are more common in adults who were abused or neglected or are currently victims of domestic violence. These factors may impair a caretaker's ability to provide appropriate childcare. Domestic violence also includes isolation and control of the victim by the perpetrator [45], which may impair appropriate initial care seeking for significant medical and dental disease and result in erratic follow-up. For example, a victim of domestic violence may be prevented from using the telephone, which prevents office staff from contacting that parent.

Neglect

Child neglect may present to the primary care dentist as extensive decay. Normally caring but uninformed parents may leave a bottle in bed with an infant or nurse them every few minutes to calm them, which causes baby bottle decay. The upper central incisors and lower molars are most affected. Such practices and decay may be only the most visible consequence of child neglect, however. Neglect can lead to the dental disease in the first place but also may impair efforts to treat established disease. As for adults, other barriers to dental care may include lack of information by parents on the importance of dental care, lack of access to dental services, or dental phobia on the part of parents or child.

It is often easy to blame parents for neglect, but a child-centered definition of neglect is "failure of the child's basic needs to be met" [46]. Basic needs include nutrition, clothing, shelter, safety, supervision, emotional nurture, education, and health needs. Failure of a caretaker to provide these needs can arise from problems in the parent, lack of means to provide, or environmental/societal barriers. The reasons are often multifactorial and usually require teamwork to understand and intervene. One of the difficulties in defining what is neglect and what warrants intervention is that it is not dichotomous but is rather a continuum from minimal to severe. If one divides neglect into physical, psychological, and environmental forms (ie, societal or community milieu), there is moderate co-occurrence of types, primarily for physical and psychological neglect [47]. Families that live in deprived environments often provide adequate nurture despite adverse circumstances. Some families can provide neither physical nor psychological nurture in a beneficent environment, however. All varieties of neglect often fail to reach protective services' notice, and society's role in failing to nurture children is ignored [47].

Psychological neglect has been associated with development of unstable and dysfunctional attachment [48]. Abused and neglected children develop coping strategies in response to their parents' behavior that are self-protective, but the behaviors limit a child's ability to interact appropriately with others or learn from normal environments. Many children become passive/compliant with the aggressor parent while becoming anxious in new situations and aggressive with peers. Although the injuries of physical abuse are most vivid, it is perhaps the lack of a safe, predictable environment and emotional nurture that are most harmful to a child's future well-being.

Social workers can assist in understanding the problems and barriers to care. After evaluation, it is helpful to develop a written contract with the family for the child's care. Community "eyes" (eg, public health nurses) can help understand the challenges families face and may be able to assist families. In cases in which initial efforts to understand and ameliorate barriers to care have failed, protective services can aid in evaluation and planning for services.

Child protective services

All 50 states in the United States have laws mandating that medical and dental personnel report suspected child abuse. Many state laws refer to "reasonable suspicion" as the criterion for reporting. Each state has an agency to receive, assess, and investigate reports. States commonly use a risk assessment instrument to assist decisions of whether to open a case for investigation. These instruments include severity of the injury, risk of significant harm, age of child, and contributing factors, such as parental mental illness or substance abuse. Reports can be made anonymously, but they are regarded as less reliable. Reports made by professionals are more likely to be investigated.

Medical providers may be reluctant to report suspected abuse because they believe it will lead to a child's removal from the home. Placing a child in foster care or in care with a relative is one of many responses to confirmed child abuse, but only when less radical approaches are insufficient. Protective services is more likely to organize services to stabilize a child in his or her own home. In Washington State in 2003, only 7.5% of new referrals resulted in removal of a child [49]. Even then, 82% of these children were returned home after less than 12 months in care.

In many states, policies or laws also require mandatory reporters to submit a written report and communicate further in response to suspected abuse. HIPAA (The federal Health Insurance Portability and Accountability Act of 1996), which established criteria for protection of medical records, clearly allows an exception in cases of suspected child abuse and neglect—(Section 45 CFR 164.512(b)(1)(ii) [50].

Protective services must know the specific injury, the child's age, the basis for the concern of abuse, and how the family can be contacted. A report should include a description of the type of force that would be necessary to cause the injury, an assessment of the probable time frame of injury, and the consistency or lack of consistency with the caretaker's history. Although the clinician is not required to tell the family that he or she is making a report, it is good practice to do so. Simply stating, "With this type of injury, I am required by law to inform the authorities" should be sufficient. It is not reasonable or wise for a clinician to attempt to unilaterally determine the veracity of the parental report or ascertain who might have inflicted the injury. Lengthy discussion with or interrogation of the parents is not helpful.

When the oral surgeon is subpoenaed in a child abuse case

Although medical providers may receive subpoenas, testimony is rarely required [51]. Cases are usually settled out of court through negotiation and plea agreements. Child abuse cases may be pursued through the civil (family or juvenile) courts or the criminal courts or both.

A clinician may be contacted by an attorney for the state or by an attorney for the parent or caregiver. Either the attorney presents a subpoena or the legal guardian of the child must sign consent for release of information. A "subpoena duces tecum" is a request for medical records. The legal custodian of records is usually the medical records department of the hospital or medical group. Medical records often suffice for civil cases, especially if they are legible and clearly written and contain complete information and interpretation of injuries.

Attorneys for the state or for the parent may subpoena the medical provider as a witness. These subpoenas typically formidably read, "You are commanded to appear." The date on the subpoena is a preliminary date; many cases are settled out of court. The clinician should call the attorney or paralegal listed on the subpoena and request a meeting in advance of testimony to discuss the significance of the clinical findings. According to legal "discovery," the defense is also entitled to interview potential witnesses.

The medical or dental clinician is an "expert witness," defined in law as a person who has specialized knowledge. Although the medical or dental expert is subpoenaed for only one side in the adversarial system, it is ethically responsible for the expert to present knowledge and opinions without bias or prejudice. The expert should bill for time spent in testimony and meetings with attorneys. This fee should reflect the usual charges for clinical practice. Rates should be presented in advance to the attorney who issued the subpoena.

It is certainly preferred that in-person testimony be scheduled to be least disruptive to the clinician's work schedule. This choice may not always be possible, but collegial and ongoing communication with the attorney should be helpful in arranging it. In testifying, the expert should be courteous, unbiased, and complete. Communication in advance with other clinicians experienced in testifying in these cases may provide helpful preparation.

Summary

Contemplating, recognizing, and responding to child abuse is professionally and emotionally challenging for the health care provider. Facial and oral structures are frequently involved, and the expertise of the oral surgeon is invaluable in this arena. Collaboration with other specialists and with other professionals is essential to providing the best care for these most vulnerable children.

References

[1] US Government Department of Health and Human Services. Child maltreatment 2002: reports from the states to the National Child Abuse and Neglect Data Systems. Available at: http://www.acf.hhs.gov/programs/cb/publications/cmreports.htm. Accessed February 7, 2005.

[2] McMahon P, Grossman W, Gaffney M, et al. Soft-tissue injury as an indication of child abuse. J Bone Joint Surg Am 1995;77A(8):1179–83.

[3] Becker DB, Needleman HL, Kotelchuck M. Child abuse and dentistry: orofacial trauma and its recognition by dentists. J Am Dent Assoc 1978;97(1):24–8.

[4] da Fonseca MA, Feigal RJ, ten Bensel RW. Dental aspects of 1248 cases of child maltreatment on file at a major county hospital. Pediatr Dent 1992;14(3):152–7.

[5] Naidoo S. A profile of the oro-facial injuries in child physical abuse at a children's hospital. Child Abuse Negl 2000;24(4):521–34.

[6] Duhaime AC, Christian C, Moss E, et al. Long-term outcome in infants with the shaking-impact syndrome. Pediatr Neurosurg 1996;24(6):292–8.

[7] Ellaway BA, Payne EH, Rolfe K, et al. Are abused babies protected from further abuse? Arch Dis Child 2004;89(9):845–6.

[8] Pascoe JM, Hildebrandt HM, Tarrier A, et al. Patterns of skin injury in nonaccidental and accidental injury. Pediatrics 1979;64(2):245–7.

[9] Sugar NF, Taylor JA, Feldman KW. Bruises in infants and toddlers: those who don't cruise rarely bruise. Puget Sound Pediatric Research Network. Arch Pediatr Adolesc Med 1999;153(4):399–403.

[10] Labbe J, Caouette G. Recent skin injuries in normal children. Pediatrics 2001;108(2):271–6.

[11] Feldman KW. Patterned abusive bruises of the buttocks and the pinnae. Pediatrics 1992;90(4):633–6.

[12] Bariciak ED, Plint AC, Gaboury I, et al. Dating of bruises in children: an assessment of physician accuracy. Pediatrics 2003;112(4):804–7.

[13] Stephenson T, Bialas Y. Estimation of the age of bruising. Arch Dis Child 1996;74(1):53–5.

[14] Schwartz AJ, Ricci LR. How accurately can bruises be aged in abused children? Literature review and synthesis. Pediatrics 1996;97(2):254–7.

[15] Betz P, Eisenmenger W. Morphometrical analysis of hemosiderin deposits in relation to wound age. Int J Legal Med 1996;108(5):262–4.

[16] Stricker T, Lips U, Sennhauser FH. Oral bleeding: child abuse alert. J Paediatr Child Health 2002;38(5):528–9.

[17] Nanda SK. Age related changes in dental arches. In: The developmental basis of occlusion and malocclusion. Chicago: Quintessence Books; 1983.

[18] Feldman KW. Evaluation of physical abuse. In: Helfer MEK, Krugman RD, editors. The battered child. 5th edition. Chicago: University of Chicago Press; 1997. p. 175–247.

[19] Bays J, Feldman KW. Child abuse by poisoning. In: Reese RL, editor. Child abuse: medical diagnosis and management. 2nd edition. Philadelphia: Lippincott Williams & Wilkins; 2001. p. 405–41.

[20] Levin AV. Retinal hemorrhages in child abuse. In: David T, editor. Recent advances in pediatrics. London: RSM Press; 2002. p. 151–219.

[21] Jenny C, Hymel KP, Ritzen A, et al. Analysis of missed cases of abusive head trauma. JAMA 1999;281(7):621–6.

[22] Feldman KW, Bethel R, Shugerman RP, et al. The cause of infant and toddler subdural hemorrhage: a prospective study. Pediatrics 2001;108(3):636–46.

[23] Hymel KP, Jenny C, Block RW. Intracranial hemorrhage and rebleeding in suspected victims of abusive head trauma: addressing the forensic controversies. Child Maltreat 2002;7(4):329–48.

[24] Starling SP, Patel S, Burke BL, et al. Analysis of perpetrator admissions to inflicted traumatic brain injury in children. Arch Pediatr Adolesc Med 2004;158(5):454–8.

[25] Ledbetter DJ, Hatch Jr EI, Feldman KW, et al. Diagnostic and surgical implications of child abuse. Arch Surg 1988;123(9):1101–5.

[26] Cooper A, Floyd T, Barlow B, et al. Major blunt abdominal trauma due to child abuse. J Trauma 1988;28(10):1483–7.

[27] Merten DF, Radkowski MA, Leonidas JC. The abused child: a radiological reappraisal. Radiology 1983;146(2):377–81.

[28] American College of Radiology. ACR standard for skeletal surveys in children. Available at: http://www.acr.org. Revised 2001. Accessed July 20, 2005.

[29] Jaudes PK. Comparison of radiography and radio-

nuclide bone scanning in the detection of child abuse. Pediatrics 1984;73(2):166–8.
[30] Kleinman PK. Diagnostic imaging in infant abuse. AJR Am J Roentgenol 1990;155(4):703–12.
[31] Kleinman PK, Nimkin K, Spevak MR, et al. Follow-up skeletal surveys in suspected child abuse. AJR Am J Roentgenol 1996;167(4):893–6.
[32] Bell TA, Stamm WE, Wang SP, et al. Chronic Chlamydia trachomatis infections in infants. JAMA 1992;267(3):400–2.
[33] Ingram DM, Miller WC, Schoenbach VJ, et al. Risk assessment for gonococcal and chlamydial infections in young children undergoing evaluation for sexual abuse. Pediatrics 2001;107(5):E73.
[34] Syrjanen S, Puranen M. Human papillomavirus infections in children: the potential role of maternal transmission. Crit Rev Oral Biol Med 2000;11(2):259–74.
[35] Watts DH, Koutsky LA, Holmes KK, et al. Low risk of perinatal transmission of human papillomavirus: results from a prospective cohort study. Am J Obstet Gynecol 1998;178(2):365–73.
[36] Mant C, Kell B, Rice P, et al. Buccal exposure to human papillomavirus type 16 is a common yet transitory event of childhood. J Med Virol 2003;71(4):593–8.
[37] Kojima A, Maeda H, Kurahashi N, et al. Human papillomaviruses in the normal oral cavity of children in Japan. Oral Oncol 2003;39(8):821–8.
[38] Anderson KM, Perez-Montiel D, Miles L, et al. The histologic differentiation of oral condyloma acuminatum from its mimics. Oral Surg Oral Med Oral Pathol Oral Radiol Endod 2003;96(4):420–8.
[39] Rosenberg NM, Meyers S, Shackleton N. Prediction of child abuse in an ambulatory setting. Pediatrics 1982;70(6):879–82.
[40] Appel AE. The co-occurrence of spouse and physical child abuse: a review and appraisal. J Fam Psychol 1998;12(4):578–99.
[41] Coohey C. Battered mothers who physically abuse their children. J Interpers Violence 2004;19(8):943–52.
[42] Kernic MA, Wolf ME, Holt VL, et al. Behavioral problems among children whose mothers are abused by an intimate partner. Child Abuse Negl 2003;27(11):1231–46.
[43] Dong M, Anda RF, Felitti VJ, et al. The interrelatedness of multiple forms of childhood abuse, neglect, and household dysfunction. Child Abuse Negl 2004;28(7):771–84.
[44] Spertus IL, Yehuda R, Wong CM, et al. Childhood emotional abuse and neglect as predictors of psychological and physical symptoms in women presenting to a primary care practice. Child Abuse Negl 2003;27(11):1247–58.
[45] Hartley CC. The co-occurrence of child maltreatment and domestic violence: examining both neglect and child physical abuse. Child Maltreat 2002;7(4):349–58.
[46] Dubowitz H, Giardino A, Gustavson E. Child neglect: guidance for pediatricians. Pediatr Rev 2000;21(4):111–6.
[47] Dubowitz H, Pitts SC, Black MM. Measurement of three major subtypes of child neglect. Child Maltreat 2004;9(4):344–56.
[48] Crittenden PM. Children's strategies for coping with adverse home environments: an interpretation using attachment theory. Child Abuse Negl 1992;16(3):329–43.
[49] Washington State Department of Social and Health Services. Children's administration performance report 2003. Available at: http://www1.dshs.wa.gov/ca/pubs/2003perfrm.asp. Accessed February 7, 2005.
[50] United States Department of Health and Human Services. Health Insurance Portability and Accountability Act of 1996. Disclosures for public health activities. Available at: http://www.hhs.gov/ocr/hipaa/guidelines/publichealth.rtf. Accessed February 7, 2005.
[51] Palusci VJ, Hicks RA, Vandervort FE. You are hereby commanded to appear: pediatrician subpoena and court appearance in child maltreatment. Pediatrics 2001;107(6):1427–30.

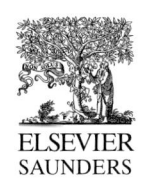

Condyle and Ramus-Condyle Unit Fractures in Growing Patients: Management and Outcomes

Thomas B. Dodson, DMD, MPH

Department of Oral and Maxillofacial Surgery, Massachusetts General Hospital, Harvard School of Dental Medicine, 55 Fruit Street, Warren 1201, Boston, MA 02114, USA

Mandibular fractures in growing patients are uncommon (ie, <10% of all mandibular fractures) [1–3], but when they occur, approximately 50% involve the condyle or ramus-condyle unit (RCU) [1,2,4–6]. The site of the RCU fracture may be age related; in younger children (age <6 years), most condylar fractures are intracapsular (58%), whereas in older children they are located inferior to the condyle and usually include the neck or ramus (78%) [7]. Sex and injury etiology are not related to fracture location [7]. Because pediatric mandibular fractures are uncommon and may present to a number of different surgical specialists, an individual clinician is unlikely to see a large volume of patients and may have a general lack of experience managing these injuries.

Controversy exists regarding the best management of RCU fractures, with treatment recommendations including observation (with or without physiotherapy or use of functional appliances), maxillomandibular fixation (MMF) (for varying durations of time), and open reduction internal fixation (with varying degrees of MMF postoperatively). Some unique complications also may occur after RCU fractures, including asymmetric mandibular growth and temporomandibular joint (TMJ) ankylosis. The purpose of this article is to review the evaluation and management of RCU fractures in growing patients with an emphasis on treatment outcomes.

Evaluation of ramus-condyle unit fractures in growing patients

History and physical examination

Obtaining a history and physical examination can be difficult in pediatric patients. The parents or witness to the injury may be a resource for ascertaining the details of the traumatic event. It is valuable to determine the cause and maintain a high degree of suspicion for other injuries. It is helpful to know the direction of the blow because trauma to the chin is associated with an increased risk of bilateral condylar fractures [8,9] and cervical spine injuries [9]. Alternatively, a unilateral blow to the mandibular body region should raise the suspicion of a contrecoup injury to the contralateral condyle. If necessary, general anesthesia may be necessary to obtain an adequate physical examination in an uncooperative child [10].

Clinical findings

A patient with a unilateral RCU fracture typically presents with preauricular swelling and pain on the affected side. There is usually limitation of jaw motion, with deviation on opening to the affected side and there may be no translation of the fractured condyle. Although malocclusion is a common finding in mandibular fractures, it is not always seen in patients who have RCU fractures, and in some cases radiographic evidence may be the only objective

E-mail address: tbdodson@partners.org

finding of such an injury. The malocclusion associated with a unilateral RCU fracture is an open bite on the unaffected side, which is caused by shortening of the injured RCU and results in premature occlusal contacts on that side. In the setting of bilateral RCU fractures, there may be an anterior open bite caused by bilateral RCU shortening.

Diagnostic imaging

Because a thorough examination of an injured child can be difficult, a clinician may need to rely on radiographic studies to complement the history and limited physical examination to establish the diagnosis. Plain films are generally inadequate for evaluating pediatric maxillofacial injuries. CT imaging is the current standard for assessing these fractures, including the RCU. Chacon and colleagues [11] compared the sensitivity, specificity, and accuracy of panoramic radiographs with CT scans for diagnosing condylar fractures in children. The overall accuracy of CT imaging was 90%, whereas that of panoramic radiographs was 73%. If plain films are the only technology available, one should obtain a panoramic radiograph, Towne view, and bilateral lateral oblique views.

Management of ramus-condyle unit fractures

Most RCU fractures in growing patients may be treated with observation and physiotherapy or a brief period, (<2 weeks) of MMF. The use of internal fixation techniques is rarely indicated (eg, concurrent facial laceration permitting ready access to the RCU). Some practitioners advocate the use of functional orthopedic therapy for treatment of RCU injuries. The data to support routine use of functional appliances to manage RCU fractures are weak (ie, isolated case reports, small case series, or poorly controlled retrospective cohort studies) [12–22]. Because of the generally good outcomes associated with supportive care or MMF, it is difficult to measure the incremental benefit of functional orthopedic therapy administered routinely to manage RCU fractures. There may be a role for functional orthopedic therapy in the setting of an evolving mandibular asymmetry or deficiency after RCU injuries, however.

Children with RCU fractures with normal motion and occlusion may be managed with supportive care (eg, observation, soft diet, physiotherapy, and long-term monitoring of growth and function). In the setting of a malocclusion or significant alternation of jaw function, a short period of MMF (<2 weeks) and guiding elastics (<8 weeks after MMF release) is generally adequate. After injury, physiotherapy (eg, passive jaw exercises) is recommended for an extended period ($\leq$7 months). Comminuted and intracapsular condyle fractures can be managed with supportive care.

There are few indications for open reduction of RCU fractures. One may consider open reduction in the rare circumstances of condylar displacement into the middle cranial fossa, if the displaced condyle interferes with jaw opening or movement, if there is ready access from a pre-existing laceration, or the fracture is associated with loss of ramus height and a persistent malocclusion. Other relative indications for open reduction and rigid internal fixation include seizure disorders, developmental delay, inability to tolerate MMF, severe upper airway obstruction, and facilitating oral and airway hygiene in the setting of a severely injured or disabled patient.

Given the unknown, unpredictable, but documented risk of ankylosis and asymmetry after RCU fractures, a critical aspect of managing these injuries is regular monitoring until cessation of mandibular growth. One recommended monitoring protocol is clinical examination at 1 and 4 weeks followed by clinical and radiographic examinations at 2, 6, and 12 months after injury [23]. Alternatively, if there are no clinical findings, radiographs may be deferred for 1 year and then obtained to assess remodeling. The child should be followed annually with clinical and, if indicated, radiographic examinations until cessation of growth and stabilization of the permanent dentition occur [16,23].

During follow-up visits, a clinician should ascertain if any symptoms are present (eg, pain, joint noise with or without pain, abnormal function, and malocclusion). The physical examination should include measures of range of motion, lateral and protrusive excursions, deviation with opening, assessment of the mandibular midline position, and occlusion. Routine radiographic examination should include a panoramic radiograph to document condylar anatomy and remodeling after injury and a posteroanterior cephalogram to assess mandibular symmetry. If during follow-up mandibular asymmetry or deficiency becomes apparent, functional appliances may help support mandibular growth [22]. If growth is complete, however, then conventional orthodontics or orthognathic surgery may be necessary to correct residual mandibular deformities.

Outcomes after ramus-condyle unit fractures

RCU fracture outcomes (Table 1) are divided into two categories: functional/developmental and radiographic. Functional/developmental studies address TMJ function (eg, range of motion or deviation with opening), symptoms (eg, pain), signs (eg, noise), and mandibular development (eg, asymmetry, hypoplasia, or ankylosis). Radiographic studies address condylar remodeling after injury and measures of mandibular growth (ie, ramus height or mandibular length). Although radiographic studies can indicate mandibular developmental problems, they are not adequate to predict functional outcomes in growing children [24]. Given the poor predictive value of radiographic assessment as a means for evaluating function, additional radiographic imaging of the RCU after the first year is not indicated in a child who has excellent function, occlusion, and symmetry [25–27]. If, however, abnormal clinical signs and symptoms were present, imaging of the RCU is appropriate.

Functional outcomes

Lindahl [24] reported on functional outcomes after RCU fractures in 24 children with a mean age of 7.5 years (range, 3–11) at the time of injury, with a follow-up of 48 months. Clinically significant TMJ dysfunction was rare in growing children after RCU injuries [24,28]. The most important predictor of TMJ motion after RCU fracture is preinjury TMJ function. Asymmetric mandibular movements, deviation on opening, and excursive movements were found to resolve in growing children after 24 months. Persistent TMJ symptoms, such as joint noise or muscle tenderness, were uncommon. Notably, incomplete RCU remodeling did not influence mandibular function or dysfunction ($P > 0.05$) [24].

Developmental outcomes

Lund [29] documented mandibular growth radiographically in 27 children who had unilateral RCU fractures with a mean follow-up of 3 years. On average, the mandibular length of the fractured side (FS) grew 3.3 ± 0.8 mm more than the nonfractured side (NFS) ($P < 0.001$), but growth was variable. In 21 cases, the FS grew more than the NFS. In one case, the growth was equal on both sides. In five cases, the NFS grew more than the FS. Clinically, differences in mandibular growth may translate into deviation of the mandibular midline from the facial midline. In this study, 6 of 27 subjects (22%) had mandibular deviation from the midline >2 mm, but in no cases was an occlusal abnormality (ie, crossbite) noted. In two cases, the deviation was toward the FS, and in four cases, deviation was toward the NFS. Compensatory growth of the FS was related to the subject's age at the time of injury but was unrelated to sex, fracture location, or amount of condylar remodeling.

Similarly, Lindahl [30] reported results in 21 patients who had unilateral RCU fractures at a mean age of 6.9 years (range, 3–11). Chin deviation (14/27 cases) was a common finding: it was ≤ 2 mm and it was toward the FS in eight cases and toward the NFS in six cases. Notably, occlusal disturbances were reported as "rare" but were not quantified.

Ankylosis after RCU fractures is a known, serious complication; fortunately, however, its frequency seems to be rare. No cases of ankylosis were documented in any of the case series reviewed in this article. Purported risk factors for ankylosis are age (young), injury type (intracapsular/crush), and a long duration of MMF. Because ankylosis is a rare, unpredictable outcome, expectant monitoring to detect early decreases in range of motion or growth inhibition is indicated. Aggressive physiotherapy may limit or prevent ankylosis.

Radiographic outcomes

After RCU fractures, the condyle may remodel and achieve a near normal radiographic appearance, or there may be evidence of incomplete remodeling characterized by an irregular condylar appearance or displacement at the fracture site. Normalization of the RCU-fossa relationship occurs within 2 to 3 years in growing subjects (age ≤ 11 years) [31]. In a sample of 38 subjects who had 27 unilateral and 11 bilateral RCU fractures (total number of fractures = 49), Lund [29] found that 37 (76%) condyles had radiographic evidence of complete remodeling by the end of follow-up (mean, 23 months; range, 5–49 months). Age was a prognostic variable for complete condylar remodeling after injury. Injuries that occurred before or during the puberal growth maximum were likely (83%) to have complete remodeling. At the end of adolescence, it was unlikely that a fractured RCU would show complete remodeling (0%). Fractures in which the condyle remained within the fossa had 100% evidence, whereas fractures located outside the fossa had a 57% chance of demonstrating complete radiographic remodeling. Fracture location (high versus low), side of fracture (unilateral versus bilateral), and gender were not associated with remodeling status.

Table 1
Outcomes after ramus-condyle unit injuries in growing children

Descriptive statistics					Functional outcomes					Developmental outcomes			Radiographic outcomes
Reference	n[a] k[b]	Age[c]	Treatment[d]	FU[g]	MIO[h]	Dev[i]	Exc[j] FS	NFS	Malocclusion	Ankylosis	Asymmetry	Remodeling[k]
[12]	55 55	(2.5–9.75)	Functional appliance (4–6 mo)	≥72 w	NR; reported no functional or occlusal abnormalities	NR	NR		NR	0/55	0/55	49/55 (complete) incomplete remodeling noted in the 7–10 age group
[20]	19 19 9 18	8.7 (2.3–14.2)	MMF (<23 d) PT	15.1	47.8 (uni) (34.3–57.4) 44.5 (bi) (35.1–54.4)	NR	NR		NR	0/28	0/28	20/37 (complete)
[26]	15 15 5 10	(2.5–12)	Obs	(0.2–17)	NR	0/20	NR		0/20	0/20	0/20	NR
[27]	27 27 11 22	(4–7)	Obs or MMF ORIF: 3 cases	3.7 (2.0–5.4)	NR	NR	NR		NR	NR	6/27 (>2mm)	37/49 (complete)
[28]	21 21	6.9 (3–11)	Obs or MMF	3.5	NR	NR	NR		rare[p]	0/24	14/27[q] (≤2 mm)	NR
[29][n]	13 13 1 2	(3–11)		15	51.9	9.1	9.3		NR	0/14	NR	13/14[o] (complete)
[30]	29 29 8 16	9.4 (3.1–15.1)	MMF 17.2 (7–26)	4.1 (1–12)	2/37 (5%) noted limited opening	8/37 (21%)	NR		NR	0/37	0/37	20/45 (complete)

| [31] | 15 | 15 | 7.7 (4–11) | MMF[e] (12–17 d) PT[f] | 4.7 (3–6) | 38.3 (34–43) | 4/18 (22%) <2 mm | 8.4 | 7.8 | 0/18 | 0/18 | 0/18 | 17/21 (good) |
| [32] | 22 | 22 | 8.7 (3–16) | Obs or MMF (≤2 w) | 15 (5–24.5) | 49.3 (40–61) | NR[l] | 10.1 | 9.6 | NR | 0/25 | 4/22[m] (18%) | 12/28 (good) no functional or aesthetic consequences |

Abbreviations: bi, bilateral; MMF, maxillomandibular fixation; NR, not reported; Obs, observation; ORIF, open reduction with internal fixation; PT, physiotherapy; uni, unilateral.

[a] Sample size (subjects), number of subjects with unilateral fractures is reported as the first number, with number of subjects with bilateral fractures reported second.
[b] Sample size (RCU fractures).
[c] Age (year) at time of injury: mean (range).
[d] Treatment.
[e] Maxillomandibular fixation: mean (range) of treatment duration (if reported).
[f] Physiotherapy.
[g] Duration of follow-up (year, unless noted otherwise): mean (range).
[h] Maximal incisal opening (mm) at the end of follow-up: mean (range).
[i] Deviation with opening.
[j] Lateral excursions (mm).
[k] Radiographic evidence of remodeling.
[l] Not reported.
[m] Asymmetry evaluations limited to subjects with unilateral RCU fractures.
[n] Limited analyses to the sample age 3–11.
[o] Outcomes reported by subject (n), not RCU fractures (k).
[p] Occlusal disturbance reported as rare, but not quantified.
[q] Of the 14 subjects with evidence of chin deviation 3–4 years after unilateral RCU fractures, in all cases the deviation was ≤2 mm. In eight cases, the deviation was toward the fractured side. In the remaining cases, the chin point deviation was toward the nonfractured side.

Feifel and colleagues [20] assessed remodeling in a sample of 28 children with 37 RCU fractures and a mean age of 8.7 years at the time of injury. Mean follow-up was 15.1 years. In most cases there was complete remodeling of the fractured condyle (20/37). Patients with incomplete remodeling were 1.1 years older than patients with complete remodeling (9.4 versus 89.3 years, respectively). In unilateral cases, the FS was 11% shorter than the NFS and the ramus was 4% shorter on the FS when compared with the NFS.

Lindahl and Hollender [25] reported on radiographic remodeling in a sample of 67 subjects with 76 RCU fractures. The sample was grouped by age: 3 to 11, 12 to 15, 16 to 19, and ≥ 20 years. The sample was followed for 36 to 48 months after injury. The authors reported that the subjects in the 3- to 11-year-old age group had excellent capacity for remodeling regardless of fracture location or displacement. With age, the remodeling capacity decreased such that there was minimal remodeling in adults and more functional adjustment to the abnormal RCU.

Various risk factors are related to incomplete remodeling [12,19,31,32]. Fracture location and displacement variably were associated with incomplete remodeling [19,32]. It seems that the older a patient is at the time of injury, the greater the likelihood for incomplete remodeling. Evidence suggests that before age 10, complete remodeling occurs [19,25].

Summary

Nonoperative management of RCU fractures in a growing child is generally agreed to be adequate in most cases and consists of supportive care and physiotherapy or a short course of MMF (<14 days) if there is evidence of a malocclusion or significant functionally abnormality (deviation on opening) and physiotherapy of variable duration after MMF release (≤ 7 months). Although some clinicians advocate the use of functional appliances for RCU fractures, based on the available data, I have little enthusiasm in supporting the routine use of functional appliances in the acute management of RCU fractures.

Serial examinations and radiographs until completion of growth are recommended to monitor for any functional or developmental abnormalities. In the setting of an evolving mandibular asymmetry or deficiency in a growing child, there may be a role for interceptive therapy using functional appliances to attempt to alter growth. If interceptive therapy fails, orthodontics or orthognathic surgery may be necessary to address any posttraumatic developmental abnormalities. The management of an evolving ankylosis, beyond aggressive physiotherapy, is unclear and speculative.

Outcomes after RCU fractures in growing children are generally good. There are occasional reports of TMJ symptoms after injury (eg, pain and joint noise), but whether this is more common than in the general population is unclear. Some studies report deviation with mouth opening, but it is subclinical, (≤ 2 mm), and range of motion seems to be normal except in the rare instance of ankylosis. In the studies reviewed, malocclusion was not reported. Mandibular asymmetry was as high as 52%, but the magnitude of chin deviation was ≤ 2 mm in most cases. The direction of the asymmetry (toward or away from the fractured side) was varied and unpredictable. Radiographic outcomes, judged by degree of RCU remodeling after injury, documents complete remodeling 2 to 3 years after injury. The degree of remodeling did not correlate well with either functional or developmental outcomes.

Risk factors associated with outcomes were age and fracture location and displacement. The relationships, however, between age and fracture location and displacement and outcomes of interest were varied and inconsistent. Generally speaking, increasing age was associated with poorer outcomes. Low or displaced fractures also were variably associated with poorer outcomes. Given the inconsistently reported associations among the various risk factors and outcomes, one may conclude that outcomes most likely are related to some interaction among age, fracture location and displacement, and inherent developmental responses. Absent good predictors of adverse outcomes, long-term monitoring of growing subjects is the practical management suggestion.

References

[1] Iida S, Matsuya T. Paediatric maxillofacial fractures: their aetiological characters and fracture patterns. J Craniomaxillofac Surg 2002;30(4):237–41.

[2] Demianczuk AN, Verchere C, Phillips JH. The effect on facial growth of pediatric mandibular fractures. J Craniofac Surg 1999;10(4):323–8.

[3] Zachariades N, Papavassiliou D, Koumoura F. Fractures of the facial skeleton in children. J Craniomaxillofac Surg 1990;18(4):151–3.

[4] Siegel MB, Wetmore RF, Potsic WP, et al. Mandibular fractures in the pediatric patient. Arch Otolaryngol Head Neck Surg 1991;117(5):533–6.

[5] Cossio PI, Galvez FE, Gutierrez Perez JL, et al. Mandibular fractures in children: a retrospective study

of 99 fractures in 59 patients. Int J Oral Maxillofac Surg 1994;23(6 Pt 1):329–31.
[6] Kaban LB, Mullikan JB, Murray JE. Facial fractures in children: an analysis of 122 fractures in 109 patients. Plast Reconstr Surg 1977;59:15–20.
[7] Thoren H, Iizuka T, Hallikainen D, et al. An epidemiological study of patterns of condylar fractures in children. Br J Oral Maxillofac Surg 1997;35(5):306–11.
[8] Lee CYS, McCullom C, Balustein DI. Pediatric chin injury: occult condylar fractures of the mandible. Pediatr Emerg Care 1991;7(3):160–2.
[9] Bertolami CN, Kaban LB. Chin trauma: a clue to associated mandibular and cervical spine injury. Oral Surg Oral Med Oral Pathol 1982;53(2):122–6.
[10] Dodson TB. Mandibular fractures in children. Oral and Maxillofacial Surgery Knowledge Update 1995;1(Part II):95–107.
[11] Chacon GE, Dawson KH, Myall RW, et al. A comparative study of 2 imaging techniques for the diagnosis of condylar fractures in children. J Oral Maxillofac Surg 2003;61(6):668–72.
[12] Strobl H, Emshoff R, Rothler G. Conservative treatment of unilateral condylar fractures in children: a long-term clinical and radiologic follow-up of 55 patients. Int J Oral Maxillofac Surg 1999;28(2):95–8.
[13] Kahl-Nieke B, Fischbach R, Gerlach KL. CT analysis of temporomandibular joint state in children 5 years after functional treatment of condylar fractures. Int J Oral Maxillofac Surg 1994;23(6 Pt 1):332–7.
[14] Luck O, Harzer W. Early treatment of angle Class II, division 2 in combination with functional therapy of TMJ fracture. J Orofac Orthop 2001;62(2):157–62.
[15] Defabianis P. Treatment of condylar fractures in children and youths: the clinical value of the occlusal plane orientation and correlation with facial development [case reports]. J Clin Pediatr Dent 2002;26(3):243–50.
[16] DeFabianis P. TMJ fractures in children: clinical management and follow-up. J Clin Pediatr Dent 2001;25(3):203–8.
[17] Defabianis P. Condylar fractures treatment in children and youths: influence on function and face development (a five year retrospective analysis). Funct Orthod 2001;18(2):24–31.
[18] DeFabianis P. Rational and philosophic basis for a functional approach to TMJ fractures in children. Funct Orthod 2000;17(3):20–4.
[19] Kahl-Nieke B, Fischbach R. Condylar restoration after early TMJ fractures and functional appliance therapy. Part I: Remodelling. J Orofac Orthop 1998;59(3):150–62.
[20] Feifel H, Albert-Deumlich J, Riediger D. Long-term follow-up of subcondylar fractures in children by electronic computer-assisted recording of condylar movements. Int J Oral Maxillofac Surg 1992;21(2):70–6.
[21] Hotz RP. Functional jaw orthopedics in the treatment of condylar fractures. Am J Orthod 1978;73(4):365–77.
[22] Profitt WR, Vig KWL, Turvey TA. Early fracture of the mandibular condyles: frequently an unsuspected cause of growth disturbances. Am J Orthod 1980;78(1):1–24.
[23] Defabianis P. TMJ fractures in children and adolescents: treatment guidelines. J Clin Pediatr Dent 2003;27(3):191–8.
[24] Lindahl L. Condylar fractures of the mandible. IV. Function of the masticatory system. Int J Oral Surg 1977;6:195–203.
[25] Lindahl L, Hollender L. Condylar fractures of the mandible. II. A radiographic study of remodeling processes in the temporomandibular joint. Int J Oral Surg 1977;6:153–65.
[26] Guven O, Keskin A. Remodeling following condylar fractures in children. J Craniomaxillofac Surg 2001;29(4):232–7.
[27] Bergsma LA. Long-term results of nonsurgical management of condylar fracture in children. Int J Oral Maxillofac Surg 1999;28(6):429–40.
[28] Leake D, Doykos J, Habal MB, et al. Long-term follow-up of fractures of the mandibular condyle in children. Plast Reconstr Surg 1971;47(2):127–31.
[29] Lund K. Mandibular growth and remodeling processes after condylar fracture: a longitudinal roentgencephalometric study. Acta Odontol Scand 1974;32(Suppl 64):1–117.
[30] Lindahl L. Condylar fractures of the mandible. III. Positional changes of the chin. Int J Oral Surg 1977;6:166–72.
[31] Dahlstrom L, Kahnberg KE, Lindahl L. Fifteen years follow-up on condylar fractures. Int J Oral Maxillofac Surg 1989;18:18–23.
[32] Thoren H, Iizuka T, Hallikainen D, et al. Radiologic changes of the temporomandibular joint after condylar fractures in childhood. Oral Surg Oral Med Oral Pathol Oral Radiol Endod 1998;86(6):738–45.

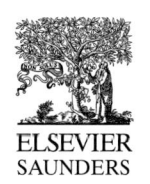

Pediatric Mandibular Hypomobility: Current Management and Controversies

Bernard J. Costello, DMD, MD[a,b],*, Sean P. Edwards, DDS, MD[a]

[a]*Division of Craniofacial and Cleft Surgery, Department of Oral and Maxillofacial Surgery, University of Pittsburgh School of Dental Medicine, 3471 Fifth Avenue, Suite 1112, Pittsburgh, PA 15213, USA*
[b]*Division of Pediatric Oral and Maxillofacial Surgery, Children's Hospital of Pittsburgh, 3471 Fifth Avenue, Suite 1112, Pittsburgh, PA 15213, USA*

Limited range of motion of the pediatric mandible (eg, mandibular hypomobility) presents many challenges. Untreated or recurrent hypomobility can cause problems with mastication, oral hygiene, speech, growth, and the airway. The difficulties that surgeons have encountered in their well-intentioned efforts to remedy this problem are reflected in the controversy found in the literature [1–19]. Treatments for ankylosis or adhesions include coronoidectomy, gap arthroplasty, costochondral rib reconstruction, prosthetic joint replacement, and transport distraction osteogenesis. Unfortunately, the literature is rather sparse with outcome studies comparing the many surgical options.

There are many different causes of mandibular hypomobility in young patients [4,9–11,16], including idiopathic (congenital), posttraumatic, infectious, inflammatory, neoplastic, and iatrogenic. A detailed evaluation and diagnosis of the limited range of motion are critical to developing an appropriate treatment strategy. This article outlines evaluation, differential diagnosis, and the current operative approaches for treating hypomobility in young patients. Controversies related to timing of various procedures and the uses of various treatment options are discussed.

Nomenclature

There are many reasons for limited mandibular range of motion in children. Hypomobility is defined as a decreased amount of maximal incisal opening. For the sake of clarity, it is important to differentiate hypomobility from temporomandibular joint (TMJ) ankylosis, which is a bony union or fusion between the glenoid fossa and condylar head of the mandible. Occasionally ankylosis is confused and used interchangeably with fibrous adhesions of the TMJ or other forms of hypomobility.

Another common nomenclature error is the use of congenital ankylosis or syndromic ankylosis for a young patient who presents with limited motion. Congenital implies an antenatal event that contributes to or causes the limited motion (eg, arthrogryposis) when in fact most hypomobility or ankylosis occurs as a postnatal event. The term "syndrome" implies a specific genetic defect that is associated with a somewhat predictable constellation of physical findings. Most syndromes are rarely associated with mandibular hypomobility, with the notable exceptions of Nager and Treacher-Collins syndromes.

The problem of hypomobility

Mandibular hypomobility has many consequences for a child, and an interdisciplinary approach is helpful in evaluating and treating these patients. Integrating the various members of the health care team to

---

* Corresponding author. Division of Craniofacial and Cleft Surgery, Department of Oral and Maxillofacial Surgery, University of Pittsburgh School of Dental Medicine, 3471 Fifth Avenue, Suite 1112, Pittsburgh, PA 15213.
E-mail address: bjc1@pitt.edu (B.J. Costello).

care optimally for the many issues associated with limited motion is essential to achieving the best result. Although mandibular hypomobility does not cause airway obstruction per se, the resultant growth restriction may lead to obstructive sleep apnea or the inability to intubate a child in an emergency. Clinicians should have a low threshold for obtaining sleep studies and airway endoscopy when evaluating these patients.

Feeding, mastication, and nutrition also may be affected, which may necessitate the help of a nutritionist, gastroenterologist, or pediatric surgeon. Children tend to be surprisingly resilient and compensate well when they wish to eat. Severe deformity of the upper aerodigestive tract easily can affect feeding and hamper nutritional intake, however, which may require a gastrostomy or other type of feeding tube.

Speech and language development is often overlooked in patients who have mandibular hypomobility. Patients may have trouble with articulation because of growth restriction and immobility. Compensatory patterns that develop during early phases of speech development are difficult to correct later in life. Patients who depend on a tracheostomy may have problems with speech development. An inability to open the mouth properly makes oral hygiene and the provision of proper dental care difficult. Carious teeth that ordinarily could be restored may need to be extracted because of difficulty in accessing the oral cavity for routine treatment.

Many children who have hypomobility develop restriction of mandibular growth. This restraint is not limited to the mandible but can affect the entire craniomaxillofacial complex. This situation is particularly relevant in unilateral cases that result in asymmetry. A carefully planned surgical orthodontic plan is essential to achieving a stable functional and aesthetic result.

Anatomy and pathophysiology

Problems that affect mandibular motion can be classified based on the anatomic location of the limiting pathology: intracapsular (within the capsule of the TMJ), extracapsular, or a combination. Intracapsular hypomobility may be related to internal derangements of the temporomandibular disc or ligaments or the development of scar in and around these structures. Patients who suffer condylar head or neck fractures may present with posttraumatic derangements associated with displacement of the

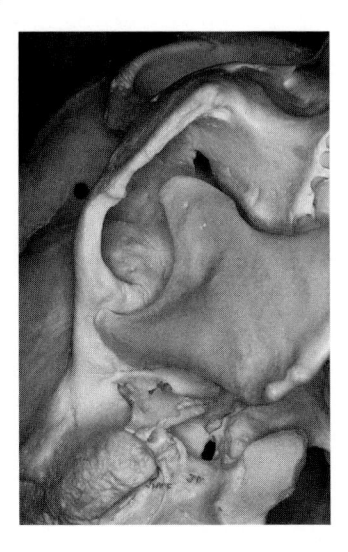

Fig. 1. Inferior view of right TMJ region highlights relationships among glenoid fossa, condyle, coronoid process, zygoma, and infratemporal fossa.

condylar head medially from the pull of the lateral pterygoid muscle. Although rare, intra-articular pathologic conditions (eg, anterior disc displacement or fibrous adhesions) and bony ankylosis do occur in children.

Hypomobility caused by extracapsular pathology includes disturbances of the muscles of mastication and the surrounding structures in the region of the TMJ. Hyperplasia, tumors, or displacement after trauma of the zygomatic arch, coronoid process, and infratemporal fossa may present physical obstructions to opening (Fig. 1). A combination of intra- and extracapsular pathology can occur. Longstanding intra-articular pathology with hypomobility can lead to degenerative changes in the muscles of mastication and their innervations [20], which contribute to limited opening even after treatment of intracapsular pathology.

History and physical examination

Obtaining a thorough history helps to determine the differential diagnosis of hypomobility. Patients born with limited opening are likely to have a different cause than patients with a later onset. Patients who have hypomobility for longer than 6 months can have intra- and extracapsular origins because longstanding disuse and limited mobility contribute to shortening and weakness of the muscles of mastication.

The presence, nature, severity, location, and chronicity of pain in association with hypomobility are important components of the history. Patients who have hypomobility without pain are more likely to have a clear anatomic obstruction that is unrelated to internal derangement (eg, tumor, contracture or fibrosis of the temporalis muscles). Painful hypomobility can be caused by internal derangement and inflamed tissue posterior to the temporomandibular disc. Patients who present with a unilateral rather than a bilateral problem usually have a different cause and progression of disease. Bilateral pathology often requires more intensive therapy and tends to be more difficult to treat. Bilateral pathology is more commonly seen with systemic conditions and syndromes.

A complete head and neck examination should be performed, as should an evaluation of other joints to evaluate for arthropathies that may have a systemic or rheumatologic origin. Some suggestive findings of generalized joint problems include warm, tender joints, effusions, and limb length discrepancies. A complete TMJ evaluation, including measuring maximal incisal opening, maximal excursions, and protrusion, is helpful in determining the severity of limitation. Deviation on opening may aid in determining if one joint is more affected than another. Joint noises should be documented, and noting any crepitus or clicking is helpful in differentiating between degenerative joint disease and internal derangement. The presence of a click that captures on closing is important when distinguishing between discs that recapture and those that are permanently anteriorly displaced. Although the anteriorly displaced disc without reduction is commonly seen in adults, it is only occasionally seen in children as a cause for hypomobility.

Palpating the movement of the lateral pole of the condyle is helpful when trying to feel for rotation and translation of the condyle as opposed to flexing of the mandible. The pediatric mandible can be flexed slightly, which is seen as opening at the incisors, without mobility of the actual condyle within the fossa. A small amount of movement at the condylar head indicates dense fibrous adhesions rather than true ankylosis (bony fusion) of the TMJ. Assisted opening is helpful in differentiating between hypomobility of differing causes. Patients who have ankylosis are not able to open during an examination despite a surgeon's gentle assistance. Patients with fibrous adhesions, myofascial pain, scarring, and internal derangements often are able to open further with manipulation. Local anesthetic blocks sometimes can be helpful if pain is a problem at a specific location.

Palpating the muscles of mastication and soft tissues of the head and neck for trigger point tenderness, spasm, and scar bands is helpful. In patients with traumatic injuries, scar bands of the soft tissue may be physical obstructions to opening. Severe traumatic scarring, radiation fibrosis, or diffuse burns may limit the normal soft tissue envelope available for motion despite perfectly normal joints and musculature. These types of limitation are often painless and there is usually no sudden, firm stop to the opening. At different examination visits, the amount of opening measured in these patients can vary. Dystonias of the muscles of mastication also may be palpated as hypertonic muscle bands with char-

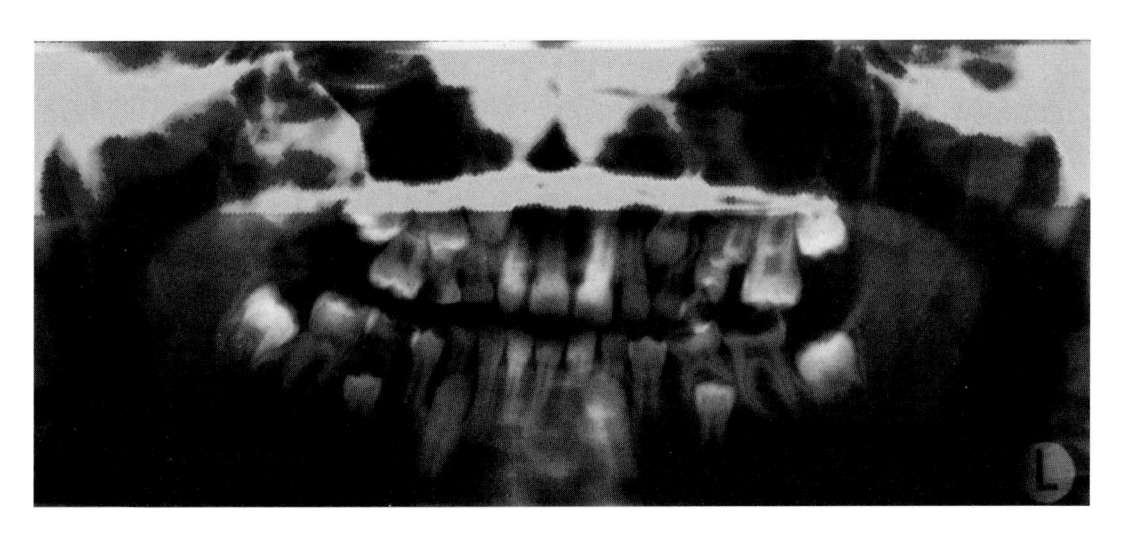

Fig. 2. Panoramic tomogram shows a tumor in right coronoid region that is limiting mandibular motion.

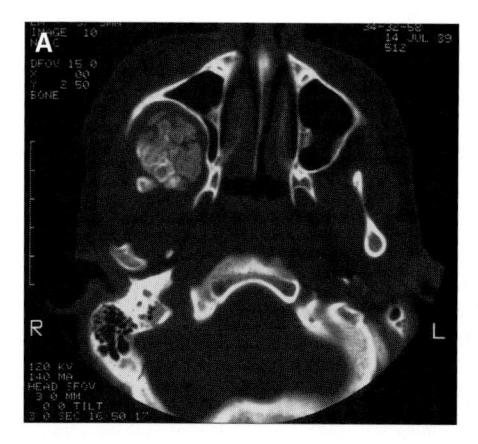

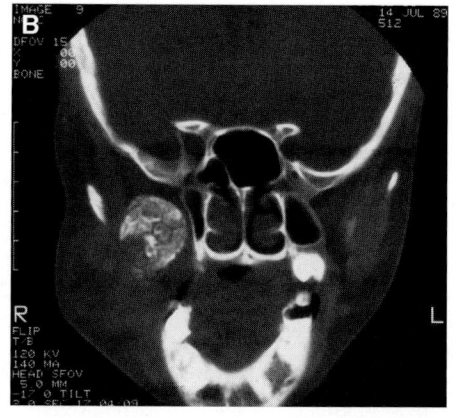

Fig. 3. (A,B) CT scans show a large tumor of the pterygoid fissure and coronoid region. Presenting symptom was hypomobility that was chronic and severe.

acteristic patterns of mandibular deviation or lack of opening.

Imaging

The panoramic tomogram is the best single view of the mandible and is excellent for imaging the condyle in a simple manner (Fig. 2). The basic condylar symmetry and form and its interface at the glenoid fossa can be appreciated using this study. Limitations of the panoramic tomogram include (1) an inability to appreciate the soft and cartilaginous tissue in and around the TMJ, (2) variations in tomogram imaging of the condylar head, (3) the fact that it provides only a two-dimensional image of the bony architecture, and (4) difficulty obtaining images on young children. Children over 5 years of age are often able to cooperate for this study, whereas younger patients are often best imaged with other modalities. Standard tomograms with or without contrast medium in the joint spaces have been used in the past but mostly have been supplanted by CT and MRI. Plain films are not helpful for evaluating most patients with hypomobility.

CT is the best study to evaluate the bony interface of the TMJ with the glenoid fossa and quickly screen for pathologic conditions in the region. The study is usually conducted without contrast unless a neoplasm is suspected (Figs. 3, 4). When the CT is of good quality and the appropriate software is available, reformatted images in the coronal and sagittal planes are helpful in determining morphology of this complex area and can help with surgical planning. Three-dimensional studies also can be generated to appreciate the anatomy further (Fig. 5).

MRI is useful for evaluating the specifics of intracapsular pathology and some tumors in the region. Neoplasms are usually imaged using contrast, but most studies that examine this area for TMJ abnormalities do not require contrast. Studies should be conducted with the patient in open and closed position using direct sagittal views. A dedicated TMJ coil is used to provide more detailed imaging when looking for purely intracapsular pathology. Imaging providers should be familiar with TMJ studies to provide the best results for interpretation.

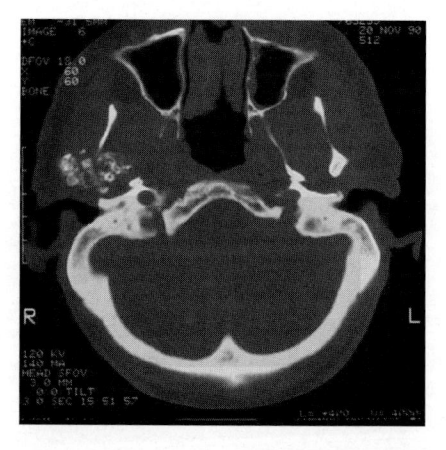

Fig. 4. CT scan shows a mixed tumor in right TMJ region in patient who presented with mandibular hypomobility.

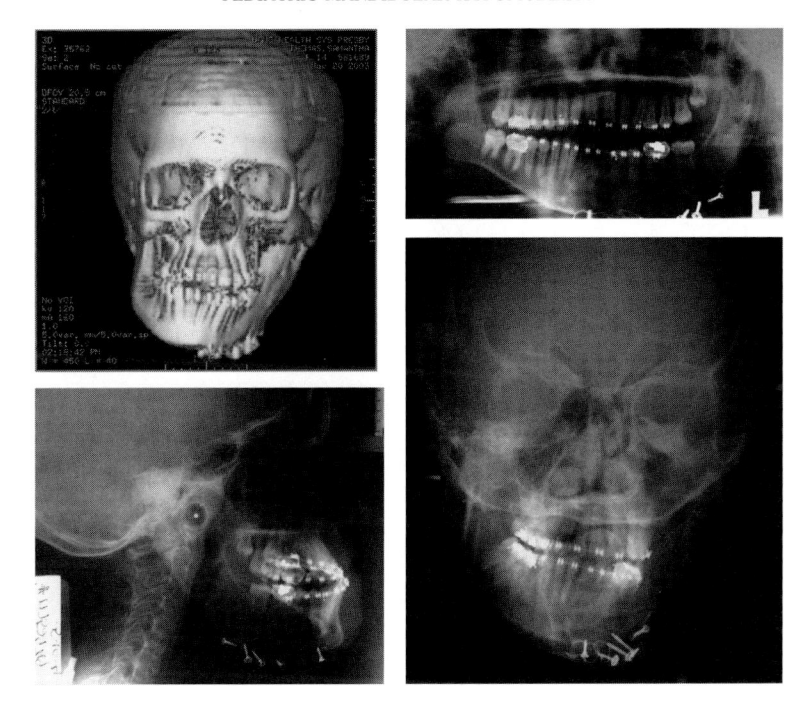

Fig. 5. Sixteen-year-old girl with type III hemifacial microsomia had costochondral graft placed at a young age and currently exhibits overgrowth with hypomobility. Three-dimensional CT reconstructions provide more information than panoramic tomogram or cephalometric studies and assist in treatment-planning definitive correction.

Bone scans that use radioactive isotope that is taken up in areas of increased blood flow (eg, inflammation or growth) are used to evaluate active inflammation or growth within the mandible, TMJ, and glenoid fossa (Fig. 6). Patients who have overgrowth of the condyle or mandible can be evaluated with this study to help determine the cessation of growth, asymmetric growth, and timing of intervention.

Extracapsular pathology

There are many extracapsular causes of hypomobility. The most common causes are related to the temporalis musculature and coronoid processes of the mandible. Hypertrophy of the coronoid process may occur and is easily seen on a panoramic tomogram. In the pathologic state the coronoid process tip is well above the zygomatic arch. Classically, these patients have greater limitation in lateral excursions toward the affected side as a result of the coronoid process impinging on the zygomatic arch and the limitation of shortened tendon attachments.

Contracture of the temporalis tendon or fibrosis of these tendons and muscles can occur, especially in patients who have been irradiated. This condition also may be seen after neurosurgical procedures that involve the temporal region if significant scarring or fibrosis occurs. Masseter muscles also can become

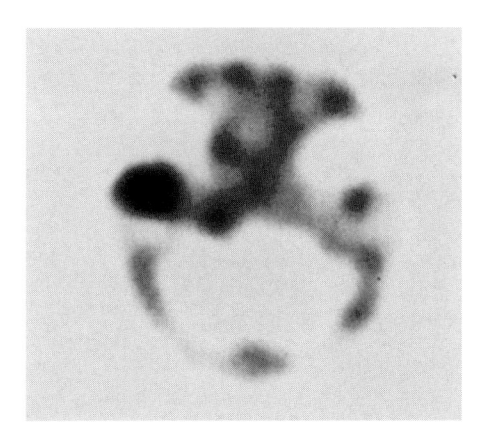

Fig. 6. Technetium 99 bone scan shows considerable uptake in patient with hypomobility and asymmetry. Uptake is caused by a tumor of the right TMJ.

fibrosed or scarred in a similar fashion. Traumatic scar bands in these areas may occur after previous surgery, infection, or ingestion of caustic substances. Atrophy of the muscles can be associated with contracture and is sometimes seen in patients with neurodegenerative disorders or severe head injuries.

Another anatomic obstruction occurs in patients who sustain trauma to the zygomatic complex or isolated arch and the displaced bones physically impede the coronoid process from rotating downward and forward during mandibular motion. A subcondylar fracture that is severely displaced also can impede opening in rare instances. It is not unusual for patients to present after these displaced fragments have healed in an inappropriate position.

Tumors of the extracapsular tissues can impede mandibular opening and should be considered when a patient presents with hypomobility. Myriad tumors—

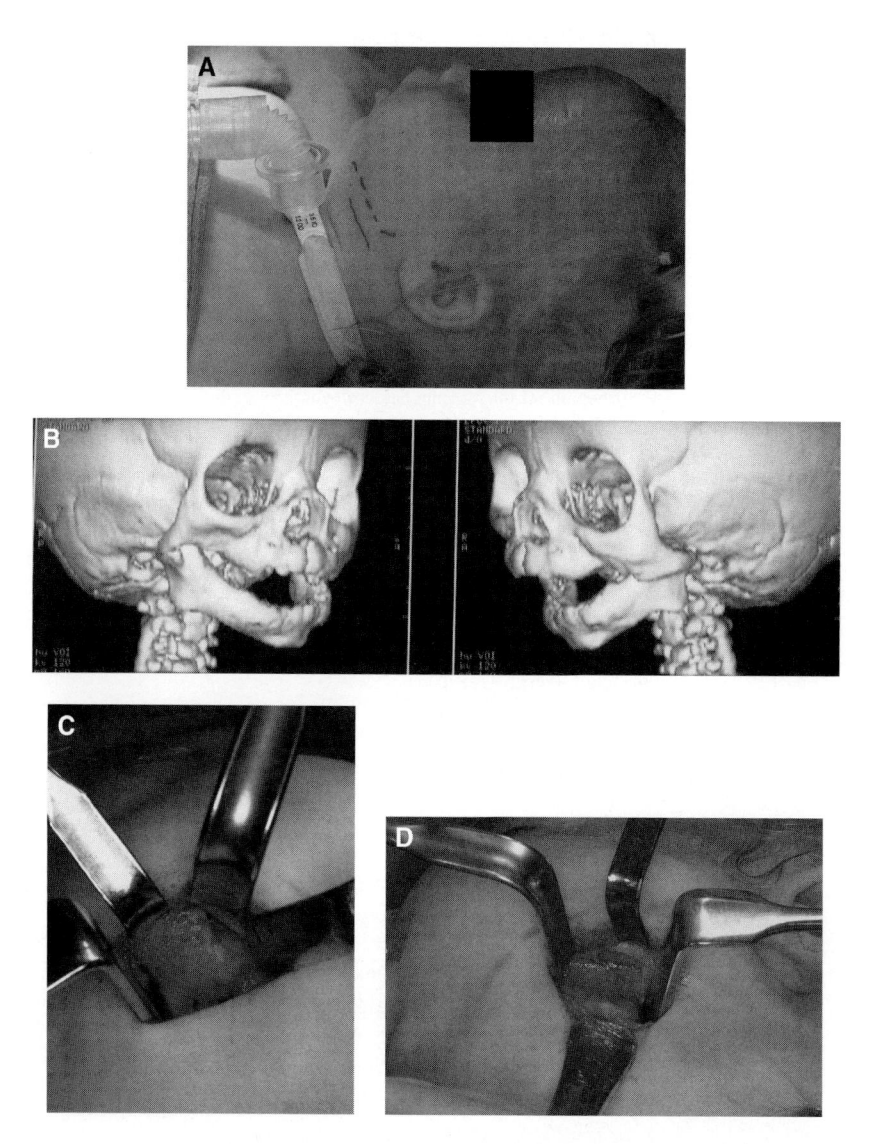

Fig. 7. (*A*) Lateral view of young child with bilateral TMJ congenital ankylosis. (*B*) Three-dimensional CT scans show bilateral fusion of glenoid fossas, TMJs, and coronoid processes. (*C,D*) Right and left views of congenital fusion to lateral cranial base. (*E,F*) Right and left views after gap arthrotomies and placement of polytetrafluoroethylene and titanium mesh. Intensive physical therapy was helpful in mobilizing this patient to more than 30 mm for 6 months. Once physical therapy was stopped, fibrous adhesions formed and the hypomobility recurred.

benign and malignant—can affect this area. Some relatively common examples are osteochondroma, fibrous dysplasia, ossifying fibroma, and ectopic bone formation. Primary tumors isolated to the coronoid process are rare. Tumors of the posterior maxillary sinus occasionally can expand to involve the coronoid process, as can tumors of the skull base and infratemporal fossa. Tumor infiltration of the muscles of mastication also can result in mobility problems.

Although rare, congenital fusion of the components of the jaws has been reported (Fig. 7) [21–24]. Patients who have this condition have no mandibular motion at birth and may have various anatomic structures fused. The maxilla may fuse to the mandible or the coronoid may fuse to either the skull base or maxilla. The condyle also may be fused to the glenoid fossa in conjunction with the other structures. Fibrosis of the pericapsular tissues after birth trauma, which results from forceps delivery, may occur and result in hypomobility.

Arthrogryposis is a term applied to a heterogeneous group of disorders characterized by multiple joint contractures, including the TMJ. The cause for these joint contractures is intrauterine akinesia. The lack of fetal movement may result from fetal (eg, muscle abnormalities) and maternal disorders, including drug and toxin exposure and infections. Intrauterine movement is essential for normal joint development. Lack of fetal movement may result in deposition of excess connective tissue around the joint, which limits its range of motion. Earlier fetal insults tend to have more severe presentations.

Intracapsular pathology

Although rare, internal derangement of the TMJ disc with anterior displacement can be seen in children, and the cause is similar to adults. Traumatic episodes may be to blame in a higher percentage of children, however, because pediatric condyle fractures are common. Systemic disorders of joint laxity also should be considered in patients who have chronic dislocation, pain, and occasional restricted motion (ie, Ehler-Danlos syndrome).

Over the last decade, surgical TMJ treatment protocols for adults have become more conservative, but they have been consistently conservative in the pediatric population for various reasons. Open joint procedures in children are not advocated because of concerns that disrupting the functional matrix of the growing TMJ could result in growth restriction and asymmetry. Some children who present with anterior disc displacement with or without reduction may be operative candidates because of the severity of their pain and dysfunction. In the author's opinion, these cases are rare, and plication procedures that are used in adults should be used only in children who present with significant functional limitation that can be correlated directly to improper disc position. For most cases of internal derangement in children, only after nonsurgical measures of treatment have been exhausted should a surgical option be considered.

Many children who present with degenerative joint disease of the TMJs have systemic disorders that are best controlled with medical therapy under the guidance of a skilled pediatric rheumatologist. Juve-

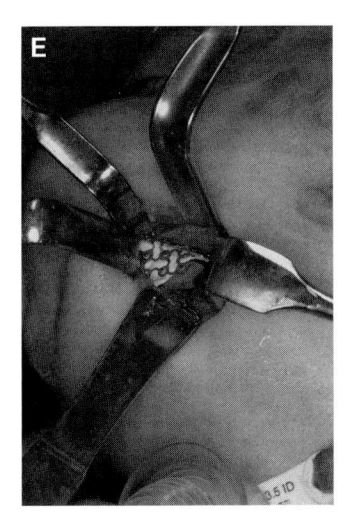

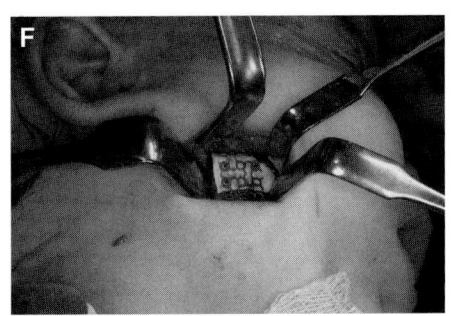

Fig. 7 (*continued*).

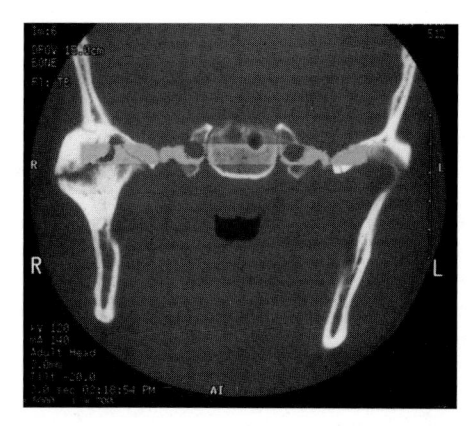

Fig. 8. CT scan shows ankylosis of right TMJ after a traumatic incident in childhood.

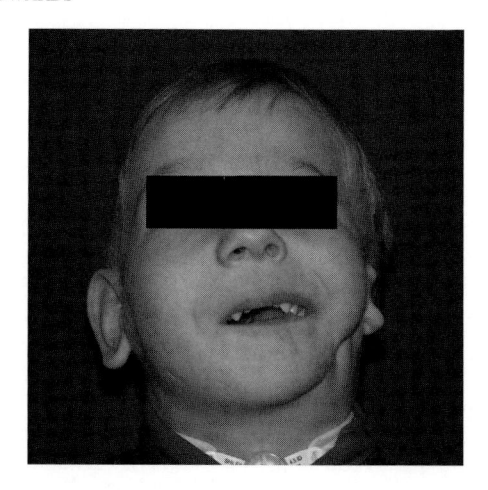

Fig. 10. Young boy who had Goldenhar syndrome had multiple attempts at distraction osteogenesis to reconstruct left type III mandibular deformity. He has asymmetry, trismus, and a tracheostomy. Limited growth is possible and should be followed over the long-term. He requires total TMJ reconstruction with a rib graft and orthognathic surgery to treat his malocclusion and skeletal imbalance.

nile rheumatoid arthritis is the most common scenario in which a child may have significant degenerative joint disease and occasionally present with pain. Operative intervention is usually not helpful in these patients because most of them have good mobility. Nonsurgical treatment is usually the best option barring severe destructive degenerative joint disease that requires reconstruction. Growth and development of the facial skeleton should be checked yearly because many children with rheumatoid arthritis of the TMJ develop mandibular hypoplasia with a reduced vertical height of the ramus. Most of these patients benefit from combined surgical orthodontic treatment once they are skeletally mature if their rheumatoid disease stabilizes.

True ankylosis of the intracapsular condyle to the glenoid fossa occurs for various reasons. Although trauma, such as a fall with an unrecognized condyle fracture, is often to blame in young children, other incidents may occur. Trauma to the TMJ at birth also may cause a hemearthrosis and bony fusion of the joints (Fig. 8) [1,3,9–11,16]. Infection of the joints, typically caused by local extension of an otitis media or mastoiditis, may produce such significant inflammation that calcification occurs and causes fusion of the joint [25]. Fortunately, such infectious complications are rare today. In 1964, Topazian [4] reviewed the causes and outcomes of pediatric patients who had some form of ankylosis/hypomobility. In his review, the causes were 40% inflammatory and 40% traumatic, and the remaining 20% were caused by various other disorders. Other intracapsular pathologic conditions include tumors, congenital fusion, and iatrogenic causes (Figs. 9, 10). True congenital fusion has been reported in only a few cases and has an unclear origin. Complications caused by scarring from lateral cranial base surgery or previous TMJ surgery are occasionally seen as reasons for hypomobility in children.

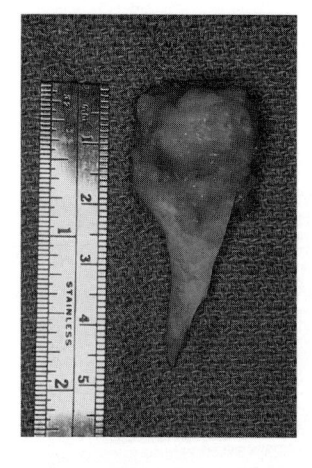

Fig. 9. Intracapsular tumor of TMJ that limited mandibular motion. Ipsilateral posterior open bite developed over several months.

Interdisciplinary treatment

Treatment decisions must be made with careful consideration of the biologic consequences of intervening in a child's growth. Patients who have severe limitation as a result of pathology that is intracapsular, extracapsular, or a combination of the two usually benefit from early release and reconstruction for various reasons. Successful treatment optimizes a patient's condition for feeding, speech, and language development. Inadequate mastication may cause nutritional deficiencies and resultant growth and developmental abnormalities. The inability to move the mandible, tongue, teeth, and lips completely may affect speech and language development, which further impacts a child's ability to communicate and learn.

Airway problems may occur because of limited growth of the mandible. When the mandible does not function completely, the delicate balance between the functional structures is disturbed. This imbalance often results in a hypoplastic mandible and may be associated with obstructive sleep apnea in young children (Fig. 10). Patients who have severe hypomobility may not be able to be intubated easily, whether for an emergency (eg, respiratory failure) or for a routine procedure (eg, myringotomy tube placement or appendectomy). In some cases, treatment may allow for decannulation of a tracheostomy or resolution of obstructive sleep apnea caused by tongue base collapse and an inefficient, obstructed airway.

Hypomobility that presents in young children may contribute to growth disturbances that are particularly severe. In addition to obvious functional problems when left untreated, there are also psychosocial concerns with respect to self-esteem and personal appearance. Although most definitive corrections for skeletal discrepancies are performed at maturity, some patients with severe deformities may benefit from earlier correction for other reasons (Fig. 11) [26–29].

One of the more commonly overlooked interdisciplinary concerns in children with hypomobility is poor oral hygiene. A rather unfortunate and common scenario is a patient with hypomobility who presents in young childhood with a severe dental infection and who may require intubation because of airway compromise. This situation usually can be avoided with regular preventive dental care. The involvement of a skilled pediatric dentist who has access to a facility that has experience intubating children with hypomobility is important. In younger children who have severe hypomobility, parents often have significant difficulty cleaning teeth in the posterior oral cavity.

Critical to the success of any of the surgical modalities used is physical therapy. Physical therapy is at least as important—if not more so—in determining the eventual outcome of the operation. It is paramount to ensure that appropriate physical therapy can and will be done postoperatively before attempting any surgical correction. Physical therapy for young children is especially difficult because they are often unable to perform the necessary exercises themselves and require parental assistance. Physical therapy, especially in the immediate postoperative period, is painful and only makes cooperation that much more difficult. Comorbidities also should be taken into consideration. For example, a young adult who has arthrogryposis that involves the upper extremities or has severe contractures from juvenile rheumatoid arthritis does not possess the dexterity necessary to perform the needed exercises adequately. It is essential to ensure that these children have the support system available that is necessary to maintain the opening achieved with an operation. Various commercially available appliances can be used to optimize opening and resist scarring in the early phase and contracture in the late phase of healing. Physical therapy should be continued for a long period of time after the surgical procedure, and patients must be seen on a regular basis to ensure that best compliance possible.

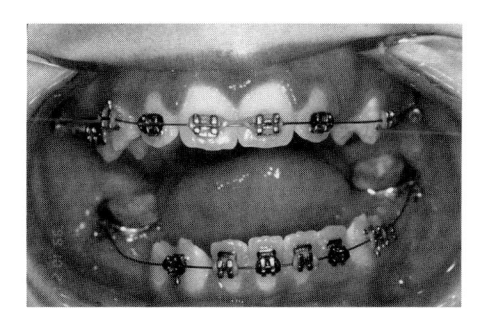

Fig. 11. The consequences of a undiagnosed condyle fracture are shown in this young girl. Left-sided ramus shortening caused by growth restriction, mandibular canting, and hypomobility is seen in this patient, who is in the stage of mixed dentition. Definitive reconstruction of the asymmetry and malocclusion is best performed at skeletal maturity.

Surgical management

Extracapsular causes of hypomobility are treated by removing the impeding elements, such as a tumor, displaced zygoma, or hyperplastic coronoid process. Most patients with chronic hypomobility also benefit from coronoidectomies as an adjunct to treatment.

One of the common operations for true ankylosis or severe fibrosis of the TMJ is gap arthrotomy, which usually involves excision of bone or fibrous tissue of the condyle and glenoid fossa, although occasionally the coronoid notch and coronoid process are also included. Patients benefit from coronoidectomies because of contracture of the temporalis tendons from disuse. Gap arthrotomy is an effective treatment, but there is an overwhelming tendency in children for healing to occur between the two segments despite physical therapy. For this reason, many surgeons have used synthetic spacers or grafts to keep this space open during early healing. These techniques have had limited success, because the ability for a child to heal this defect seems to overcome most attempts to prevent fusion with a spacer. One approach is to use a spacing material, such as poly-tetra-fluoro-ethylene, in conjunction with titanium mesh to prevent bone healing between the segments. No matter which material is used, physical therapy is the key element for avoiding early fusion after a successful arthrotomy.

Kaban and colleagues [15] reviewed the success of a protocol showing good results using a liner within the TMJ after arthroplasty/arthrotomy. Fourteen patients were reviewed and all had good results, but the ages varied, as did the causes of the disease. Posnick and Goldstein [16] reported their experience with a similar protocol and tracked quantifiable data on nine patients after TMJ reconstruction. They found an average of 5 mm of maximal incisal opening preoperatively and an average of 25 mm postoperatively, with a mean follow-up of 2 years. Of note was the poor outcome in patients who had bilateral involvement, longstanding disease, muscle disuse arthropathy, and Nager or Treacher-Collins syndrome.

Total reconstruction of the TMJ is an option for many patients who have complete ankylosis or have had multiple failed attempts at reconstruction. Costochondral grafting continues to be the preferred method for TMJ reconstruction in children, although a temporary custom total prosthesis can be used in some patients before definitive reconstruction in a fully grown child.

Treatment of the pathologic condyle must address various issues to maintain function. Rowe [9–11] described his goals in treatment for patients with ankylosis in a series of papers for the Royal College of Surgeons in 1982. These concepts are still adhered to currently, although many experts readily admit that treatment of limited mobility in children continues to be a difficult problem even after decades of diligent effort and advances. Rowe's goals included establishing mandibular mobility and function, preventing recurrence of the ankylosis, and restoring the functional growth matrix.

Additional goals include reconstitution of vertical dimension, preservation of the occlusion, and improvement of facial symmetry. Multiple materials have been used to replace the condyle. Ideally, materials must be well tolerated by patients, have a low lifetime risk of infection, and provide a long-lasting and dynamic reconstruction to achieve the stated treatment goals. The costochondral graft replaces not only the vertical bony portion of the ramus but also the cartilage of the condyle and disc articulation. In the case of pediatric patients, it may be considered advantageous to have a graft that continues to grow with a patient. Reconstruction with costochondral grafts generally provides good functional and cosmetic results. The timing of the procedure should take into consideration functional and aesthetic issues and the effects of surgery on further growth.

Costochondral grafting in a growing child is not without its drawbacks. An otherwise successful graft still may grow at a different rate or not at all, which has been shown by many authors, with much of the data demonstrating overgrowth as being the most common scenario [27,28,30]. Some surgeons have attempted to correlate the degree of graft overgrowth with the amount of costal cartilage included with the graft, although it is still unpredictable.

When treating ankylosis, the prevention of reankylosis is a concern. Ross [31] reviewed the experience over 12 years at Toronto's Hospital for Sick Children and found successful results to be associated with earlier rib grafting (ages 3–9), fewer surgeries, and a diagnosis of hemifacial microsomia, as opposed to Goldenhar syndrome, ankylosis, or pathology. Recurrent ankylosis or hypomobility is a concern in most of these patients. It remains a difficult problem to treat effectively in young children, who have excellent healing capabilities and a hard time complying with recommended physical therapy regimens. For this reason the timing of repeat operations in young children should be considered carefully if failure has occurred in the past. Patients who have grafting performed at ages younger than 5 years tend to have higher complication rates (eg, resorption of the graft and reankylosis). Children who are slightly older and have completed more growth may have a greater chance of success and definitive reconstruction if the endeavors are delayed. The balance between functional needs of the patient and the likely success of the procedure at that time must be weighed carefully.

Distraction osteogenesis

Distraction osteogenesis is a technique that has been used to lengthen bones. Use of the technique in the craniofacial skeleton received much attention in the 1990s, but currently the overall enthusiasm has been curbed significantly. This waning enthusiasm is partly the result of difficulty in achieving a stable and long-lasting result that is as predictable and accurate as traditional techniques of osteotomies with or without bone grafting. Some attempts have been made to use gradual distraction after gap arthrotomy to transport a regenerate "disc" of tissue back into the TMJ fossa in the hopes that the tissue would work as a condyle by histologically changing and becoming a neo-joint with cartilaginous tissue interposed between the bony segments of the glenoid fossa and new ramus of the mandible [32–34].

Stucki-McCormick was one of the first to describe the technique in the late 1990s, and several case reports have followed [32–34]. Hijihi and colleagues [35] reported the histologic changes of bone to cartilaginous-type tissue after transport distraction, but the value of this change is unknown. These reports have claimed initial success with creating a neocondyle that functions, but no data have been reported regarding retained maximal incisal opening, reankylosis, pain, need for additional operation, or other long-term data.

Once the gap arthrotomy is complete, an additional osteotomy is made in the remaining ramus for transport superiorly into the joint space. Vector planning can be difficult when trying to have the transport disc approximate the glenoid fossa, and as with all other techniques, physical therapy is important in the postoperative phase. Manipulation of the transport disc after arthrotomy is difficult when one considers the possible consequences on mandibular position of the distal segment. Occlusion may be altered and salvage osteotomies are often required later.

Potential advantages include the possible transformation of the neocondyle into one with a cartilaginous cap that conforms to the glenoid fossa and simultaneous ankylosis resection and condyle reconstruction without the need for a donor site. Potential disadvantages include a less predictable result, external pin tracks with scarring when external devices are used, the need for multiple anesthetic agents and operations, and other complications reported with distraction osteogenesis [36]. Although the technique is still reported anecdotally to have had success in some pediatric patients, the authors cannot endorse its widespread use without more published supporting data. As the devices and techniques are refined, this procedure may become a viable alternative or a preferred modality of treatment for some patients. Given the difficult nature of the problem, the authors recommend considering the most predictable and proven techniques.

Summary

Hypomobility of the mandible in pediatric patients is, and has been, a vexing problem for surgeons. The goals initially described by Rowe remain as important currently no matter which technique is used. Physical therapy is an important part of the success of any surgical endeavor. The choice for intervention and reconstruction techniques should be based primarily on functional needs, but one also should consider aesthetic and psychosocial concerns. The timing of intervention should be thought out carefully based on the immediate needs of patients and the likely long-term success of the technique.

References

[1] Beavis JO. Intra-articular bony ankylosis of the temporomandibular articulation. J Am Dent Assoc 1928;15:874.

[2] Risdon F. Ankylosis of the temporomandibular joint. J Am Dent Assoc 1933;21.

[3] Burket LW. Congenital bony temporomandibular ankylosis and facial hemiatrophy: review of the literature and report of a case. JAMA 1936;106:1748.

[4] Topazian RG. Etiology of ankylosis of temporomandibular joint: analysis of 44 cases. J Oral Surg 1964; 22:227–33.

[5] Snyder CC, Levine GA, Dingman DL. Trial of a sternoclavicular whole joint graft as a substitute for the temporomandibular joint. Plast Reconstr Surg 1971; 48:447–52.

[6] Ware WH. Growth center transplantation in temporomandibular joint surgery. In: Walker RV, editor. Oral surgery: transactions of the third international conference in oral surgery. Edinburgh: E & S Livingstone; 1970. p. 148.

[7] Ware WH, Brown SL. Growth center transplantation to replace mandibular condyles. J Maxillofac Surg 1981;9:50–8.

[8] MacIntosh RB, Henny FA. A spectrum of application of autogenous costochondral grafts. J Maxillofac Surg 1977;5:257–67.

[9] Rowe NL. Ankylosis of the temporomandibular joint. J R Coll Surg Edinb 1982;27:67–79.

[10] Rowe NL. Ankylosis of the temporomandibular joint. J R Coll Surg Edinb 1982;27:167–73.

[11] Rowe NL. Ankylosis of the temporomandibular joint. J R Coll Surg Edinb 1982;27:209–18.
[12] Politis C, Fossion E, Bossuyt M. The use of costochondral grafts in the arthroplasty of the temporomandibular joint. J Craniomaxillofac Surg 1987;15: 345–54.
[13] Munro IR, Chen YR, Park BY. Simultaneous total correction of temporomandibular ankylosis and facial asymmetry. Plast Reconstr Surg 1986;77(4):517–29.
[14] Raveh J, Vuillemin T, Ladrach K, et al. Temporomandibular joint ankylosis: surgical treatment and long-term results. J Oral Maxillofac Surg 1989;47:900–6.
[15] Kaban LB, Perrott DH, Fisher K. A protocol for management of temporomandibular joint ankylosis. J Oral Maxillofac Surg 1990;48:1145–51.
[16] Posnick JC, Goldstein JA. Surgical management of temporomandibular joint ankylosis in the pediatric population. Plast Reconstr Surg 1993;91:791–8.
[17] Perrot DH, Umeda H, Kaban LB. Costochondral graft reconstruction/reconstruction of the ramus/condyle unit: long term follow-up. Int J Oral Maxillofac Surg 1994;23:321–8.
[18] Svensson B, Adell R. Costochondral grafts to replace mandibular condyles in juvenile chronic arthritis patients: long term effects on facial growth. J Craniomaxillofac Surg 1998;26:275–85.
[19] Ko EW, Huang CS, Chen YR. Temporomandibular joint reconstruction in children using costochondral grafts. J Oral Maxillofac Surg 1999;57:789–98.
[20] El-Labban NG, Harris M, Hopper HM, et al. Degenerative changes in masseter and temporalis muscles in limited mouth opening and TMJ ankylosis. J Oral Pathol Med 1990;19(9):423–5.
[21] Domarus H, Scheunemann H. Congenital prearticular temporomandibular ankylosis in two siblings. J Craniomaxillofac Surg 1990;18:299–303.
[22] Komorowska A. Congenital temporomandibular joint ankylosis: a case report. European Journal of Orthodontics 1997;19:243–8.
[23] Wittbjer J, Sarnas K, Rune B. Displacement of the mandible in a child with congenital unilateral temporomandibular joint ankylosis treated with two-stage condylar replacement: a long-term study with the aid of roentgen stereometric analysis. Cleft Palate Craniofac J 2001;38:636–44.
[24] Nwoku A, Kekere-Ekun TA. Congenital ankylosis of the mandible: report of a case noted at birth. J Maxillofac Surg 1986;14:150–2.
[25] Guilhem P, Cadenat E. Etiology of so-called congenital temporomandibular joint ankylosis. Oral Surg 1955; 8:449.
[26] Costello BJ, Shand JM, Ruiz RL. Craniofacial and orthognathic surgery in the growing patient. Selected Readings in Oral and Maxillofacial Surgery 2003;11(5).
[27] Guyuron B, Lasa C. Unpredictable growth pattern of costochondral graft. Plast Reconstr Surg 1992;90: 880–6.
[28] James DR, Irvine GH. Autogenous rib grafts in maxillofacial surgery. J Craniomaxillofac Surg 1983;11: 201–3.
[29] Proffit WR, Vig KW, Turvey TA. Early fracture of the mandibular condyles: frequently an unsuspected cause of growth disturbances. Am J Orthod 1980;78:1–24.
[30] Peltomaki T, Vahatalo K, Ronning O. The effect of unilateral costochondral graft on the growth of the marmoset mandible. J Oral Maxillofac Surg 2002;60: 1307–14.
[31] Ross RB. Costochondral grafts replacing the mandibular condyle. Cleft Palate Craniofac J 1999;36:334–9.
[32] Stucki-McCormick SU. Reconstruction of the mandibular condyle using transport distraction osteogenesis. J Craniofac Surg 1997;8(1):48–53.
[33] Stucki-McCormick SU, Fox RM, Mizrahi RD. Reconstruction of a neocondyle using transport distraction osteogenesis. Semin Orthod 1999;5:59–63.
[34] Papageorge MB, Apostolidis C. Simultaneous mandibular distraction and arthroplasty in a patient with temporomandibular joint ankylosis and mandibular hypoplasia. J Oral Maxillofac Surg 1999;57(3): 328–33.
[35] Hikiji H, Takato T, Matsumoto S, et al. Experimental study of reconstruction of the temporomandibular joint using a bone transport technique. J Oral Maxillofac Surg 2000;58(11):1270–7.
[36] Costello BJ, Ruiz RL. The role of distraction osteogenesis in orthognathic surgery of the cleft patient. Selected Readings in Oral and Maxillofacial Surgery 2001;10(3):1–27.

Dealing with the Effects of Juvenile Rheumatoid Arthritis in Growing Children

Brett A. Ueeck, DMD, MD*, Nina A. Mahmud, BS, Robert W.T. Myall, BDS, FRCD, FDS, MD

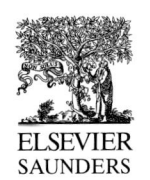

Oral and Maxillofacial Surgery, Oregon Health and Science University, 611 SW Campus Drive, Portland, OR 97239, USA

Juvenile rheumatoid arthritis (JRA) affects an estimated 250,000 children in the United States and constitutes one of the five most common classes of chronic illness in childhood [1]. The diagnosis is clinical and is defined as swelling or limitation of motion of a joint accompanied by heat, pain, or tenderness for at least 6 weeks duration with other identifiable causes of arthritis excluded. JRA is characterized by unpredictable flairs during which children may experience an abrupt exacerbation of symptoms, including joint swelling, pain, and limitation of function [2].

The effects of JRA on growth are multifactorial and include not only the disease itself but also side effects of medications, altered nutrition, and mechanical problems [3]. Local growth disturbances occur because of inflammation, and the accompanying increase in vascularity may result in over- or undergrowth of the affected site. In the maxillofacial region, micrognathia and malocclusion are common sequelae. In addition to changes in vascularization, growth can be disturbed owing to the destruction of a growth center or site, as seen in micrognathia.

Several subtypes of JRA exist. The order of frequency is as follows: pauciarticular, 50% to 60%; polyarticular, 30% to 35%; and systemic onset disease, 10% to 20% [2,4]. These subtypes are recognized based on the clinical features observed during the first 6 months of the disease process. A child is deemed to have pauciarticular JRA if fewer than five joints are involved during the first 6 months of the disease. Polyarticular JRA affects more than five joints. Children with systemic onset disease typically have 2 weeks of high spiking fever, classically with two peaks daily. During these episodes, fevers and chills are common and the child appears ill; however, when the fever breaks, the child appears well (Fig. 1). There is also an attendant evanescent rash. In addition to growth retardation, delayed puberty is a common occurrence in JRA [2].

Examination of children and adolescents with JRA needs to be undertaken in a particular fashion dependent on their age. In infants and toddlers, one uses observational skills, whereas school age children are likely to participate actively in the examination. In adolescents, the degree of chronic discomfort and disability caused by the disease can make relating with this age group difficult. The surgeon must overcome this difficulty before committing to a definitive plan of care. Once a relationship is established, the patient will be clearly elated and grateful postoperatively (Figs. 2 and 3).

The objectives when treating JRA include controlling pain and inflammation, preserving function, and promoting normal growth and overall development. During the past few years, remarkable advances have been made with the advent of disease modifying antirheumatic agents (DMARDS) and biologic therapy. Control of the disease is of utmost importance when planning surgery. Destruction of the mandibular condylar growth sites must be arrested before embarking on surgical orthodontic treatment. Approximately 50% of children show remission of the disease after 5 to 10 years. The

* Corresponding author.
E-mail address: ueeckb@ohsu.edu (B.A. Ueeck).

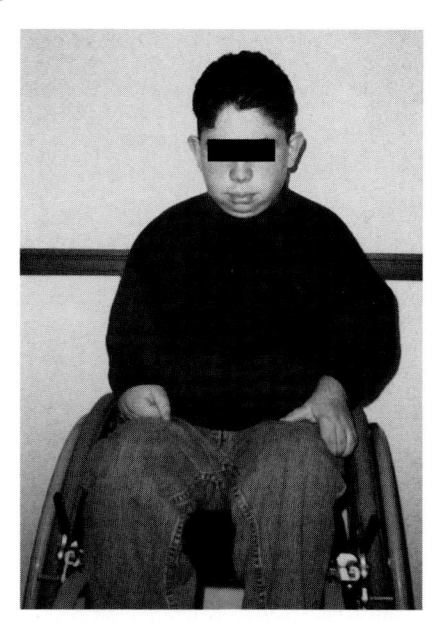

Fig. 1. A wheel chair–dependent patient with severe systemic onset JRA. Note the moon face and flushing from prolonged steroid use.

prognosis is most favorable for children with the pauciarticular form [5].

Growth and development

The most important growth center of the mandible is located in the head of the condyle. Early destruction of its fibrocartilage cap can seriously affect mandibular development and growth. Asymmetry between the two condyles is a common finding in JRA, especially at the onset of disease [6]. As the disease progresses, radiographic lesions are found in approximately 60% of children. There is a higher instance in children with polyarticular onset when compared with those with pauciarticular or systemic onset [7,8]. The most common radiographic signs of arthritis of the temporomandibular joint are erosion and flattening of the condyle. These changes range from small erosions on the superior bony surface to almost complete absence of the condylar head (Fig. 4). Changes seemingly affect the condylar head more frequently then the temporomandibular fossa. Reduction of the joint space, anterior displacement of the condyle in the fossa, osteophyte formation, subcondylar cysts, and restricted translatory movements have been described [9]. MRI scans show arthritic changes earlier than conventional radiographic techniques, leading to the suspicion that the percentage of temporomandibular joint involvement in JRA is probably underestimated. That modality should be used early and more frequently in groups in which temporomandibular joint involvement seems most likely [6,10].

There are several effects of JRA on the growth and development of the facial skeleton. The relationship between the condylar ramus height expressed as the condylar ratio is significantly smaller in this group of children than in unaffected children with class I or class II malocclusion. The maxilla tends to be smaller in vertical dimensions and is rotated posteriorly. This effect occurs as a reaction to the decreased growth of the mandible or an altered loading on the posterior regions of the maxilla. When there is

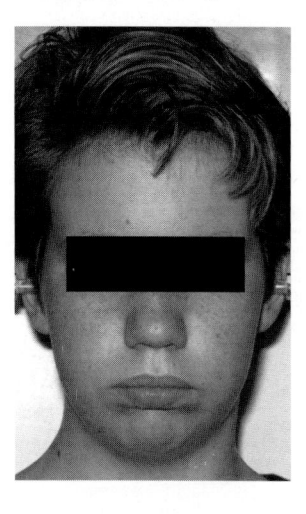

Fig. 2. Patient with JRA shown preoperatively. Note patient's deviantly unhappy appearance.

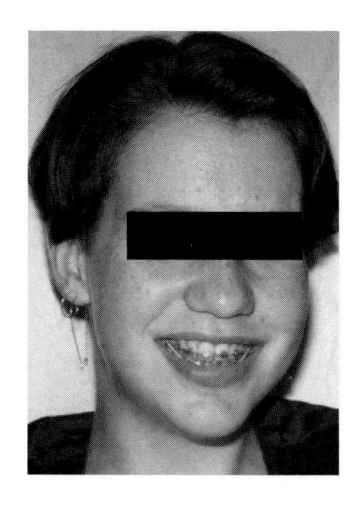

Fig. 3. Same patient in Fig. 2 postoperatively showing a glowing appearance. The patient's mother described how her daughter went from a recluse to a "social butterfly."

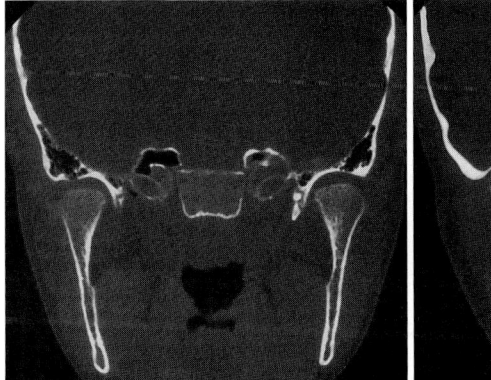

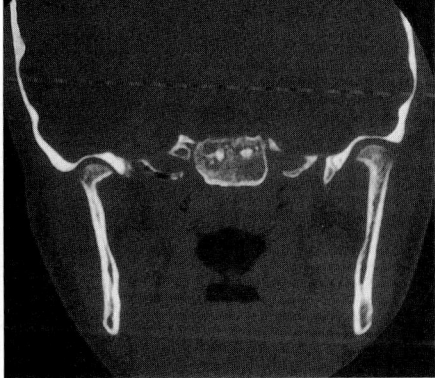

Fig. 4. A comparison of normal condyle heads with those affected by JRA. Note the cortication on the articular surfaces of the affected condyles, suggesting that the disease is quiescent.

unilateral condylar destruction, asymmetry develops with the chin deviating to the affected side. It also results in a shorter vertical dimension on the affected side [5].

A higher degree of mandibular retroposition and smaller mandibular dimensions are found in children with complete destruction of the head of the condyle when compared with those with partial destruction. Solow and Kreiborg [11] have suggested that the lack of forward growth of the mandible initiates an increased extension of the head in relation to the cervical column to maintain an adequate airway (Fig. 5). They propose that this results in soft-tissue stretching that also has a restraining effect on facial development [12]. The earlier onset, long duration, and degree of severity of the disease are directly correlated to the temporomandibular joint abnormality. Nevertheless, Stabrun and coworkers [13] found reduced mandibular growth in affected children without visible condylar lesions. It is likely that early inflammatory changes that caused no conventional radiographic changes occurred in the jaw joints of these children. This finding further underlines the need to consider the use of MRI when jaw growth lags [5].

Other soft-tissue structures that are impacted by this disease process are the muscles of mastication. Maximum molar bite force is reduced in children with JRA to about 60% of that recorded in healthy children. This reduction, in turn, might influence the craniofacial morphology during growth [5].

The effect of therapy on the temporomandibular joints has been investigated by several researchers. Ince and coworkers noted that methotrexate therapy was effective in minimizing temporomandibular joint destruction and craniofacial dysmorphology in a group of patients with the polyarticular form of the disease [3]. Pedersen noted that the inflammatory activity could be controlled by intra-articular steroid injections, but no controlled studies of this procedure to the temporomandibular joint have been performed in growing children [8]. Such therapy will be an important modality if inflammation can be detected and treated early, avoiding destruction of the joint and the ensuing effects on the growth of the mandible. Pedersen has noted that, because the temporomandibular joint is histologically different from other joints in regards to its embryology, bone formation, maturation, growth, type of cartilage, and loading, it is difficult to transpose the experience of intra-articular injections in other joints to the temporomandibular joints. The use of intra-articular steroids in joints other than the temporomandibular joint in children with pauciarticular JRA is an accepted

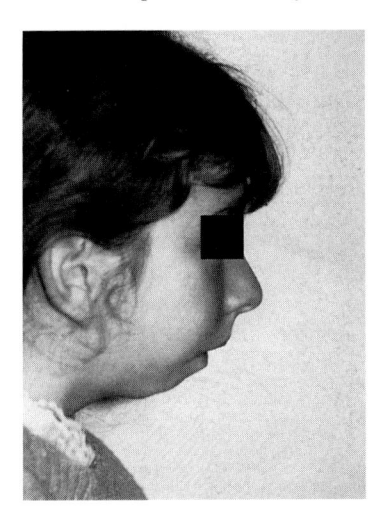

Fig. 5. Patient adopting the "sniffing" position to facilitate breathing.

therapeutic option. In recent survey, the use of these injections was second only to nonsteroidal anti-inflammatory drugs (NSAIDs) in the treatment of pauciarticular JRA. These steroids quickly reduce inflammation, and the effect can last for up to a year. Apparently, the steroids reduce the inflammation and pannus without deleteriously affecting the hyaline cartilage. Petersen noted that functional appliances were helpful to reduce the load on the joint during active arthritis, minimizing the detrimental effect of the disease. The corollary to such use is that, if much of the condyle is already destroyed, subsequent abnormal growth is already present, and simple orthopedic principles cannot be used [8,14].

Wenneberg and coworkers [15] performed an 8-year study on the effects of intra-articular injection of steroids into the temporomandibular joint on the subjective and clinical dysfunction and radiographic appearance in 16 patients. Suggestive symptoms and clinical signs were significantly reduced at follow-up examinations. Erosions of the bony articular margins that could be seen on standard radiographic techniques were found to be remineralized and associated with bony remodeling. These results suggest that the long prognosis of intra-articular steroid injections is beneficial and that such therapy radiographically demonstrates an improvement rather than an adverse effect.

Anesthesia

Children with JRA have several problems that can challenge the anesthetist; therefore, a preoperative evaluation is mandatory. Restricted neck movement owing to fused vertebrae, unstable cervical vertebrae,

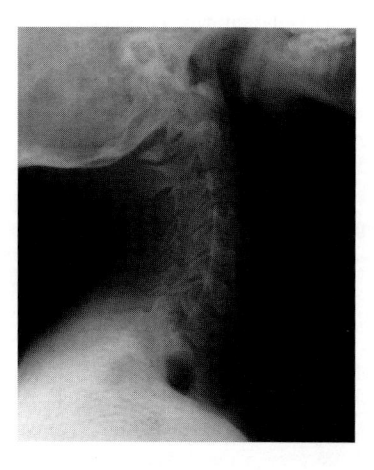

Fig. 6. Extension radiographic view of the cervical spine.

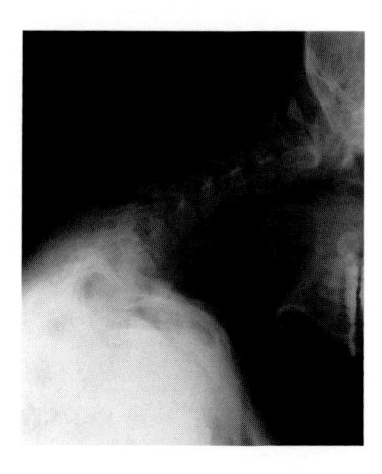

Fig. 7. Flexion radiographic view of the cervical spine.

laxity at the atlantoaxial joint, minimal mouth opening, and micrognathia make intubation a special challenge. Extension and flexion radiographs of the cervical spine have a useful role in preoperative assessment (Figs. 6 and 7). In patients in whom some instability of the spine at the atlantoaxial joint is suspected, the use of intraoperative sand bags or similar means to support the neck and cranium is recommended. At the preoperative visit, the anesthetist should also evaluate the more global problems found in children with JRA, such as pericarditis, pluritis, anemia, and the side effects of medications they might be taking. The comfort of the patient on the table must be addressed. Pads, rolled towels, sand bags, and other stabilizing materials can prevent overrotation of the neck, overextension of the deformed joints, and neurovascular compression. Not all anesthetists will realize that the jaw lengthening will facilitate early extubation postoperatively, and this factor should be discussed early on. If, after conferring, the anesthetist and surgeon have doubts about the propriety of extubation, the child can be left intubated overnight in the intensive care unit [16–18].

Surgical technique

As is true for any facial deformity, congenital or acquired, the application of surgical technique requires a thorough understanding of each of the deformities. Every aspect must be appreciated separately as well as on the whole to predict what can be accomplished successfully. Often, the focus is narrowed to simply the skeleton; however, the joints and soft tissues need equal consideration. Furthermore, the systemic, variable, and chronic nature of JRA can add to the difficulty in predicting the outcome and stability of surgery.

Mandible

The facial deformity associated with JRA has been described as a "bird face." The deformity involves the entire mandible in form and size and the associated soft tissues. The cranial base and dentition are secondarily affected. Overall, these defects are appreciated as a short posterior facial height and a short corpus length. A retruded chin position, steep mandibular plane angle, and antegonial notching are common. The deformity progresses with age, and the continued clockwise rotation around the first and second molar results in further steepness of the mandibular plane and resulting apertognathia with increased anterior lower facial height. As a result, the musculature is shortened and hypotonic and the facial soft tissues hypoplastic (Figs. 8 and 9).

Surgery to correct the mandibular micrognathia involves lengthening the mandible with standard osteotomies with or without the aid of distraction, or the use of costochondral grafts to replace the arthritic condyle to allow for renewed growth potential. Sagittal split osteotomy for use in JRA was first described by Turpin and West [19] in 1978. They described a case in which an 11-year-old girl was treated successfully and have since published a 14-year follow-up discussing the outcome. The technique was reasonably stable over time for this patient and, most importantly, was stable through her teenage years and psychosocial development [20]. Since that report, others have employed the sagittal split osteotomy successfully in the treatment of

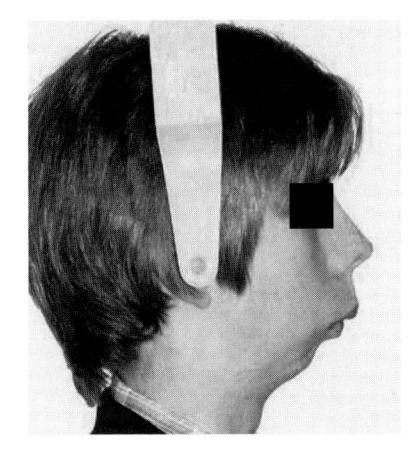

Fig. 8. Typical patient with "bird face" deformity.

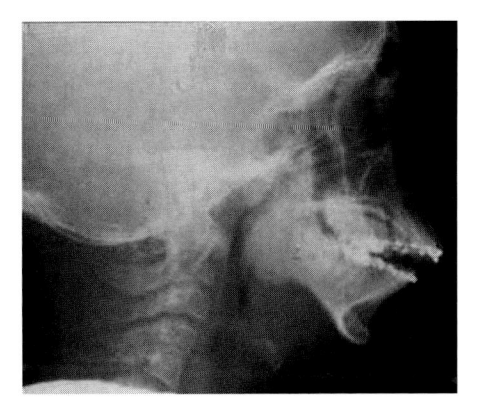

Fig. 9. Lateral cephalometric film of patient.

patients with JRA. The goal of the operation includes increasing vertical and horizontal length of the mandible. A counterclockwise rotation of the mandible is often needed to correct the mandibular plane angle and anterior open bite. The authors recommend the use of rigid internal fixation for this technique.

Inverted L-osteotomies with bone grafting can also be used to correct the mandible deformity. This technique allows for large movements, increasing posterior facial height and closing the open bite. The drawback of this osteotomy is the resulting facial scar and the need for a donor site. Unfortunately, there has been little documentation of this technique in patients with JRA in the literature.

Genioplasty is required in nearly all patients and can include osteotomy techniques or augmentation with alloplastic materials, although alloplastic materials often lead to the appearance of relapse as they resorb into the mandible. In the patient in whom there is lack of angle show, augmentation with alloplastic material may be beneficial. These implants can be custom made or preformed. The decision to place the implants at the time of the sagittal split or secondarily is made according to surgeon and patient preference.

Costochondral grafting is performed in an attempt to correct the deformity by allowing a new growth center to provide a mature mandibular length. This technique entails resecting the involved condyle and insetting a costochondral graft. As in costochondral grafts for hemifacial microsomia, it is critical to include the correct amount of cartilage cap in the graft to allow for growth. This amount can be difficult to predict as demonstrated in a case series by Svensson and Adell [21]. Under- and overgrowth is a problem, as is asymmetric growth as a result of the two grafts growing at differing rates and amounts.

The use of distraction techniques has been reported when lengthening the vertical and horizontal mandibular rami. Advocates of distraction promote the concept of "histiogenesis," claiming that soft as well as hard tissues are treated. Nevertheless, there have been reports of condylar resorption with the use of distractors [22,23]. The use of distraction for JRA has not been studied and is not advocated as an accepted technique for these patients.

Maxilla

The decision to perform maxillary surgery depends on the effect the mandibular deformity has had on the maxilla. There may be little to no deformity of the maxilla, because the maxilla is not affected by JRA primarily. Addressing the mandible early may obviate the need for maxillary surgery; however, if vertical maxillary growth has occurred and excess has resulted, surgery to reduce this effect should be considered. Intrusion of the maxilla, reducing the middle facial height, is the method most commonly employed.

The timing of surgery in relation to the growth of the child is largely a preference of the surgeon, and the decision is made by conferring with the family. The question as to when growth is complete is one of semantics, because, often, the destruction of the condylar growth center occurs before the child has truly stopped growing. Surgical intervention enjoys success regardless [24,25]. It is the preference of the authors to wait until the second molars have erupted before intervening surgically.

Overall, several conventional techniques have been employed successfully in the treatment of patients with JRA; however, there are no randomized clinical trials and limited long-term data to guide technique selection. The difficulty comes in reconciling the deformity, the disease process, the growth status of the patient, and the planned surgical technique. Keeping in mind the differences between a child who has JRA and one who does not will place the issues of the elaborate preoperative assessment, the choice of surgical technique, the outcome, and the stability of surgery in perspective.

Summary

JRA is a chronic childhood disease associated with multiple effects on the growth and development of the facial skeleton as well as the possibility of severe systemic issues. These patients present with a unique subset of skeletal facial deformities and surgical-orthodontic cases. A solid understanding of the disease in general and of the intricacies of therapy is necessary for successful surgical-orthodontic care.

References

[1] Sandstrom MJ, Schanberg LE. Peer rejection, social behavior, and psychological adjustment in children with juvenile rheumatic disease. J Pediatr Psychol 2004;29(1):29–34.

[2] Weiss JE, Ilowite NT. Juvenile idiopathic arthritis. Pediatr Clin North Am 2005;52(2):413–42.

[3] Ince DO, Ince A, Moore TL. Effect of methotrexate on the temporomandibular joint and facial morphology in juvenile rheumatoid arthritis patients. Am J Orthod Dentofacial Orthop 2000;118(1):75–83.

[4] Bakke M, Zak M, Jensen BL, et al. Orofacial pain, jaw function, and temporomandibular disorders in women with a history of juvenile chronic arthritis or persistent juvenile chronic arthritis. Oral Surg Oral Med Oral Pathol Oral Radiol Endod 2001;92(4):406–14.

[5] Kjellberg H. Craniofacial growth in juvenile chronic arthritis. Acta Odontol Scand 1998;56(6):360–5.

[6] Kuseler A, Pedersen TK, Gelineck J, et al. A 2-year follow-up study of enhanced magnetic resonance imaging and clinical examination of the temporomandibular joint in children with juvenile idiopathic arthritis. J Rheumatol 2005;32(1):162–9.

[7] Karhulahti T, Ylijoki H, Ronning O. Mandibular condyle lesions related to age at onset and subtypes of juvenile rheumatoid arthritis in 15-year-old children. Scand J Dent Res 1993;101(5):332–8.

[8] Pedersen TK. Clinical aspects of orthodontic treatment for children with juvenile chronic arthritis. Acta Odontol Scand 1998;56(6):366–8.

[9] Pedersen TK, Jensen JJ, Melsen B, et al. Resorption of the temporomandibular condylar bone according to subtypes of juvenile chronic arthritis. J Rheumatol 2001;28(9):2109–15.

[10] Kuseler A, Pedersen TK, Herlin T, et al. Contrast enhanced magnetic resonance imaging as a method to diagnose early inflammatory changes in the temporomandibular joint in children with juvenile chronic arthritis. J Rheumatol 1998;25(7):1406–12.

[11] Solow B, Kreiborg S. Soft-tissue stretching: a possible control factor in craniofacial morphogenesis. Scand J Dent Res 1977;85(6):505–7.

[12] Peltomaki T, Ronning O. Interrelationship between size and tissue-separating potential of costochondral transplants. Eur J Orthod 1991;13(6):459–65.

[13] Stabrun AE, Larheim TA, Hoyeraal HM, et al. Reduced mandibular dimensions and asymmetry in juvenile rheumatoid arthritis: pathogenetic factors. Arthritis Rheum 1988;31(5):602–11.

[14] Sherry DD, Stein LD, Reed AM, et al. Prevention of leg length discrepancy in young children with pauciarticular juvenile rheumatoid arthritis by treatment with

intra-articular steroids. Arthritis Rheum 1999;42(11): 2330–4.
[15] Wenneberg B, Kopp S, Grondahl HG. Long-term effect of intra-articular injections of a glucocorticosteroid into the TMJ: a clinical and radiographic 8-year follow-up. J Craniomandib Disord 1991;5(1):11–8.
[16] Kohjitani A, Miyawaki T, Kasuya K, et al. Anesthetic management for advanced rheumatoid arthritis patients with acquired micrognathia undergoing temporomandibular joint replacement. J Oral Maxillofac Surg 2002;60(5):559–66.
[17] Skues MA, Welchew EA. Anaesthesia and rheumatoid arthritis. Anaesthesia 1993;48(11):989–97.
[18] Smith BL. Anaesthesia and Still's disease [letter]. Anaesthesia 1985;40(2):209.
[19] Turpin DL, West RA. Juvenile rheumatoid arthritis: a case report of surgical/orthodontic treatment. Am J Orthod 1978;73(3):312–20.
[20] Turpin DL. Juvenile rheumatoid arthritis: a 14-year posttreatment evaluation. Angle Orthod 1989;59(3): 233–8.
[21] Svensson B, Adell R. Costochondral grafts to replace mandibular condyles in juvenile chronic arthritis patients: long-term effects on facial growth. J Craniomaxillofac Surg 1998;26(5):275–85.
[22] Azumi Y, Sugawara J, Takahashi I, et al. Positional and morphologic changes of the mandibular condyle after mandibular distraction osteogenesis in skeletal class II patients. World Journal of Orthodontics 2004; 5(1):32–9.
[23] Van Strijen PJ, Breuning KH, Becking AG, et al. Condylar resorption following distraction osteogenesis: a case report. J Oral Maxillofac Surg 2001;59(9): 1104–7 [discussion: 1107–8].
[24] Turvey TA, Simmons K. Orthognathic surgery before completion of growth. Oral and Maxillofacial Surgery in Children and Adolescents 1994;6(1):121–35.
[25] Wolford LM, Schendel SA, Epker BN. Surgical-orthodontic correction of mandibular deficiency in growing children (long-term treatment results). J Maxillofac Surg 1979;7(1):61–72.

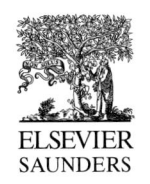

Mandibular Distraction Osteogenesis in Children

Ramon L. Ruiz, DMD, MD[a,*], Timothy A. Turvey, DDS[b], Bernard J. Costello, DMD, MD[c]

[a]*Division of Pediatric Craniofacial Surgery, Department of Oral/Maxillofacial Surgery, Southwest Florida Oral and Facial Surgery, Children's Hospital of Southwest Florida, 5285 Summerlin Road, Suite 101, Fort Myers, FL 33919, USA*
[b]*Department of Oral and Maxillofacial Surgery, University of North Carolina at Chapel Hill, Chapel Hill, NC, USA*
[c]*Division of Craniofacial and Cleft Surgery, Department of Oral and Maxillofacial Surgery, University of Pittsburgh, Pittsburgh, PA, USA*

The concept of distraction osteogenesis is not new. As early as 1905, Codvilla [1] described a limb-lengthening procedure using a plaster cast–retained device for the application of traction to healing long bones. In 1927, Abbott [2] performed similar procedures to produce gradual lengthening of the tibia and fibula following an osteotomy. Orthopedic surgeons interested in the lengthening of bones continued to refine these methods, but the modern era of distraction osteogenesis did not begin until the 1950s, when Ilizarov reported the use of an external fixator for gradual lengthening of long bones [3].

In 1973, the first published report applying distraction to the facial skeleton appeared when Snyder and colleagues [4] used an extraoral approach for lengthening of the canine mandible. Michieli and Miotti [5] also described lengthening of the mandibular body in canines but applied tooth-borne distraction devices and a transoral approach for the creation of the bone cuts. Although these early experiments involved animal subjects only, the authors suggested that distraction be applied in the human mandible and even described specific incisions, surgical approaches, mandibular body osteotomy design, and distractor constructs for use in humans. Later, Karp demonstrated how distraction techniques created new bone during mandibular lengthening in skeletally mature and growing animals [6].

The use of distraction osteogenesis for the lengthening of congenitally deficient mandibles in children with craniofacial microsomia was first described by McCarthy and coworkers in 1992 [7]. During the 13 years since that initial report, others have reported on the use of distraction techniques for the reconstruction of various maxillofacial problems [8,9].

Today, the use of distraction osteogenesis is considered a useful treatment option for the correction of specific facial skeletal deformities. Growing numbers of clinicians have advocated the use of distraction of the jaws through published reports that largely consist of isolated case reports or small case series. Although it is apparent that distraction may have significant potential and broader application in the management of maxillofacial problems, very few comprehensive scientific data exist, making it difficult to describe its exact role in the reconstructive oral and maxillofacial surgeon's armamentarium.

In this article, the biological basis for distraction osteogenesis, potential applications, and current surgical approaches are presented. Because the role of distraction for lengthening of the neonate mandible and correction of midfacial problems is presented elsewhere in this issue, the scope of the manuscript will be limited to the role of mandibular distraction in children. Our goal is to place the role of distraction within a context relative to established orthognathic surgical techniques.

Biological basis for distraction osteogenesis

The process of distraction osteogenesis involves the formation of new bony regenerate at the site of

* Corresponding author.
E-mail address: pedmaxillofacial@aol.com (R.L. Ruiz).

an osteotomy. This occurs when a controlled fracture (ie, osteotomy) is created and gradual, intentional forces are directed away from the fracture gap. The biological mechanisms of fracture healing are important for bone formation during distraction osteogenesis. When a fracture occurs, four distinct stages of bone healing may be observed: (1) inflammatory phase, (2) formation of a soft callus, (3) conversion of the soft callus into a hard callus, and (4) bony maturation and remodeling.

The first stage of bone repair involves the formation of a hematoma in the space between the bone segments. Histologically, an inflammatory cell infiltrate is seen as part of this initial response to the injury.

In the second stage of fracture healing, a malleable bony soft callus forms. During this period, cellular activity continues with the recruitment of fibroblasts and mesenchymal cells, and increased angiogenesis. The result is a soft fibrovascular structure (ie, soft callus) that bridges the fracture gap.

Next, mineralization of the soft callus forms a hard callus. This process takes approximately 2 weeks and results in an immature bony matrix composes of woven, poorly organized bone.

The final phase of bone repair consists of extensive remodeling of the young bony matrix. The hard callus is replaced by a mature segment of bone with the return of an organized lamellar structure.

Distraction osteogenesis is correlated with the specific histologic events seen in normal fracture healing. Essentially, the application of slow, controlled traction forces to the fractured bone ends gradually stretches and proliferates the soft callus while delaying complete calcification across the fracture gap. The technique is divided into three distinct clinical phases:

1. Latency phase: The latency phase is the time between performance of the osteotomy and activation of the device. This phase generally lasts 5 to 7 days and allows for the development of an adequate hematoma/granulation tissue plug within the distraction gap at the osteotomy site. The intervening granulation tissue exhibits activity of inflammatory cells, proliferation of fibroblasts that provide a collagen network, the development of vascular channels, and invasion of capillaries. The quality of this fibrovascular structure is influenced by the regional blood supply and overlying soft tissue and periosteum. Ideally, the latency phase must be long enough to permit formation of a good quality soft callus, but brief enough to prevent its mineralization into a hard callus that would prematurely consolidate the fracture site.

2. Activation phase: The active phase is the period when application of traction to the bone segments produces actual bone lengthening. Active distraction occurs with a specified rhythm and rate. In the maxillofacial skeleton, the distraction appliance is activated a total distance of 1 mm/d. Ideally, this is done during two to four intervals of 0.5 mm or 0.25 mm each, respectively. If distraction is too slow or is interrupted, calcification may cause premature consolidation of the bones before the desired length has been achieved. The regenerate (soft callus) continues to proliferate as long as an appropriate rate and rhythm are maintained. If distraction is too fast, then the soft, malleable regenerate may become overstretched with subsequent thinning or nonunion [11].

3. Consolidation phase: The consolidation phase is from the end of active distraction until the device is removed. During this phase, bony union between the osteotomized, separated segments is completed by calcification of the regenerate. Throughout this period, the distraction device acts as a fixation device. Total immobilization is necessary for calcification of the regenerate and the successful union of the distracted segments. Typically, a consolidation phase of 6 to 8 weeks is required following mandibular advancement. Although bony union is obtained at the conclusion of the consolidation phase, it is important to note that bony remodeling and maturation continue for up to 1 year following the initial surgical procedure.

Distraction osteogenesis is thought to capitalize more on membranous bone growth than endochondral bone growth. Cartilaginous components have been seen in some distraction regenerates, but the process is primarily membranous (ie, without cartilaginous intermediates). Developing collagen is oriented in the direction of the distraction forces, and the matrix is subsequently calcified by populations of osteoblasts that form along the collagen bundles. Immobilization allows for uninterrupted angiogenesis and callus formation.

Indications for mandibular distraction

General considerations

To *appropriately* apply distraction techniques for the correction of mandibular problems in children, the treating clinician must first understand what is possible using "conventional" orthodontic and surgical techniques. Proffit and White [11] previously described an "envelope of discrepancy" to illustrate the amount of three-dimensional change in tooth or skeletal position that can be introduced using various treatments. Specifically, in the growing patient, the amount of correction possible depends on whether the treatment involves orthodontic tooth movement alone, orthodontic tooth movement in combination with growth modification techniques, or orthodontic tooth movement and orthognathic surgery. It is important to note that the exact limits for each treatment modality may be influenced by factors including the patient's age, regional blood supply, existing scar tissue, and the quality of the overlying soft tissue envelope. Where exactly distraction osteogenesis techniques belong within the spectrum of these treatment modalities remains an important question. We know that facial deformities are frequently the result of conditions characterized by undergrowth or overgrowth of the involved skeletal components (ie, maxilla, mandible). Because distraction is a technique that results in the lengthening of bone, its applications are limited to conditions characterized by deficient growth (eg, class II discrepancies, retrognathia, and so forth).

Currently, the indications and limitations of conventional orthognathic surgical techniques are well understood. In addition, a large body of published data has provided practitioners with important insights about the long-term stability of surgical–orthodontic treatment [12]. It is well-known that mandibular ramus osteotomies (ie, bilateral sagittal split osteotomies or inverted "L") for mandibular advancements up to 10 mm in length are among the most stable orthognathic maneuvers used in the correction of dentofacial deformity. As the degree of mandibular advancement exceeds 10 mm, the predictability and long-term stability decreases. From the perspective of being able to predictably achieve those larger movements and the degree of long-term skeletal stability, the potential roles for orthognathic procedures and mandibular distraction become increasingly clear.

As contemporary orthognathic surgery has evolved, a central principle has been the meticulous control of skeletal movements, which allows for the precise correction of occlusal discrepancies and facial dysmorphology. The standard approach now involves coordinated phases of care with presurgical orthodontic preparation to eliminate dental compensations, the surgical procedures themselves, and postsurgical orthodontic detailing. In fact, the achievable surgical movements are so specifically measured that that preoperative "model surgery" is done using dental casts of the maxilla and mandible so that the three-dimensional position of the corrected jaw segment can be planned and performed with extreme precision. This information is then transferred to the patient through the use of model tables, articulators, and acrylic surgical splints [13]. With the current technology, the most serious unresolved problem associated with maxillofacial distraction is the inability to achieve equally precise movements. Most available distraction appliances allow for only unidirectional (lengthening) movements, making it difficult to address a complex malformation. Although multidirectional distraction devices are being developed, most require a more bulky external assembly attached to the mandible using pins. For now, the lack of precise three-dimensional control limits the use of the distraction technique to clinical situations where the occlusal correction is not the primary goal or where the patient/parents are willing to accept the likely need for a secondary orthognathic surgical procedure later for normalization of the occlusion.

As distraction techniques have been described, significant consideration has been given to the effects of distraction on the surrounding soft tissue structures. The rate of distraction is critical to the adaptation of any tissue at the distraction site [10]. For example, nerve tissue generally does not tolerate distraction rates greater than 1 or 2 mm/d, and inferior alveolar nerve function can be significantly compromised at higher distraction rates [14,15]. More research is required to establish the effects of the localized inflammation of the peripheral tissues associated with distraction osteogenesis. A number of authors have used the term *distraction histiogenesis* to describe the creation of soft tissue volume at the same time that bone lengthening is occurring via distraction [16]. Unfortunately, this promising advantage of distraction osteogenesis has not yet been documented convincingly by clinical studies, and there is no documentation of volumetric increases in soft tissue as a result of distraction. Despite this, there is often significant benefit to the gradual lengthening of the soft tissues. This is especially true when large skeletal advancements are performed and a high degree of soft tissue pull must be overcome. In cases where limited soft tissue envelope exists or there is extensive scarring, distraction may help achieve the desired skeletal advancement. It is likely that soft tissues such as skin, subcutaneous connective tissue, muscle, nerves, and blood vessels simply adapt to the tensile stress in a manner similar to what occurs with a tissue expander, rather than by actually generating new tissue around the distraction site.

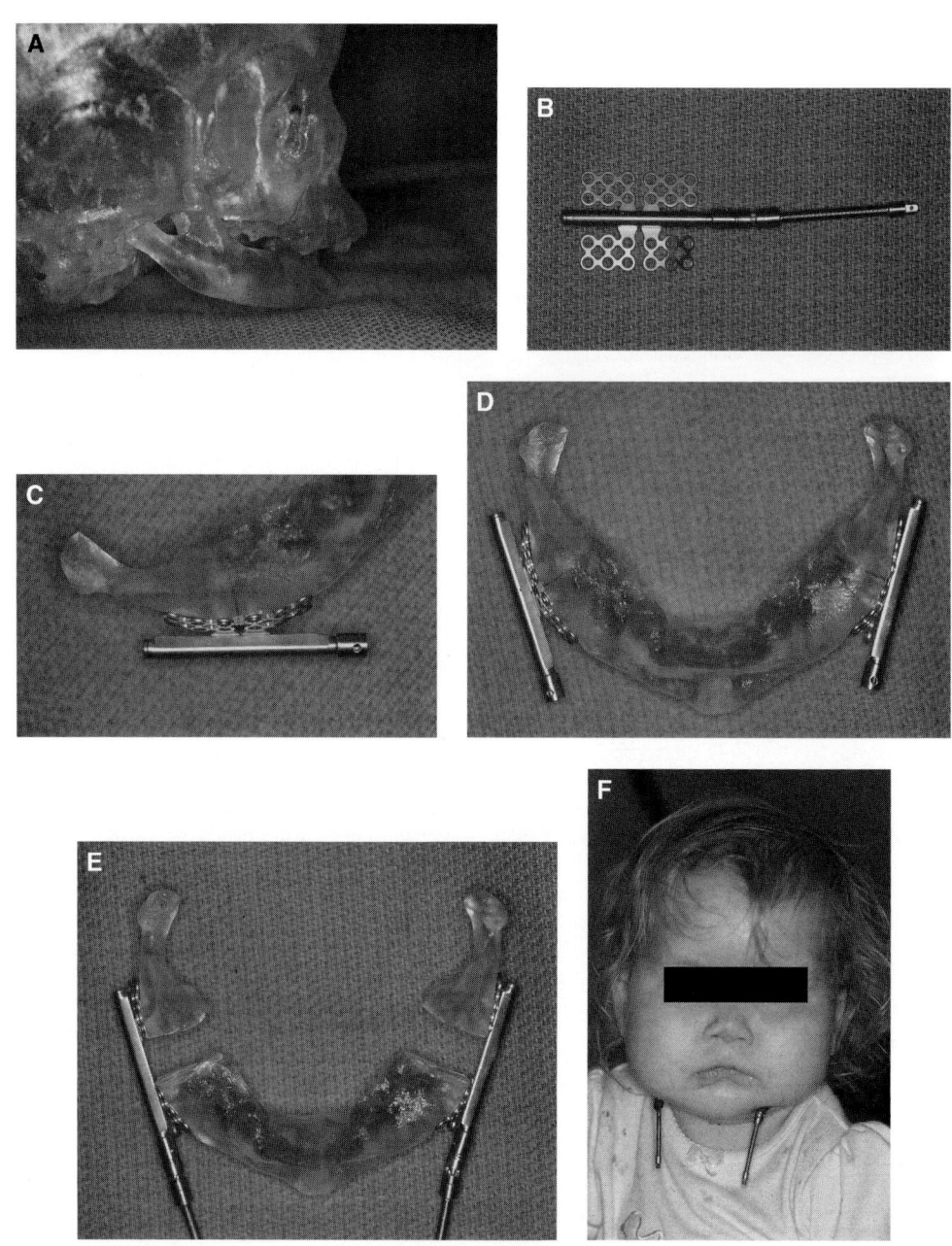

Fig. 1. Bilateral mandibular distraction in a 2½-year-old female child with a history of severe obstructive sleep apnea, upper airway obstruction, and persistent feeding difficulties requiring gastric feeding tube placement. (*A*) A stereolithographic model was fabricated for surgical planning and contouring of distraction appliances. Presurgical measurements revealed a severe class II discrepancy with approximately 14 mm of overjet. (*B*) Internal distraction device (KLS Martin Company, Jacksonville, Florida). (*C–E*) The device is contoured and applied to the mandibular model before the surgical procedure. In addition, the actual osteotomies are created on the stereolithographic model and the distractor is applied and activated. These maneuvers provide useful insights regarding potential interferences and the new morphology of the corrected/elongated mandible. (*F*) Patient with distractors in place during the activation phase of distraction treatment. Flexible activation arms are exposed through separate percutaneous sites. (*G, H*) Frontal and three-quarter view of patient during the consolidation phase. Note that the activation arms of the distraction appliances have been removed. (*I*) Intraoperative view of distraction appliance at the time of removal. Right and left distractors have been fully activated with appliance footplates 20 mm apart. (*J*) Intraoperative view of new bone within the distraction gap.

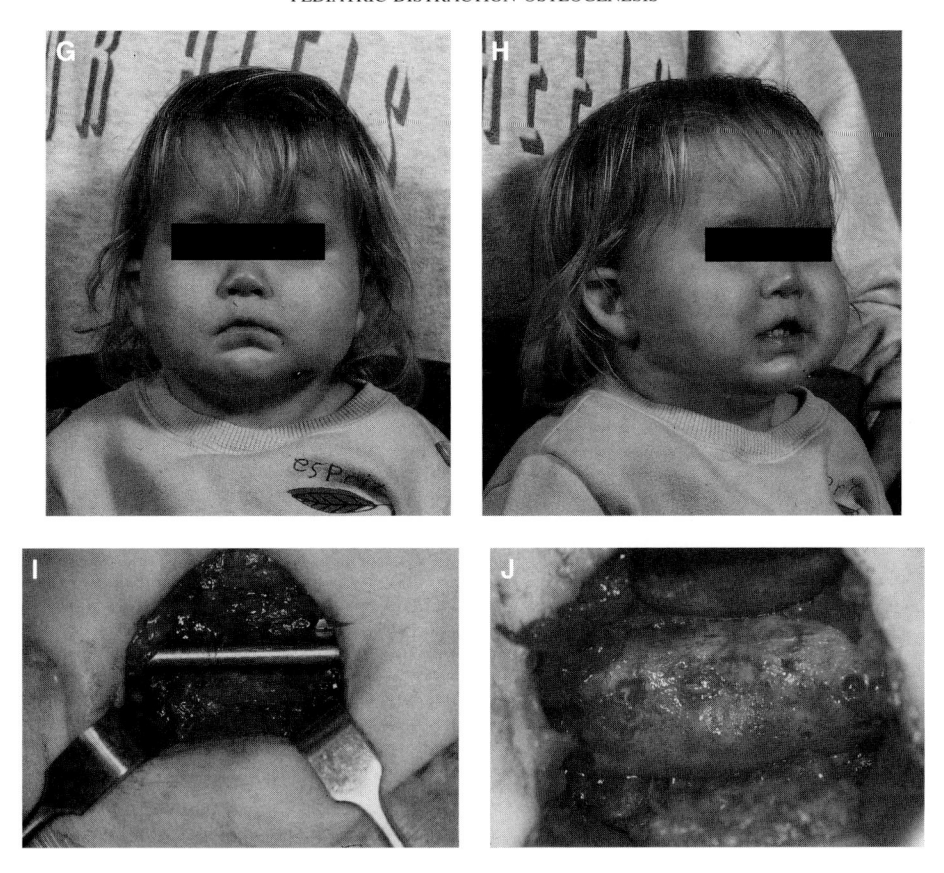

Fig. 1 (continued).

Finally, it is important to realize that when the distraction techniques are employed, many of the advantages of the conventional orthognathic approach are lost [17]. When mandibular surgery is undertaken using contemporary orthognathic techniques, precision movements and ideal results are typically achieved immediately in the operating room. Isolated mandibular advancements are usually completed in a short 60- to 90-minute procedure involving small transoral incisions that are closed with resorbable suture material, minimal blood loss, and a brief period of postsurgical observation. In many centers, patients undergoing isolated mandibular orthognathic surgical procedures are discharged home on the same day. With the advent of rigid internal fixation devices, maxillomandibular fixation is not routinely used and patients may return to a normal diet and activity level at 6 weeks. Although orthognathic surgery patients are followed closely following surgery and remain on a limited diet, the postoperative course is typically straightforward and requires limited cooperation from the patient or family. In contrast, most distraction procedures using internal devices require broader surgical excess for placement of a semiburied apparatus. In cases where external devices are used, the necessary surgical access my be less extensive, but the patient must tolerate an external distraction assembly that may be cumbersome and prone to trauma or dislodgement. The postsurgical regimen is more complicated and patients require daily device activation of the device and subsequent procedures for removal of distraction hardware. These are important practical considerations, especially in when applying distraction techniques in young children.

For children with facial skeletal deformities, it is obvious that the most appropriate applications of mandibular distraction techniques are those clinical situations where the desired skeletal change cannot be attained with conventional treatment modalities, including orthodontic treatment, growth modification, and orthognathic surgical procedures. Presently, the specific indications for mandibular distraction are all related to cases of severe deficiencies of mandibular length or width.

Mandibular hypoplasia/micrognathia

Mandibular hypoplasia is the most commonly encountered dentofacial deformity in the United States. [11] Severe mandibular deficiency may be an isolated, nonsyndromic finding or a morphologic component of some underlying craniofacial condition (eg, Pierre Robin Sequence, Treacher Collins Syndrome, Nager Syndrome, and so forth). Functional consequences of severe mandibular hypoplasia include acute and chronic upper airway obstruction, obstructive sleep apnea, speech difficulties, and impaired feeding. In the long term, affected children may suffer failure to thrive, adverse cardiopulmonary changes (eg, pulmonary hypertension, right-sided heart failure), and death.

Although surgery for early mandibular advancement is a viable option in the management of infants and children who have severe micrognathia, it is rarely the first-line treatment modality. This is because most patients with congenital, nonsyndromic micrognathia will undergo substantial catch-up growth early in the postnatal period, which obviates the need for any surgical intervention. Similarly, patients born with isolated Pierre Robin Sequence (ie, no specific syndrome) frequently demonstrate substantial catch-up growth early in life and outgrow their airway difficulties [18,19]. In these patients, all of the morphologic components of the mandible are present at birth, but these parts are deficient in size. The likely explanation is that the mandibular structure and surrounding soft tissue matrix are capable of significant growth and that the original etiology was at least partially related to some intra-uterine deformation. Interestingly, the amount of growth that patients with congenital mandibular deficiency (eg, Pierre Robin Sequence) demonstrate early in life frequently gets them out of trouble in terms of airway difficulties, but the total magnitude of that "catch-up" growth in the long term is often not enough to eliminate the need for comprehensive orthodontics and orthognathic surgery later in life to normalize their facial profile and occlusion.

When infants and children present with severe deficiency of the mandible that is associated with functional (airway, speech, feeding) consequences, the use of distraction osteogenesis for early mandibular advancement may be appropriate (Fig. 1) [20,21]. Distraction is reserved for severe cases where nonsurgical means (ie, positioning, nasopharyngeal airway) have failed and tracheostomy is required. Although some surgeons advocate the use of distraction to avoid tracheostomy, we believe that tracheostomy, when indicated, remains the gold standard for airway control in the acute period. Once the airway is secure, distraction osteogenesis can be used to lengthen the mandible, improve the upper airway space, and facilitate early decannulation.

In infants and very young children (<6 years), distraction osteogenesis techniques have allowed surgeons to carry out mandibular advancement procedures that were previously difficult if not impossible. In children older than 6 years of age, both distraction osteogenesis and conventional osteotomy techniques may be viable options with the specific treatment choice largely based on the magnitude of the necessary advancement and other factors such as the mandibular morphology, bone quality, soft tissue envelope, and developing dentition.

Irrespective of the type of procedure used, the effect of early surgical intervention on subsequent growth and the effect of growth on the initial surgical result must be considered as part of the long-term treatment plan for the patient. Because most children with disproportionate growth preoperatively will maintain disproportionate growth postoperatively, it is unrealistic to suggest that one surgical procedure performed early in life will definitively correct maxillomandibular proportions and occlusion. The reality is that early mandibular advancement is typically undertaken to address some serious underlying functional problem (ie, airway, feeding, speech) and not for definitive occlusal treatment. Similarly, early surgery may also be indicated in cases where no functional problem is present, but the affected child is suffering adverse psychosocial consequences from a facial deformity. In these cases, the biological interests (ie, growth) must be weighed against the psychosocial benefits of early surgery. Decisions to treat children before skeletal maturity must include an open discussion with the family so that parents understand that additional, definitive corrective surgery will likely be required once growth is complete.

In patients who have severe mandibular deficiency and an underlying syndromic diagnosis (eg, Treacher Collins syndrome), the use of distraction osteogenesis for elongation of the mandible has been frequently reported [22]. Early decannulation of the tracheostomy is often a realistic objective if the mandible can be successfully lengthened. Before early mandibular advancement is undertaken, a detailed evaluation of the entire airway is mandatory. Children with craniofacial syndromes frequently demonstrate airway obstruction at various levels. If a complex airway obstruction with anomalies at multiple levels goes unrecognized and distraction is performed to lengthen the mandible, the child will remain tracheostomy-dependent. It must also be realized that successful early mandibular advancement during early childhood does not eliminate the need for definitive orthognathic surgical reconstruction when the child is at or near skeletal maturity.

Distraction techniques may also be of significant value in the management of acquired (eg, posttraumatic, postablative) mandibular deformities. Simultaneous release of the bony ankylosis and application of a distraction appliance for correction of the mandibular deformity has been reported [23]. Our preferred approach involves the completion of a mandibular osteotomy with application of the distraction appliance during an initial procedure and then release of the bony ankylosis performed during a second surgical stage. Delaying the surgical release of the ankylosis allows for improved anchorage of the distraction device and avoids reciprocal displacement of the ramus (proximal) segment during the mandibular lengthening phase (Fig. 2).

Craniofacial microsomia

The application of distraction osteogenesis for correction of the skeletal facial deformity associated with craniofacial microsomia remains a topic of interest among reconstructive surgeons [7,20,24,25]. Despite multiple published reports, there is little consensus regarding which patients would most

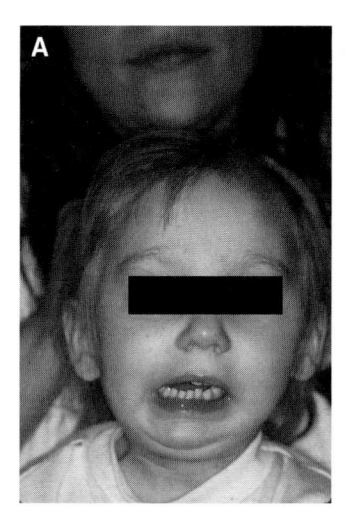

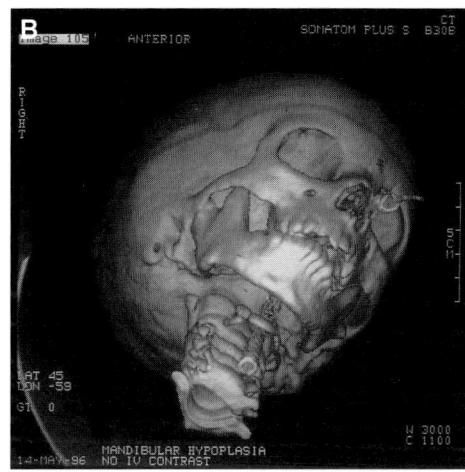

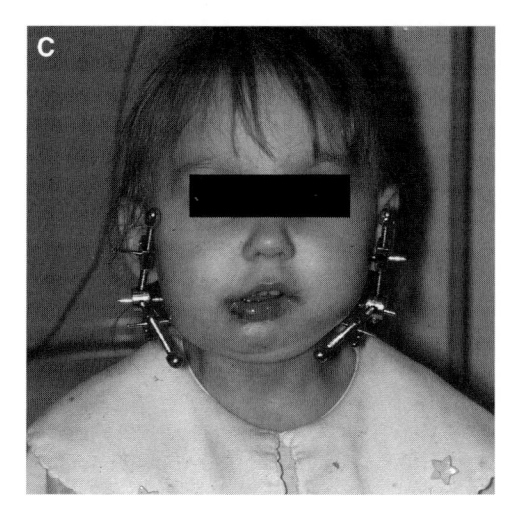

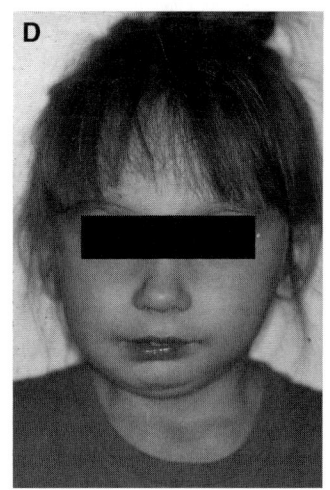

Fig. 2. A 3-year-old child with right-sided temporomandibular ankylosis and severe growth restriction of the mandible. The patient suffered from upper airway obstruction with severe obstructive sleep apnea. (*A*) Preoperative view with inability to open mouth and mandibular deficiency. (*B*) Preoperative three-dimensional CT scan. (*C*) Patient with bilateral external distractors in place. (*D*, *E*) Frontal and profile views of patient 20 months following distraction of mandible and release of TMJ ankylosis.

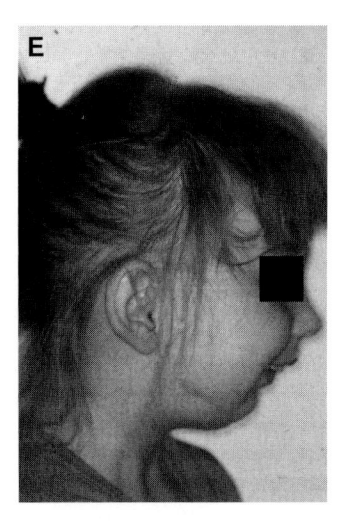

Fig. 2 (*continued*).

benefit from this treatment approach and few long-term data to suggest any improvement in overall treatment outcomes.

The reconstructive approach for the maxillomandibular complex in patients who have craniofacial microsomia varies depending on the severity of the skeletal dysmorphology. In patients with type I and IIA (Kaban modification of Pruzansky Classification System) [26] mandibular deformities, early treatment is typically limited to growth surveillance and an initial phase of orthodontic treatment with growth modification. These children will benefit from definitive correction consisting of orthodontic treatment and bimaxillary surgery later in life as they reach or near skeletal maturity. There is little role for early surgery in patients with mild (Type I and IIA) deformities.

In patients with more pronounced hypoplasia of the condyle-ramus complex (type IIB), an initial phase of reconstructive surgery is undertaken during childhood (age 5–8 yr). Traditionally, this has consisted of an inverted "L" type osteotomy of the affected ramus with bone grafting to allow for lengthening of the affected side. More recently, the use of distraction techniques for this purpose has shown promise. The purpose of this early surgical procedure includes lengthening of the affected condyle-ramus complex, concomitant stretching of the soft tissue envelope (including whatever components of the pterygomassateric sling are present), and the creation of a posterior open bite on the affected side [27]. This unilateral open bite is maintained using an occlusal splint or bite-block and then gradually eliminated over the 6 to 9 months following the surgical procedure. This is done in an effort to facilitate downward growth and development of the maxillary dentoalveolar structures on the affected side with leveling of the occlusal plane. If this is done successfully, there is a possibility that the need for additional maxillary (Le Fort I) osteotomy later in life will be eliminated. Sometimes, the degree of condyle-ramus hypoplasia seen in type IIB patients is so se-

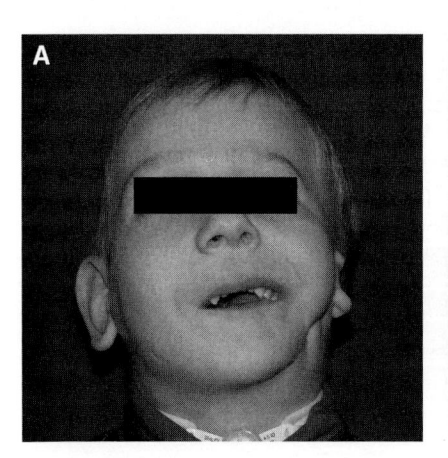

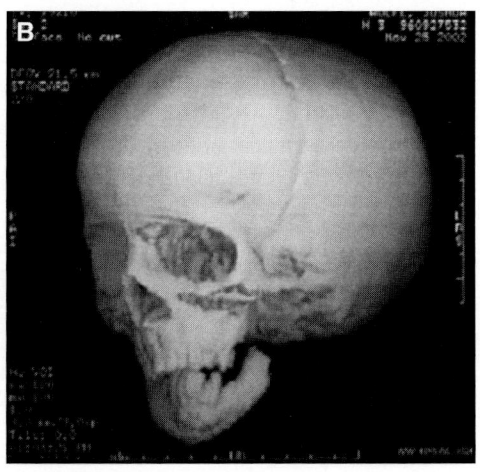

Fig. 3. A 7-year-old child with Kaban type III left sided mandibular deformity. The patient underwent previous bilateral mandibular distraction procedures (performed by another surgeon) in an attempt to create a condyle from the bone of the left mandibular body. (*A*) Facial view demonstrates persistent lower facial asymmetry with deviation of the chin toward the left, lack of posterior facial height on the affected side, and soft tissue hypoplasia. (*B*) Three-dimensional CT scan view demonstrates type III deformity with absence of the condyle-ramus complex on the affected side.

vere that the temporomandibular joint is not functionally viable and consideration is given to joint reconstruction using a costochondral graft [28]. However, if the joint structures present are dysmorphic, but functional, then we prefer maintaining the working joint and carrying out the initial phase of reconstruction at the level of the ramus. Definitive orthognathic surgery is then performed later in life as the child approaches skeletal maturity.

In their current state, distraction osteogenesis techniques have little place in the treatment of the most severe (type III) mandibular deformities associated with craniofacial microsomia. Patients who have type III deformities are congenitally missing the entire ramus-condyle complex. An initial phase of surgical treatment is undertaken at 5 to 8 years of age using of a costochondral graft. The benefits of this reconstructive step include the construction of missing anatomic components, stretching of the soft tissue envelope, favorable repositioning of the mandible to improve facial symmetry, and the creation of a posterior open bite to facilitate maxillary dentoalveolar development. Although some have advocated for the use of distraction to create a "neocondyle" from the posterior aspect of the mandibular body, no evidence exists to support this maneuver as a responsible reconstructive alternative. Although distraction is useful in the lengthening of bones, it is not possible to distract a congenitally missing skeletal component into existence (Fig. 3). In a search for other potential surgical applications for this new technique, some centers have even proposed the use of distraction to lengthen previously placed costochondral grafts. The logic of this thinking is difficult to follow. Most of the published data related to the use of distraction for elongation of the constructed condyle-ramus complex (rib graft) indicates that it is associated with a number of serious complications including fracture, graft resorption and devitalization, and fibrous nonunion [29–31]. Overall complication rates range from 30% to more than 60%, with no evidence to suggest that postgraft distraction improves outcomes in any meaningful way. It is even more difficult to understand the motivation for such treatment when one considers the fact that these children will still go on to require definitive orthognathic surgery as they near skeletal maturity.

Summary

Contemporary orthognathic procedures have well-defined, known applications and known limitations.

Although interest in techniques for maxillofacial distraction osteogenesis has increased over the course of the past decade, the exact role of these procedures in dento-facial surgery remains unclear. For the foreseeable future, it seems that the use of distraction is most appropriate in cases where an ideal result is not achievable using conventional techniques. If distraction is to occupy a more prominent role in the oral and maxillofacial surgeon's armamentarium, then its current limitations must be overcome in the form of multidirectional device designs, technical refinements related to surgical placement, and improved distraction protocols. In the meantime, surgeons must critically evaluate each potential indication and surgical outcome so that distraction is not treated as a new procedure "in search of applications."

References

[1] Codvilla A. On the means of lengthening in the lower limbs, the muscles, and tissues, which are shortened through deformity. Am J Orthop Surg 1905;2:353.

[2] Abbott LC. The operative lengthening of tibia and fibula. J Bone Joint Surg 1927;9:128.

[3] Ilizarov GA. The tension-stress effect on the genesis and growth of tissues. I. The influence of stability of fixation and soft tissue preservation. Clin Orthop 1989; 238:249–80.

[4] Snyder CC, Levine GA, Swanson HM, et al. Mandibular lengthening by gradual distraction. Plast Reconstr Surg 1973;51:506–8.

[5] Michieli S, Miotti B. Lengthening of mandibular body by gradual surgical-orthodontic distraction. Oral Surg 1977;35:187–92.

[6] Karp NS, Thorne CHM, McCarthy JG, et al. The lengthening of the craniofacial skeleton. Ann Plast Surg 1990;24:231–6.

[7] McCarthy JG, Schreiber JS, Karp NS, et al. Lengthening of the mandible by gradual distraction. Plast Reconstr Surg 1992;89:1–10.

[8] Rachmiel A, Levy M, Laufer D. Lengthening of the mandible by distraction osteogenesis: a report of cases. J Oral Maxillofac Surg 1995;53:838–46.

[9] Molina F, Ortiz-Monasterio F. Mandibular elongation and remodeling by distraction: a farewell to major osteotomies. Plast Reconstr Surg 1995;96:825–40.

[10] Ilizarov GA. The tension-stress effect on the genesis and growth of tissues: II. The influence of the rate and frequency of distraction. Clin Orthop 1989;239:163.

[11] Proffit WR, White RP. Dentofacial problems: prevalence and treatment needed. In: Proffit WR, White RP, Sarver DM, editors. Contemporary treatment of dentofacial deformity. Philadelphia: Mosby; 2003. p. 2–28.

[12] Proffit WR, Turvey TA, Phillips C. Orthognathic surgery: a hierarchy of stability. Int J Adult Orthod Orthogn Surg 1996;11:191–204.

[13] Ruiz RL, Blakey GH. Model surgery for orthognathic procedures. In: Betts N, Turvey TA, editors. Fonseca oral and maxillofacial surgery. Philadelphia: WB Saunders; 2000. p. 98–107.

[14] Hu J, Tanz Z, Wang D, et al. Changes in the inferior alveolar nerve after mandibular lengthening with differential rates of distraction. J Oral Maxillofac Surg 2001;59:1041.

[15] Huang SC, Chang CW. Electrophysiological evaluation of neuromuscular function during limb lengthening by callus distraction. J Formos Med Assoc 1997; 96:172.

[16] Cope JB, Samchukov ML, Cherkashin AM. Distraction histiogenesis. In: Samachukov ML, Cope JB, Cherkashin AM, editors. Craniofacial distraction osteogenesis. St. Louis (MO): Mosby; 2001. p. 73–128.

[17] Posnick JC, Ruiz RL. Secondary orofacial cleft deformities. In: Goldwyn RM, Cohen MN, editors. The unfavorable result in plastic surgery: avoidance and treatment. Philadelphia: Lippincott; 2001. p. 349–58.

[18] Pruzansky S. Not all dwarfed mandibles are alike. Birth Defects 1969;5:120.

[19] Pruzansky S, Richmond JB. Growth of the mandible in infants with micrognathia. Am J Dis Child 1954;88:29.

[20] Shand JM, Smith KS, Heggie AA. The role of distraction osteogenesis in the management of craniofacial syndromes. Oral Maxillofac Surg Clin N Am 2004;16:525–40.

[21] Leighton S, Drake AF. Airway considerations in craniofacial patients. Oral Maxillofac Surg Clin N Am 2004;16:555–66.

[22] Posnick JC, Ruiz RL. Treacher Collins syndrome: current evaluation, treatment, and future directions. Cleft Palate Craniof J 2000;37:1–22.

[23] Rao K, Kumar S, Kumar V, et al. The role of simultaneous gap arthroplasty and distraction osteogenesis in the management of temporomandibular joint ankylosis with mandibular deformity in children. J Craniomaxillofac Surg 2004;321:38–42.

[24] Mommerts MY, Nagy K. Is early osteodistraction a solution for the ascending ramus compartment in hemifacial microsomia? A literature study. J Craniomaxillofac Surg 2002;30:201–7.

[25] Polley JW, Figueroa AA. Distraction osteogenesis: its application in severe mandibular deformities in hemifacial microsomia. J Craniofac Surg 1997;8:422–30.

[26] Kaban LB, Mulliken JB, Murray JE. Three-dimensional approach to analysis and treatment of hemifacial microsomia. Cleft Palate J 1981;18:90–9.

[27] Proffit WR, Turvey TA. Dentofacial asymmetry. In: Proffit WR, White RP, Sarver DM, editors. Contemporary treatment of dentofacial deformity. Philadelphia: Mosby; 2003. p. 574–645.

[28] Kaban LB. Congenital abnormalities of the temporomandibular joint. In: Kaban LB, Troulis M, editors. Pediatric oral and maxillofacial surgery. Philadelphia: WB Saunders; 2004. p. 302–39.

[29] Corcoran J, Hubli EH, Sayler KE. Distraction osteogenesis of costochondral neomandibles: a clinical experience. Plast Reconstr Surg 2002;100:311–5.

[30] Eppley BL. Distraction lengthening of the mandibular costochondral graft: a precautionary note. J Craniofac Surg 2000;11:350–3.

[31] Sellnicki E, Hollier L, Le C, et al. Distraction osteogenesis of costochondral bone grafts in the mandible. Plast Reconstr Surg 2002;109:925–33.

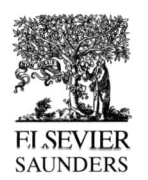

Distraction Osteogenesis of the Midface

George K.B. Sándor, MD, DDS, PhD, Dr Habil, FRCDC, FRCSC, FACS[a,b,c,d,e,f],*,
Leena P. Ylikontiola, DDS, PhD[e,f,g], Willy Serlo, MD, PhD[g,h],
Robert P. Carmichael, DMD, MSc, FRCDC[a,b,c,d],
Iain A. Nish, DDS, MSc, FRCDC[a,b,i],
John Daskalogiannakis, DDS, MSc, FRCDC[a,b,c]

[a]*University of Toronto, Toronto, Ontario, Canada*
[b]*The Hospital for Sick Children S-525, 555 University Avenue, Toronto, Ontario, Canada M5G 1X8*
[c]*Bloorview MacMillan Children's Centre, 170 Kilgour Road, Toronto, Ontario, Canada M4G 1R8*
[d]*Department of Oral and Maxillofacial Surgery, Mount Sinai Hospital, Toronto, Ontario, Canada*
[e]*Department of Oral and Maxillofacial Surgery, University of Oulu, Oulu, Finland*
[f]*Institute of Dentistry, University of Oulu, Box 5281 FIN-90014, Finland*
[g]*Oulu University Hospital, Box 23, FIN-90029 Oulu, Finland*
[h]*Department of Pediatric Surgery, University of Turku, Turku, Finland*
[i]*Lakeridge Medical Centre, Oshawa, Ontario, Canada*

The field of pediatric oral and maxillofacial surgery is continuing to evolve and is in a dynamic phase as our understanding of growth and development of the craniomaxillofacial complex expands. Bone regeneration and tissue engineering technologies have been developed to treat skeletal defects with reduced morbidity [1]. Distraction osteogenesis recently emerged as a technique that by its very nature allows changes to the vectors of growth and results in the genesis of new tissues [2]. It is a rapidly developing area with applications in the area of pediatric oral and maxillofacial surgery.

Distraction osteogenesis is a biologic process that promotes bone formation between cut osseous surfaces that are gradually separated by incremental traction [3]. This process is initiated when forces are applied to separate the segments and continues as long as the tissues of the callus that forms between the segments are stretched. Bone formation occurs parallel to the direction or vector of distraction. This process also initiates histiogenesis of the tissues surrounding the distracted bone: cartilage, ligaments, muscle, blood vessels, gingiva, and nerve tissue [2,4,5].

History of midfacial distraction osteogenesis

Distraction osteogenesis as it applies to the midface is not a new concept. Dentists have used techniques that involve the application of tensile and compressive forces to the bones of the craniomaxillofacial skeleton for almost 300 years. According to Balaji [6], Fauchard described the use of an expansion arch as early as 1728, a custom-made metallic arch applied to the crowded maxillary dentition, to widen the arches to a more physiologic form. Wescott attempted to correct a crossbite by placing two double clasps on the maxillary bicuspid teeth and a telescopic bar to apply transverse force [6]. Similarly, Angell [7] expanded a maxillary arch by using a transverse jackscrew and clasps on the bicuspid teeth.

* Corresponding author. The Hospital for Sick Children S-525, 555 University Avenue, Toronto, Ontario, Canada M5G 1X8.

E-mail address: george.sandor@utoronto.ca (G.K.B. Sándor).

Goddard is credited with standardization of the palatal expansion protocol with activation twice daily for 3 weeks followed by a period of stabilization [8]. Modern clinical distraction osteogenesis of the facial bones developed quickly once McCarthy applied the concept to mandibular lengthening in 1992 [9]. This development led to an explosion of clinical and research activity in the field of craniomaxillofacial distraction osteogenesis over the past decade [10].

Distracting tubular long bones

The mechanical manipulation of bone segments dates as far back as Hippocrates, who described the use of external devices to apply traction to bone [11,12]. Codivilla [13] is credited with using an external skeletal traction apparatus after performing an oblique femoral osteotomy to accomplish the first lower extremity lengthening. The Siberian surgeon Gavril Ilizarov was the first to describe a tissue-sparing osteotomy and reliable distraction protocol that involved the long bones of the lower extremity in 1951 [11].

Ilizarov's protocol was unique and involved a 5- to 7-day latency period after the osteotomy. This critical rest period was followed with a period of distraction applied at a rate of 1 mm per day using four incremental distractions of 0.25 mm. The most critical aspect of the technique described by Ilizarov was maximal preservation of endosteum and periosteum using a procedure he termed "corticotomy." He described a method in which he divided two thirds of the cortical bone of the femur with a narrow osteotome and finally separated the bony segments from each other by rotational osteoclasis [3]. The gradual application of traction resulted in the tension-stress effect that can stimulate the genesis, regeneration, and active growth of living tissues as long as there is an adequate blood supply [4,11,12].

Distraction osteogenesis involves five distinct periods: osteotomy, latency, distraction, consolidation, and remodeling [3,4,11,12]. Osteotomy is the surgical separation of an intact bone into two segments. It results in a loss of continuity and mechanical integrity, which triggers the process of fracture healing. A reparative callus begins to form within and around the ends of the fractured bone segments.

Latency is the period during distraction osteogenesis that begins with osteotomy of the bone segments and ends with the onset of traction. Latency permits sufficient time to elapse for a callus to form between the osteotomized bone segments [3,4].

Distraction is the period during which traction is applied to the bony segments when new bone or, more precisely, a distraction regenerate is formed within the gap between the bony segments. Two parameters can be used to tailor the distraction process: rate and frequency. Gradual traction of the soft callus disrupts fracture healing, and the tensional stress stimulates changes at the cellular and subcellular levels [2–5]. These changes include increased proliferation of fibroblasts with an altered phenotypic expression that secrete collagen fibers parallel to the vector of distraction. Bone formation begins at the termini of the bony segments and progresses toward the center of the distraction gap [3].

Consolidation begins after termination of traction [11,12]. Consolidation permits mineralization and eventual corticalization of the newly formed bone in the distraction regenerate and must be substantially complete before removal of the distraction device.

Remodeling begins at the onset of functional loading of the distracted bone. The initial bony scaffold is reinforced by parallel fibered lamellar bone. Gradually the cortical bone and marrow cavity are formed. Remodeling of Haversian systems is the last process to occur before development of completely normal bone at the site of distraction. The process of remodeling can take more than 1 year [11,12].

Distracting irregularly shaped membranous bones

Distraction osteogenesis can be applied to multiple sites in the midfacial skeleton in pediatric and adult populations. The application of the concepts described in limb lengthening and the distraction of tubular long (endochondral) bones, however, must be modified when applied to the irregularly shaped membranous bones of the midface [2]. Distraction osteogenesis can be used in several areas (Box 1), including the maxilla at the LeFort I, II, and III levels, the nasal and zygomatic bones, and the bones that comprise the cranium. Distraction osteogenesis can be applied to healed bone grafts in the craniomaxillofacial skeleton and to vertical and horizontal defects of the maxillary alveolus.

The devices required for distraction of each of these areas varies depending on the site and goals of treatment. Hardware may range from large external halo-like devices (Fig. 1) to much smaller appliances that resemble bone fixation plates (Fig. 2) to jackscrews that attach to the teeth (Fig. 3). The goals of treatment and the necessary vectors used in each of

Box 1. Midfacial distraction device classification

External: bone-borne
Internal: subcutaneous
Intraoral
- Extramucosal
    Tooth-borne
- Submucosal
    Bone-borne
    Hybrid
Classification according to distraction direction
Unidirectional
Bidirectional
Multidirectional
Classification according to site of midfacial distraction
LeFort I, II, III
Nasal bones
Zygomatic bones
Healed bone grafts
Maxillary alveolus
- Transverse
- Vertical
- Horizontal

these regions are also distinct. The direction of distraction must be well planned. Certain devices allow distraction in more than one plane or vector (see Fig. 1). At times, two appliances may be used simultaneously; however, neither the devices themselves nor their vectors of distraction should be allowed to interfere with each other (Fig. 4).

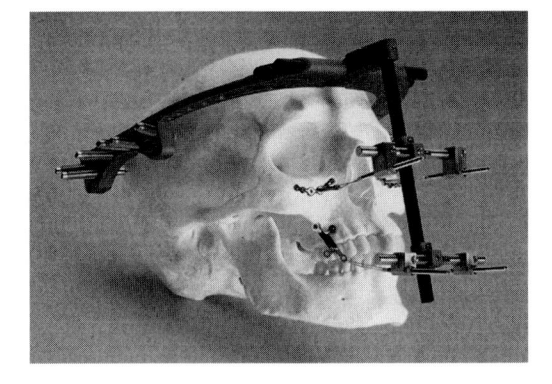

Fig. 1. A halo-like external frame device used to distract the retrusive midface (Biomet-Lorenz, Jacksonville, Florida). Such devices have become simple to apply, lightweight, and based on transcutaneous pin fixation to the skull. This device can be adapted to provide distraction vectors in more than one plane.

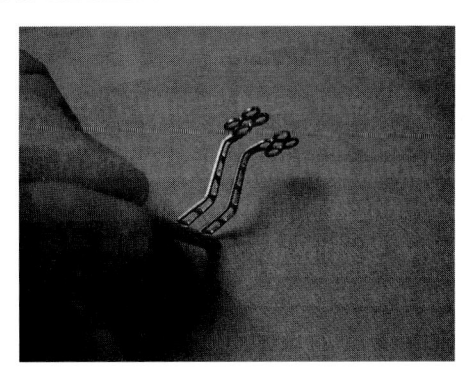

Fig. 2. Intraosseous devices configured like bone plates with a distractor rod between them are much smaller than their halo-like counterparts (KLS Martin, Jacksonville, Florida, USA).

Indications

Distraction osteogenesis is a labor-intensive and technique-sensitive treatment modality and should be reserved for specific indications. Distraction osteogenesis of the midface has two main advantages over traditional osteotomies. It can produce larger movements, and it may be associated with less relapse than traditional osteotomies. Distraction osteogenesis should be used for significant bony movements in the treatment of conditions known to have high relapse rates after traditional forms of treatment.

Distraction osteogenesis can be repeated at different phases of life. In some cases the application of a halo to the skull and a few simple titanium plates screwed into the bones of the craniomaxillofacial skeleton may be less invasive than certain osteo-

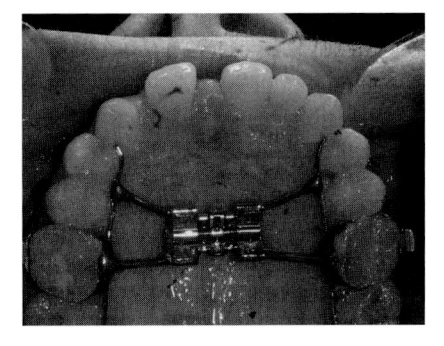

Fig. 3. Traditional tooth-borne palatal distractor. Note diastemma between maxillary central incisors, which is site of the palatal distraction osteogenesis. Same as Fig. 5.

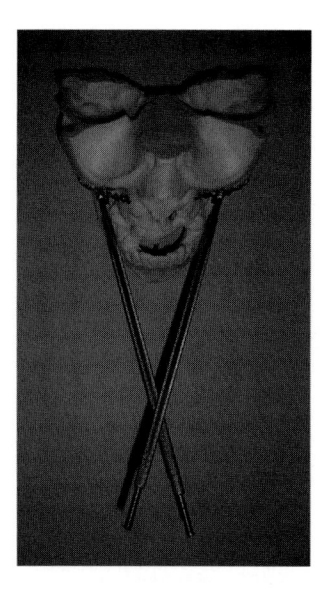

Fig. 4. Two devices are used to distract at the LeFort I level. The vectors of distraction of the devices must have minimal convergence so they do not interfere with each other (Synthes, Oberdorf, Switzerland).

tomies, and developing tooth roots can be avoided and left undamaged by the design of osteotomies.

Patients who have cleft lip and palate often require significant advancement of their midface at one or more LeFort levels. Maxillary advancement using traditional osteotomies may place these patients at risk for the development of velopharyngeal insufficiency [14,15]. It has been reported that this debilitating complication may be avoided for some of these patients if distraction osteogenesis is used to advance the maxilla [2,16], because it can leave the posterior dentition and velopharyngeal relationships undisturbed.

Distraction osteogenesis of the midface also may be applied to treat functional problems, such as obstructive sleep apnea and exposure keratitis and corneal scarring from proptosis [17–19].

Risks associated with midfacial distraction

The risks associated with distraction osteogenesis of the midfacial structures are similar to the risks encountered with traditional osteotomies. Careful preoperative planning of the vector of distraction is essential to ensure that the distracted segment advances fully in the desired direction without interference from surrounding bony structures or teeth.

Swennen and colleagues [10] reported complications in 828 patients undergoing craniomaxillofacial distraction. Complications included mechanical problems, such as pin loosening caused by accidental trauma, device failure, minor local infections, infections of the skin surrounding percutaneous pins, premature consolidation, limited skeletal advancement, asymmetric advancement, ankylosis of zygoma and coronoid process, severe infection, damage to teeth, and tooth mobility.

Distraction across the midpalatal suture

The age of the patient dictates the type of distraction that may be used to expand the maxilla. In growing children with a transverse deficiency of the maxilla and in whom the midpalatal suture has not yet fused, force analogous to physeal distraction used in orthopedics can be applied across the midpalatal suture [20]. Distraction of the midpalatal suture occurs in membranous bone across a suture, whereas physeal distraction is used in endochondral bones across an epiphyseal growth plate.

Rapid palatal expansion, also known as orthopedic rapid maxillary expansion, can be performed in girls before 15 years of age and in boys before 16 years of age [8]. If the palatal suture is fused then tipping of teeth occurs rather than transverse expansion of the maxilla [21].

Surgical widening of the maxilla must be used to correct transverse maxillary deficiency in patients with a fused midpalatal suture. This procedure has been termed surgically assisted rapid palatal expansion or surgically assisted maxillary expansion. Although it predates all other distraction osteogenesis procedures performed in the midface, it is often forgotten in the classification of midfacial distraction.

As with other distraction osteogenesis procedures, there are five distinct phases in surgical widening of the maxilla at the level of the midpalatal suture: osteotomy, latency, distraction, consolidation, and remodeling [3]. The osteotomy is performed at the LeFort I level and involves a variable combination of surgical separation of the midpalatal suture and osteotomy of the lateral and medial nasal walls, nasal septum, vomer, and pterygomaxillary junction [21–23]. The exact combination of osteotomies varies among authors [24–31]. The latency period is generally 1 to 2 days. Distraction is performed using a transverse jackscrew connected to attachments placed on the first molar and bicuspid teeth. Distraction is performed with a frequency of two increments of 0.5 mm per day (1 mm/d) until the maxilla has been widened sufficiently. The distraction device is kept in place for 3 months to allow for

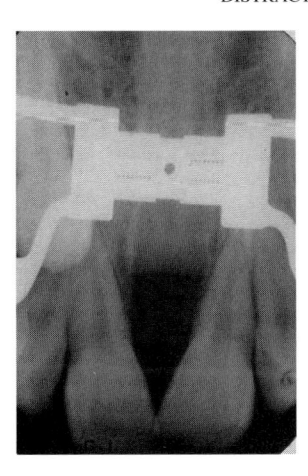

Fig. 5. Note intersegmentary bone formed in the maxillary midline after surgically assisted rapid palatal expansion on this occlusal radiograph. The device has been left on after the distraction phase to serve as a retainer during the consolidation phase.

consolidation. Active orthodontic treatment can resume during the remodeling phase.

The surgically assisted rapid palatal expansion or surgically assisted maxillary expansion procedure produces intersegmental bone (Fig. 5) and creates a stable widening of the maxillary arch, even when it is significantly constricted (Fig. 6A, B). As in other forms of distraction osteogenesis, distraction of the midpalatal suture permits a larger correction than nonsurgical orthodontic treatment could achieve.

Distraction strategies in cleft lip and palate

Distraction osteogenesis offers several advantages over conventional osteotomies in the treatment of patients who have cleft lip and palate. There is a reduced tendency for significant relapse after distraction of the maxilla than after traditional maxillary osteotomies. The soft tissue changes associated with maxillary advancement may be superior after distraction osteogenesis when compared with traditional LeFort I level advancement surgery [32]. It is also possible that deterioration of velopharyngeal function may be avoided in patients at risk for its development [2,14–16,33].

The midfacial deformities seen in patients who have cleft lip and palate include transverse maxillary deficiency, midfacial retrusion, and significant alveolar cleft defects. Transverse maxillary deficiency in a patient who has unilateral cleft lip and palate can be corrected with corticotomy and distraction in a modified procedure similar to the surgically assisted rapid palatal expansion or surgically assisted maxillary expansion technique.

Midfacial retrusion may be treated at the LeFort I, II, or III levels. LeFort I level distraction may involve advancement of segmentalized maxillary fragments or the entire maxilla [34,35]. Large alveolar cleft defects may be reduced in size using distraction osteogenesis to transport bone segments across the cleft [36]. Such a decrease in size of the cleft and associated oronasal fistula may enhance the outcome and predictability of bone grafting techniques [37].

Distraction hardware developed for anterior maxillary segmental advancement (Fig. 7A–E) has been used successfully in patients who have cleft lip and palate [38,39]. A stereolithic skull reconstructed from a three-dimensional CT scan can aid planning of such osteotomies by permitting preoperative selection and bending of plates, which reduce expenditures on distraction hardware and operating room time. Preoperative planning also ensures that a certain configuration and arrangement of the selected distraction hardware actually produce the vectors of distraction desired (Figs. 8–12).

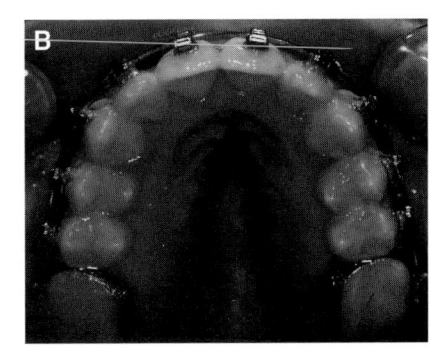

Fig. 6. (A, B) Constricted maxillary dental arch before and after surgically assisted rapid palatal expansion and orthodontic alignment.

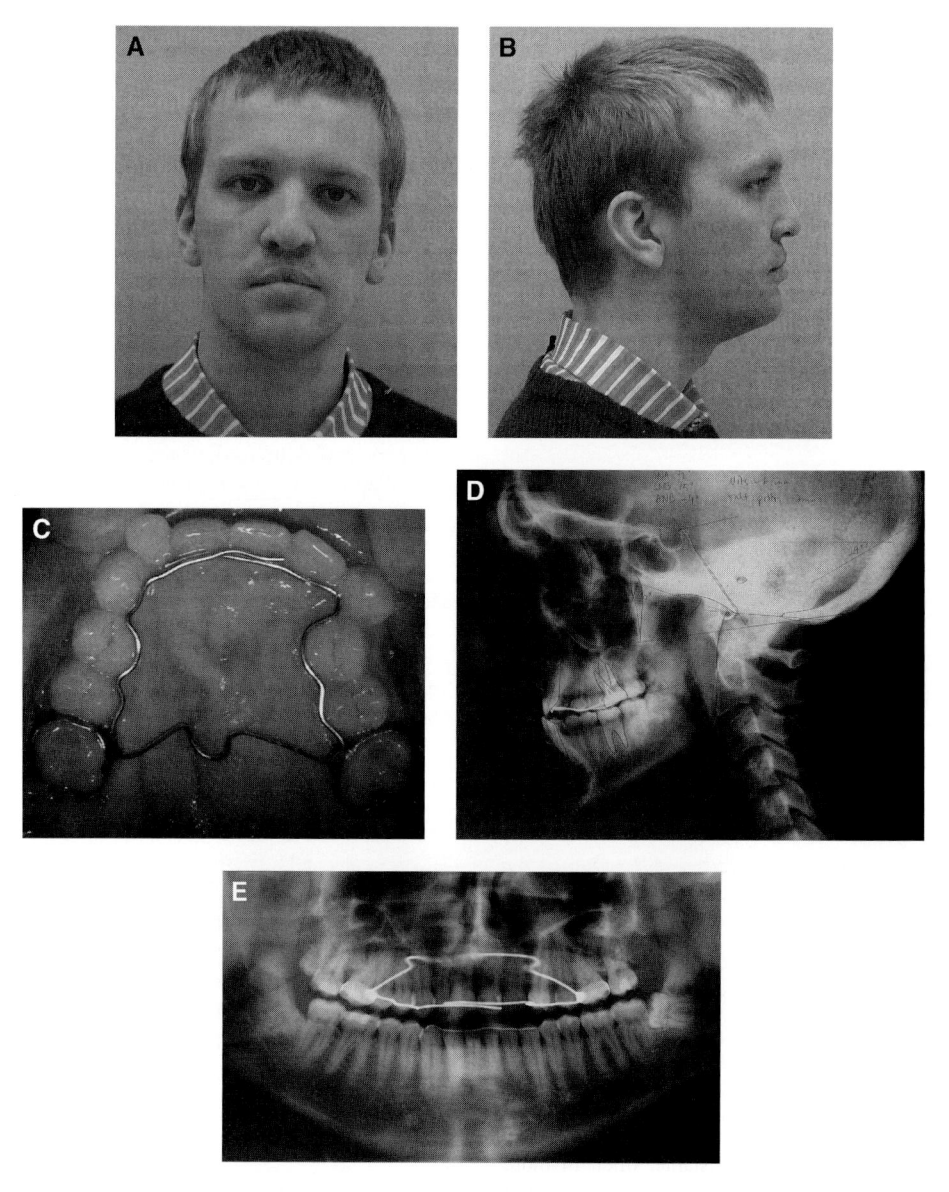

Fig. 7. Frontal (*A*) and lateral (*B*) view of 18-year-old man with bilateral cleft lip and palate and maxillary hypoplasia. (*C*) Extensive palatal scarring put the patient at risk for developing velopharyngeal insufficiency with traditional LeFort I maxillary advancement. Panoramic radiograph (*D*) and lateral cephalogram (*E*) of patient.

Distraction hardware also has been developed for LeFort I level osteotomies (Fig. 13A–C) in embodiments designed to be used submucosally and subcutaneously [40–42]. The selection of a specific device is determined by the goals of the distraction procedure, anatomic constraints, and the amount of room available to accommodate placement of the hardware. Care must be taken to avoid damaging the developing dental follicles or tooth roots when applying such devices to the lateral wall of the maxilla.

The initiation of midfacial distraction relative to creation of the corticotomy or osteotomy has been studied in growing sheep [43]. In primates, a protocol for immediate distraction that was composed of intraoperative device activation, 10 mm of acute distraction, and an additional 10 mm of distraction performed at a rate of 1 mm per day was compared with a protocol for delayed distraction that comprised a 5-day postoperative latency followed by a 20-mm distraction performed at a rate of 1 mm per day. There

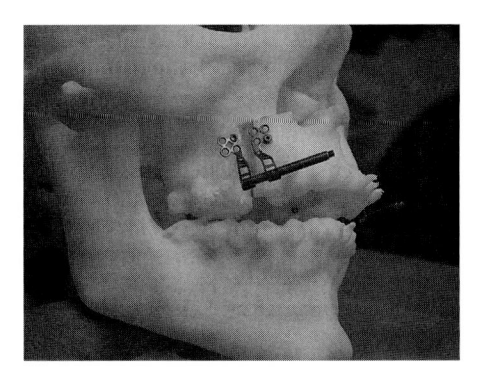

Fig. 8. Simulation of osteotomy, distractor placement, and advancement on stereolithic model.

was no evidence of relapse after immediate distraction or delayed distraction 6 months later. Neither were significant differences noted after either distraction protocol when the regenerated bone was examined histologically, ultrastructurally, or by dry skull analysis [44].

High level LeFort distraction osteogenesis

The treatment of patients with craniosynostotic syndromes (eg, Crouzon [Fig. 14A–D], Apert, Pfeiffer, and Saethre-Chotzen) includes advancement of the midface [45]. Distraction osteogenesis can be performed at all levels of the midface [46–48], zygomatic bones [49], healed facial bone grafts [50], frontal bones [51], and other bones of the cranium [52,53]. Various distractor designs are available, but essentially they can be grouped into two basic categories [54–59]: external halo-like devices (see Fig. 1) and smaller internal devices (Figs. 15–18).

Proponents of external devices point out that although these devices are large and cumbersome, they are rigid and easily adjustable, often in more than one plane of space. External appliances permit

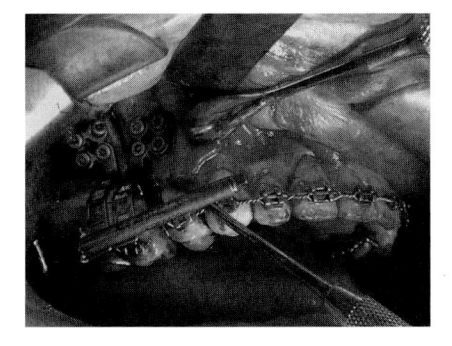

Fig. 9. Distraction device fixed in position on right maxilla.

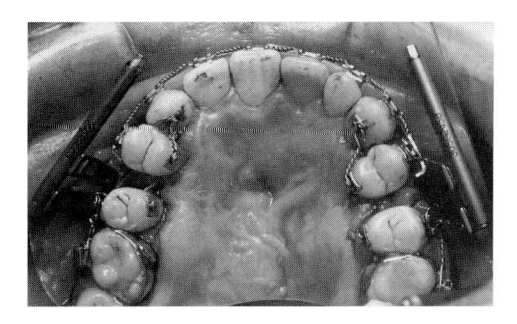

Fig. 10. Occlusal photographic view of palate shows vectors of distraction in a minimally convergent orientation.

easy control of the force and direction of distraction [55]. They can be applied easily to growing children, and they obviate the need for rigidly fixing devices on the lateral walls of the maxilla using screws where developing dental follicles and roots of the permanent dentition can be damaged. The use of these appliances is associated with the risk of the fixation pins penetrating the cranium, and pin site infections, however [56]. The social stigma associated with wearing an external device may deter its use. External devices also are prone to being accidentally dislodged [10].

Internal appliances are out of sight and have minimal impact on a patient's daily activities [59]. They are unidirectional, however, which makes distraction possible in only one plane of space. Often two internal devices must be used simultaneously on either side of the maxilla, which increases the chance for asymmetry and doubles the cost. Metal internal distraction devices are rigid but require removal after the distraction process, which can be difficult and complicated. Resorbable appliances that do not require removal recently have become available [60–62]. The tissues surrounding the transcutaneous distraction rods of the internal devices can become infected.

The results of maxillary distraction at the LeFort III level are far better than those of traditional midface advancement. Fearon [45] compared 12 children who had LeFort III distraction to an age-matched cohort of 10 children treated by osteotomy at the same level. The average horizontal advancement achieved in the LeFort III distraction group was 19 mm compared with 6 mm in the LeFort III osteotomy group. Two of the patients in the distraction group with obstructive sleep apnea demonstrated objective airway improvement and two further patients with obstructive sleep apnea were decannulated.

Fearon [45] used external and internal devices in his cohort of patients and preferred the aesthetic results accomplished using a halo over those obtained

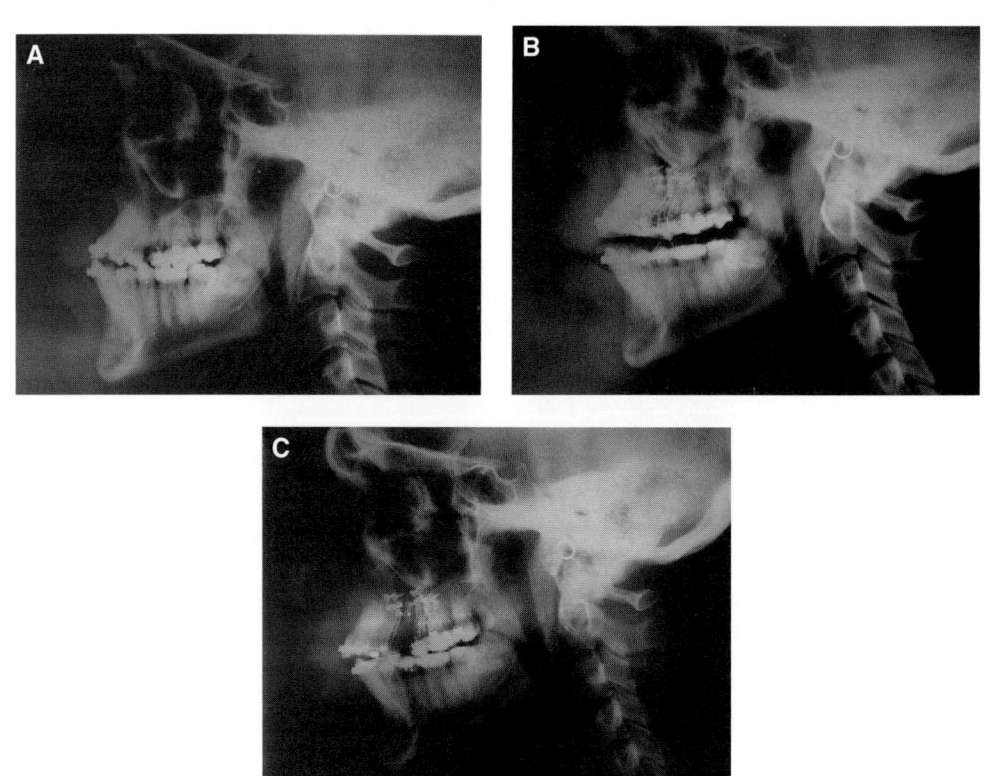

Fig. 11. (*A*) Preoperative lateral cephalogram. (*B*) Lateral cephalogram taken immediately after operation. (*C*) Lateral cephalogram taken at end of distraction phase, at beginning of consolidation phase. Note presence of bone gaps between roots of bicuspid teeth.

with internal distractors because the halo allows the vector of distraction to be focused on the facial midline, which helps to reposition the concave midface and provides a more convex facial profile.

Osteotomies can be tailored to the specific aesthetic and functional needs of a patient. Distraction osteogenesis can be executed at multiple levels to correct the occlusion and the midfacial retrusion independently using separate devices and vectors [63]. This is because the teeth, the nasofrontal region, and the orbital rims may not all advance the same distance (Fig. 18). Satoh and colleagues [63]

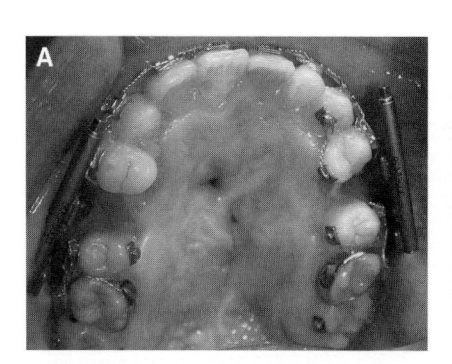

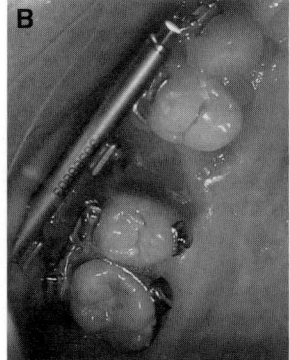

Fig. 12. (*A*) Palatal view of distractors in place. Note small fistula has opened on palate since beginning of distraction process. (*B*) Palatal view of right buccal segment shows distraction gap.

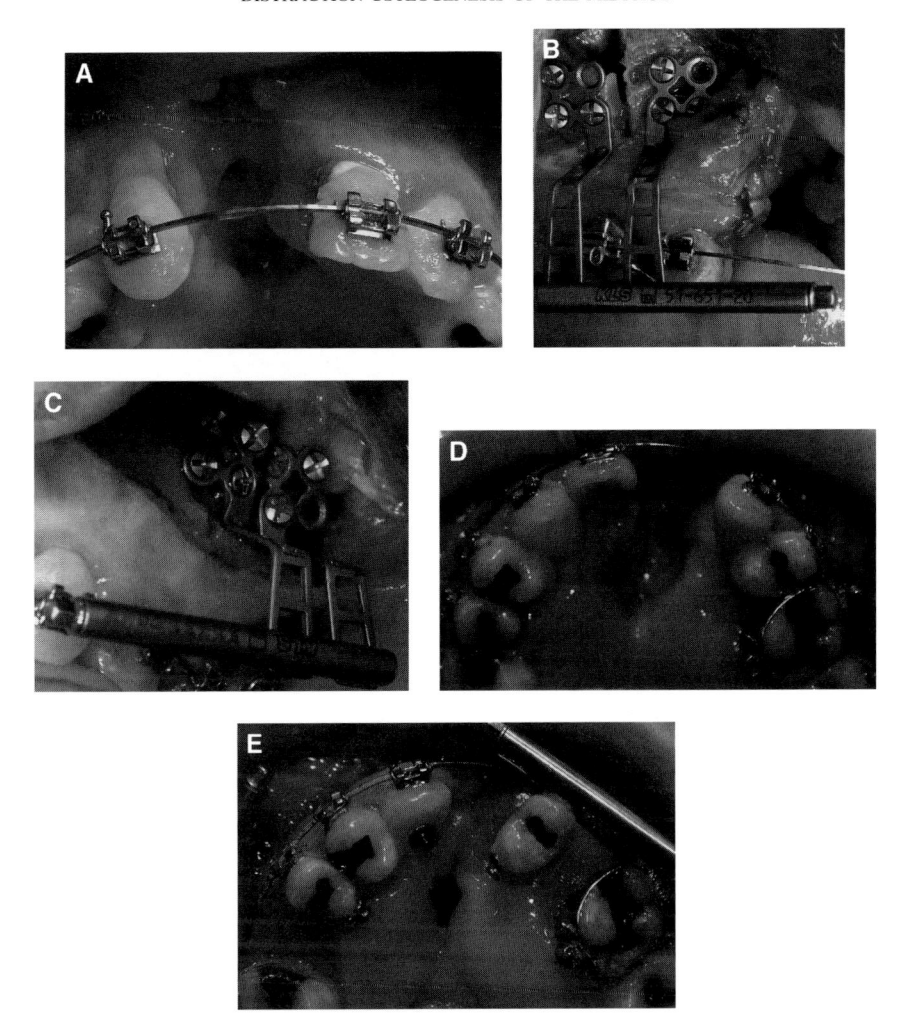

Fig. 13. (A) Anterior view of large alveolar cleft with oronasal fistula. (B, C) Internal distractor is applied to right and left osteotomized segment. (D) Occlusal view of alveolar defect preoperatively. Note two failing cleft adjacent teeth were removed before start of distraction. (E) Postoperative occlusal view of alveolar cleft and oronasal fistula, both of which have been reduced in size. More soft tissue is available for closure of oronasal fistula and reconstruction of alveolar defect.

recommend that the final position of the midface be governed subjectively by the position of the nasal bones, malar complexes, and orbital rims relative to the rest of the face [45,63], whereas the occlusion should be governed by an occlusal splint [63]. They also recommend osteotomizing the midface into two portions and distracting them separately using independent vectors and different amounts of distraction [63].

Alveolar distraction in the maxilla

Congenital absence of teeth (eg, oligodontia and alveolar clefting) is usually accompanied by bony defects of the maxillary alveolus. Acquired bony defects occur after tooth extraction, periodontal disease, maxillofacial trauma, and tumor ablation. The configuration of alveolar defects can be primarily horizontal or vertical in nature—or a combination of each—and can limit the restoration of missing teeth with dental implants.

The treatment of alveolar defects includes guided bone regeneration using various membranes, onlay autogenous bone grafts, connective tissue grafts, and alloplastic augmentation. Vertical alveolar defects are difficult to overcome in a predictable manner using autogenous bone grafts, and they often lead to aesthetic shortcomings [64,65]. Distraction osteogenesis

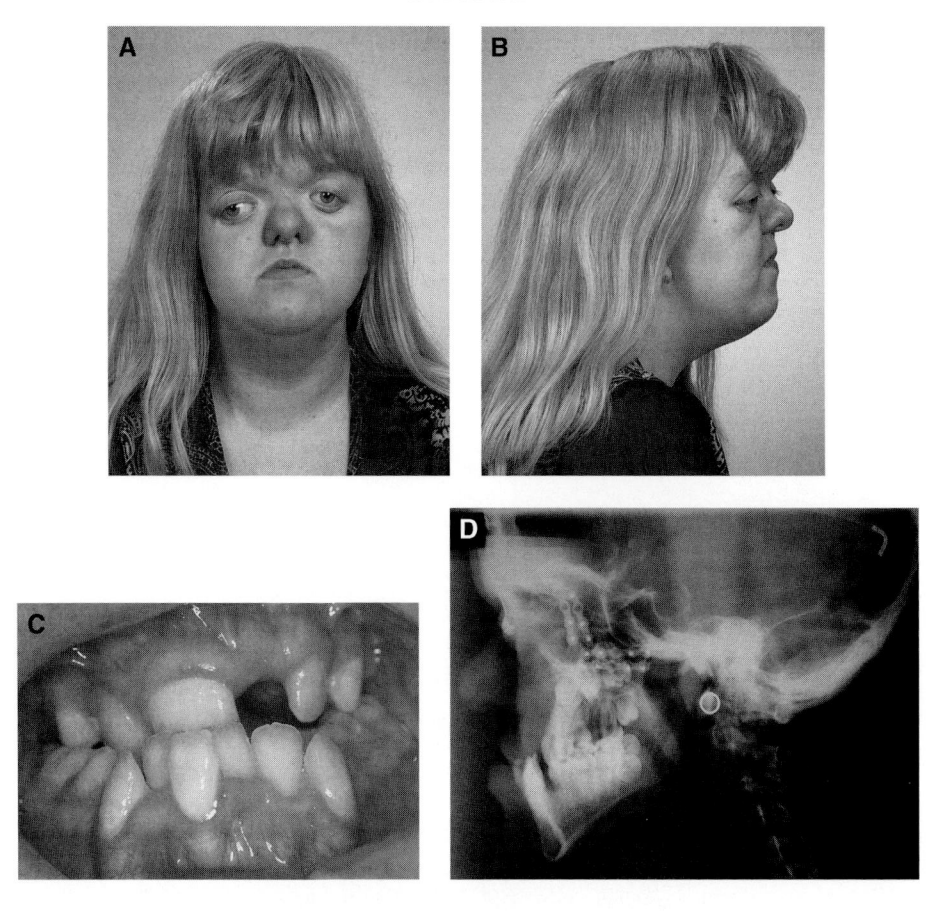

Fig. 14. Frontal (*A*) and lateral (*B*) view of 16-year-old girl with Crouzon syndrome and midface retrusion. (*C*) Occlusal view demonstrates severely retrusive maxilla and crowded dentition. (*D*) Lateral cephalogram shows significant midfacial retrusion despite previous osteotomy to advance the midface.

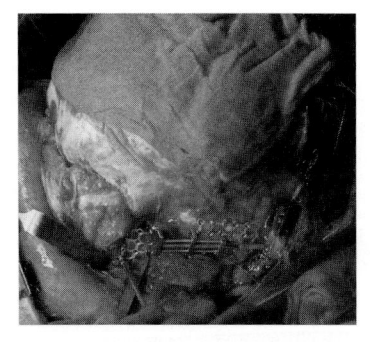

Fig. 15. Position of distraction devices after LeFort III osteotomy. Note foot plate secured below (frontozygomatic) osteotomy along lateral orbital wall and on temporal bone.

of the maxillary alveolus permits correction of alveolar defects often without the use of a bone graft.

Alveolar distraction osteogenesis may offer several advantages over bone grafting alone in the treatment of vertical alveolar defects because no donor site is required, distraction of bone and surrounding soft tissue occurs simultaneously, the transport segment is a form of pedicled graft that is never separated from its blood supply, and it has the potential for better control of vertical height, aesthetics, and biomechanical loading [66,67].

Alveolar distraction devices have three basic components: an upper member, a distraction rod, and a lower member/baseplate that supports the vertical force of distraction. These devices can be classified as intraosseous or extraosseous, uni-, bi- or multidirectional, nonresorbable or resorbable (ie, they do not require a second surgery to remove distractor components), and prosthetic (ie, they can remain in place to be used to support the dental

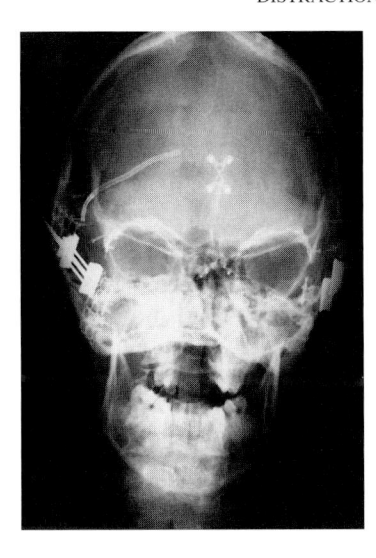

Fig. 16. Immediate postoperative anteroposterior cephalogram before onset of distraction phase.

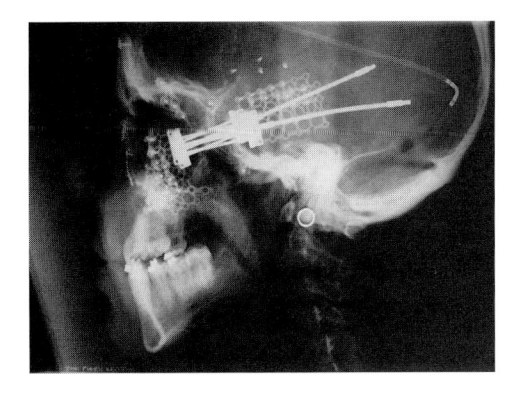

Fig. 18. Post-consolidation lateral cephalogram. Advancement at incisal level was 19 mm and 8 mm at frontonasal region.

prosthesis) or nonprosthetic (ie, they must be removed after distraction and replaced with a dental implant) [68,69].

Alveolar distraction osteogenesis is indicated for the treatment of alveolar defects in which the alveolar processes are atrophic and deficient. Alveolar distraction osteogenesis also can be used to correct vertical defects caused by ankylosis and submergence of primary teeth retained in the absence of succedaneous teeth (Fig. 19). Alveolar distraction osteogenesis is contraindicated in cases of severe atrophy in which there is insufficient bone to allow safe hardware placement between tooth roots and the floor of the nose or maxillary sinus. It also may be contraindicated in patients who have severe osteopo-

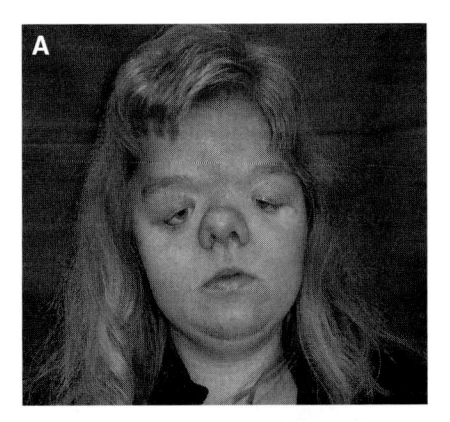

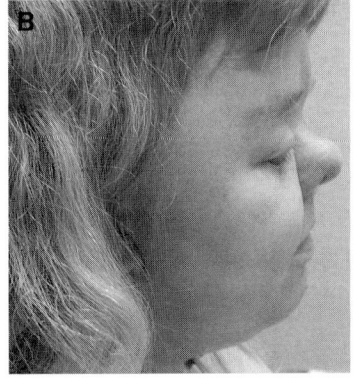

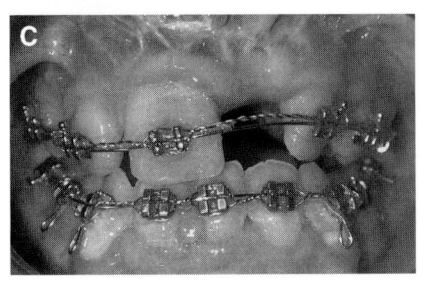

Fig. 17. Frontal (*A*) and lateral (*B*) view of patient at end of consolidation phase of distraction. (*C*) Postoperative occlusion with correction of anterior crossbite.

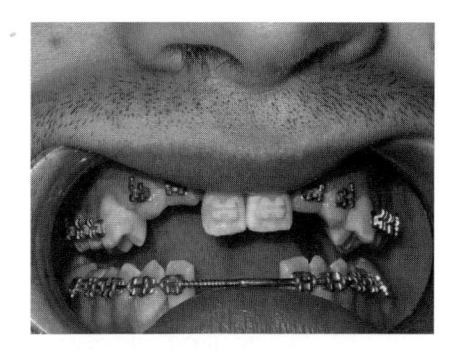

Fig. 19. Ankylosed deciduous teeth are useful anchorage units for attachment of tooth-borne distraction devices. Note submergence of deciduous lateral incisors and canines. There is a vertical discrepancy in the alveolus, which required vertical distraction osteogenesis before dental implant restoration.

rosis in which bone quality is poor, in patients of extremely advanced age, or in patients who are unlikely to demonstrate compliance with the rigors of the distraction process. The first step in alveolar distraction is to plan the vector of distraction and select a distractor that is capable of delivering that force in the proper direction. If teeth are available to anchor a distraction device then an external tooth-borne device can be used (Figs. 20, 21A–C); otherwise, an internal bone-borne device must be selected. The effect of the rigid palatal tissues on the vector of distraction should be kept in mind when treating the maxilla. Palatal tissues tend to exert pull on the distracting segment and cause it to tilt lingually away from the desired vector. If ankylosed teeth are used for anchorage of the distraction segment, they are extracted after the removal of the distraction hardware (Fig. 21C). Dental implants can be placed into the distracted alveolar segment and restored in their new ideal position (Fig. 22).

The distracting dental implant

There are clear advantages to having a device that can be used to correct vertical bony defects and can serve as the anchor for a prosthesis after completion of distraction. Such an intraosseous, prosthetic distraction device with completely internalized components is currently in the prototype stage of development (Fig. 23). The distracting implant, which is composed of a fixture connected to a footing by means of a retaining screw, is placed within the bone. When the assembly is installed completely, the proximal surface of the footing bears against the bottom of the osteotomy. After the completion of the distraction process (Fig. 24), the distracting dental implant is used to support a dental prosthesis.

Description of the alveolar distraction process using dental implants

The first step in alveolar distraction osteogenesis using a dental implant is assessment of the nature of the bony defect. The distracting dental implant should be used in a vertical defect up to 5 mm in which there is sufficient bone to distract without bone grafting. Alveolar defects with up to 10 mm of vertical loss in which there is significant horizontal loss may require bone grafting for width followed by healing before distraction.

Distracting dental implantation is a two-stage procedure in which the implant is placed and permitted to heal for some months before the distraction procedure commences. When sufficient osseointegration of the fixture and the footing have occurred, a corticotomy using an oscillating saw or bone chisel is completed. After a latency period of 5 to 12 days, active distraction is started. To commence the distraction procedure, the retaining screw is removed and the distractor rod is placed within the fixture (Fig. 24). The distractor rod is advanced along the bore of the fixture until it bears against the footing. Further rotation of the distractor rod results in the fixture moving in the distal direction relative to the footing. The segment of bone into which the fixture is integrated moves in the direction of

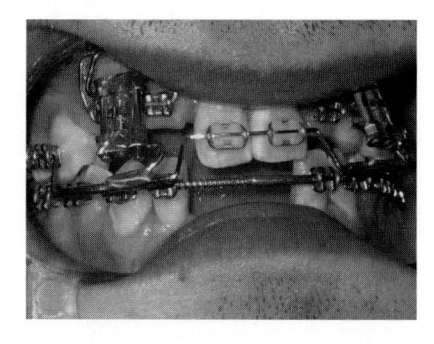

Fig. 20. Anterior view of tooth-borne distraction apparatus to vertically lengthen maxillary alveolus.

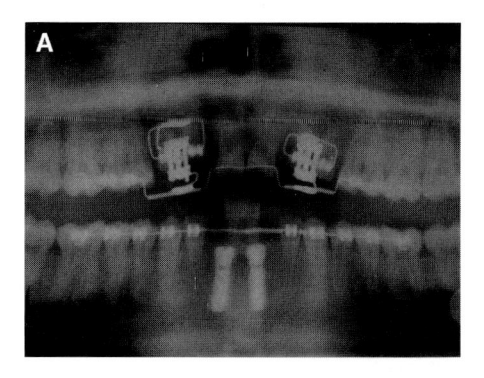

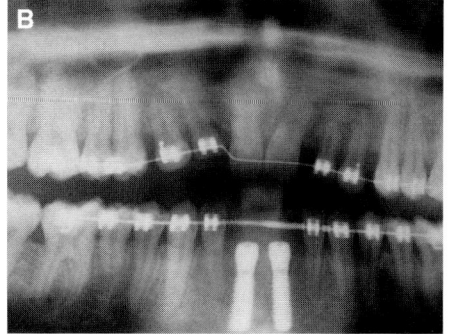

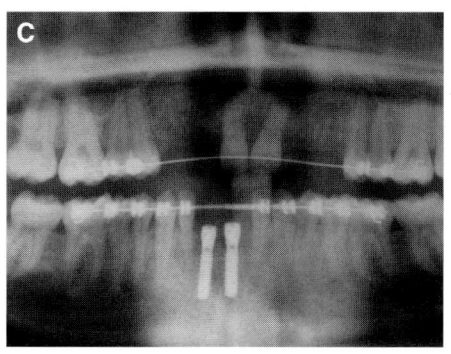

Fig. 21. (*A*) Immediate postoperative panoramic radiograph shows device position. (*B*) Panoramic radiograph after distraction device removed shows increased vertical height of alveolus and teeth. (*C*) Panoramic radiograph after extraction of deciduous teeth shows increased vertical height of alveolus.

distraction [3,4]. Depending on the length of travel along the direction of distraction, one or more distractor rods of different lengths may be used inside the implant.

Final bone healing occurs during the consolidation period. The distractor or an external support, such as orthodontic splinting, is used to stabilize the segments. Thereafter, the distractor rod is removed, which leaves a cylindrical void in the newly formed bone that also fills in with bone. Upon completion of the distraction, the fixture may remain in place, having been firmly integrated in the bone tissue, where it can be used to serve as an anchor for a prosthetic crown or bridge. With the advent of new titanium surface geometries and concomitant use of growth factors, more rapidly developing osseointe-

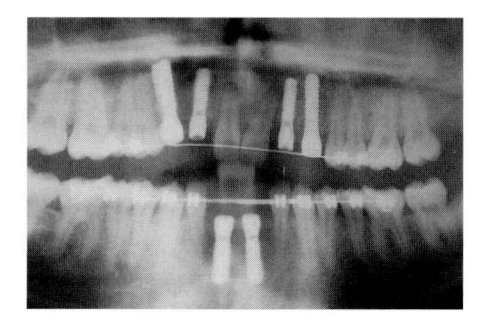

Fig. 22. Panoramic radiograph after implant fixture placement.

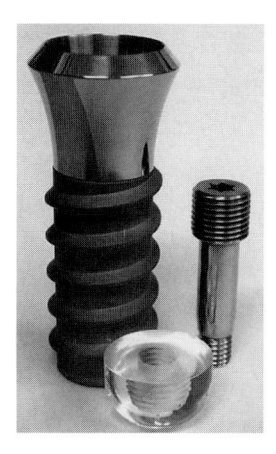

Fig. 23. Distracting dental implant including fixture body, distractor rod, and footplate represented by clear plastic disc next to implant (CSMT, Mississauga, Ontario, Canada).

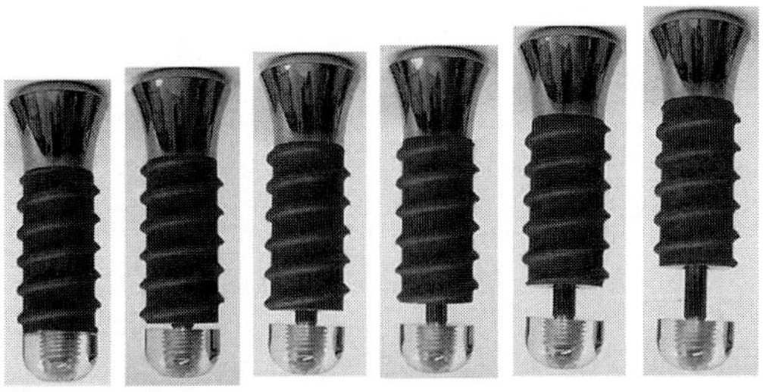

Fig. 24. Distracting dental implant activated demonstrates gradual gains in vertical alveolar height. Distracting hardware also serves as prosthetic restoration.

gration may allow for implant placement and distraction in a single stage.

Guidance of implant placement

Although the distracting dental implant is a unidirectional distraction device, its trajectory can be guided to a certain extent using orthodontic forces or a prosthodontic docking station. A further consequence of the unidirectional nature of the distracting dental implant is that the vector of distraction is defined primarily by the implant's longitudinal axis. To a certain extent, the geometry of the corticotomy can be designed to counter pull from the lingual or palatal mucoperiosteum. Because the trajectory of the distracting implant depends substantially on the vector of distraction, it is critically important to control the spatial location and axial inclination of the implant. An implant positioning device with the capability of controlling spatial location and axial inclination is currently under development.

The future of alveolar and midface distraction osteogenesis

Distraction osteogenesis is a powerful technique that already has revolutionized pediatric oral and maxillofacial surgery by providing a means of reliably lengthening the bones of the midface and mandible [48]. As an alternative or an adjunct to conventional ridge augmentation procedures, alveolar distraction osteogenesis with a distracting dental implant offers the prospect of greater control in the correction of vertical alveolar defects and better aesthetic outcomes. A distracting implant also allows for correction of some unsuccessful results that otherwise might require the use of long clinical crowns or pink porcelain, or, in the worst case, removal of the implant, revisional ridge augmentation, and reimplantation.

Distraction osteogenesis may allow for earlier implant placement in children. The most appropriate time for implant placement in growing patients has been discussed. Experiments designed to study the effect of dental implants on dentoalveolar growth and development in pigs demonstrated that implants remain stationary and do not erupt together with adjacent teeth [70]. Implants were found to inhibit local growth and development of the alveolar process, much in the same way that ankylosed teeth behave [71]. A 3-year prospective clinical study in adolescents with congenitally missing teeth verified that implants do not move during jaw growth and result in development of an infraocclusion and vertical marginal discrepancy of the prosthetic crown that is proportional to the amount of residual jaw growth after implant restoration [71,72]. One case report [73] documented a similar phenomenon occurring over a decade in an adult, putatively caused by continuing growth of the facial skeleton [74–76].

Standardization of implant capability to permit distraction osteogenesis would extend the ability to refine aesthetics in the future after late detrimental changes related to residual alveolar growth, continued growth of the dentoalveolar process through adulthood, eruption of adjacent teeth, and recession of soft tissue.

In the future, distraction osteogenesis may benefit from automation of the distraction technique by the incorporation of a micromotor controlled by a microprocessor to allow for smooth and continuous distraction. Three-dimensional treatment planning with accurate transfer will allow for proper placement of the bony segments in three dimensions. Endoscopy may be another future adjunct to the distraction procedure to facilitate minimally invasive surgery with improved visualization of the osteotomy sites [77].

References

[1] Moghadam HG, Sàndor GKB, Holmes H, et al. Histomorphometric evaluation of bone regeneration using allogeneic and alloplastic bone substitutes. J Oral Maxillofac Surg 2004;62(2):202–13.

[2] Molina F. Distraction osteogenesis for the cleft lip and palate patient. Clin Plast Surg 2004;31(2):291–302.

[3] Ilizarov GA. The tension-stress effect on the genesis and growth of tissues: Part I. The influence of stability of fixation and soft tissue preservation. Clin Orthop 1989;238(2):249–85.

[4] Ilizarov GA. The tension-stress effect on the genesis and growth of tissues: Part II. The influence of the rate

and frequency of distraction. Clin Orthop 1989; 239(2):263–85.
[5] Komuro Y, Akizuki T, Kurakata M, et al. Histological examination of regenerated bone through craniofacial bone distraction in clinical studies. J Craniofac Surg 1999;10(4):308–11.
[6] Balaji S.M. History of craniofacial distraction osteogenesis. In: Abstracts of the Second Asia Pacific Congress on Distraction Osteogenesis. Male (Maldives): 2003. p. 1–9.
[7] Angell EH. Treatment of irregularities of the permanent or adult teeth. Dental Cosmos 1860;1:540–4.
[8] Haas AJ. Rapid expansion of the maxillary dental arch and nasal cavity by opening the midpalatal suture. Angle Orthod 1961;31:73–90.
[9] McCarthy JG, Schreiber J, Karp N, et al. Lengthening of the human mandible by gradual distraction. Plast Reconstr Surg 1992;89(1):1–8.
[10] Swennen G, Schliephake H, Demf R, et al. Craniofacial distraction osteogenesis: a review of the literature. Part I. Clinical studies. Int J Oral Maxillofac Surg 2001;30(2):89–103.
[11] Ilizarov GA. Clinical application of the tension-stress effect for limb lengthening. Clin Orthop 1990;250(1): 8–26.
[12] Ilizarov GA. The principles of the Ilizarov method. Bull Hosp Joint Dis 1997;56(1):49–53.
[13] Codivilla A. On the means of lengthening in the lower limbs, the muscles and tissues which are shortened through deformity. Am J Orthop Surg 1905;2: 353–7.
[14] Sàndor GKB, Witzel MA, Posnick JC. The use of nasendoscopy in predicting velopharyngeal function after maxillary advancement. J Oral Maxillofac Surg 1990;48(8):123.
[15] Sàndor GKB, Leeper HA, Carmichael RP. Risks and benefits of orthognathic surgery: speech and velopharyngeal function. Oral Maxillofac Surg Clin North Am 1997;9(2):147–65.
[16] Karakasi D, Hadjipetrou L. Advancement of the anterior maxilla by distraction [case report]. J Craniomaxillofac Surg 2004;32(3):150–4.
[17] Uemura T, Hayashi T, Satoh K, et al. A case of improved obstructive sleep apnea by distraction osteogenesis for midface hypoplasia of an infantile Crouzon's syndrome. J Craniofac Surg 2001;12(1):73–7.
[18] Cohen SR, Holmes RE, Machado L, et al. Surgical strategies in the treatment of complex obstructive sleep apnea in children. Pediatr Respir Rev 2002; 3(1):25–35.
[19] Britto JA, Evans RD, Hayward RD, et al. Maxillary distraction osteogenesis in Pfeiffer's syndrome: to provide urgent ocular protection by gradual midfacial skeletal advancement. Br J Plast Surg 1998;51(5): 343–9.
[20] Zarzycki D, Tesiorowski M, Zarzacka M, et al. Long term results of limb lengthening by physeal distraction. J Pediatr Orthop 2002;22(3):367–70.
[21] Haas AJ. The treatment of maxillary deficiency by opening of the midpalatal suture. Angle Orthod 1965;35:200–17.
[22] Pogrel MA, Kaban LB, Vargervik K, et al. Surgically assisted maxillary expansion in adults. Int J Adult Orthodon Orthognath Surg 1992;7:37–41.
[23] Lines PA. Adult rapid maxillary expansion with corticotomy. Am J Orthod 1975;67:44–56.
[24] Kraut RA. Surgically assisted rapid maxillary expansion by opening the midpalatal suture. J Oral Surg 1984;42:651–5.
[25] Betts NJ, Vanarsdall RL, Barber HD, et al. Diagnosis and treatment of transverse maxillary deficiency. Int J Adult Orthodon Orthognath Surg 1995;10(2): 75–96.
[26] Albern MC, Yurosko JJ. Rapid palatal expansion in adults with and without surgery. Angle Orthod 1987;57:245–63.
[27] Bays RA, Greco JM, Hale RG. Stability of surgically assisted rapid palatal expansion. J Dent Res 1990; 69:296.
[28] Lehman JA, Haas AJ. Surgical-orthodontic correction of transverse maxillary deficiency. Dent Clin North Am 1990;34:385–95.
[29] Stromberg C, Holm J. Surgically assisted, rapid maxillary expansion in adults: a retrospective long tern follow-up study. J Craniomaxillofac Surg 1995; 23:222–7.
[30] Bell WH, Epker BN. Surgical-orthodontic expansion of the maxilla. Am J Orthod 1976;70:517–28.
[31] Turvey TA. Maxillary expansion: a surgical technique based on surgical-orthodontic treatment objectives and anatomic consideration. J Maxillofac Surg 1985;13: 51–8.
[32] Harada K, Baba Y, Ohyama K, et al. Soft tissue profile changes of the midface in patients with cleft lip and palate following maxillary distraction osteogenesis: a preliminary study. Oral Surg Oral Med Oral Path Endod 2002;94(6):673–7.
[33] Scheuerle J, Habal MB. Functional impact of distraction osteogenesis of the midface on expressive language development. J Craniofac Surg 2001;12(1): 69–72.
[34] Rachmiel A, Levy M, Laufer D, et al. Multiple segmental gradual distraction of facial skeleton: an experimental study. Ann Plast Surg 1996;36(1):52–9.
[35] Altuna G, Walker DA, Freeman E. Surgically assisted rapid orthodontic lengthening of the maxilla in primates: a pilot study. Am J Orthod Dentofacial Orthop 1995;107(5):531–6.
[36] Dolanmaz D, Karaman AI, Durmus E, et al. Management of alveolar clefts using dento-osseous transport distraction osteogenesis. Angle Orthod 2003;73(6): 723–9.
[37] Yen SL, Yamashita DD, Kim TH, et al. Closure of an unusually large palatal fistula in a cleft patient by bony transport and corticotomy-assisted expansion. J Oral Maxillofac Surg 2003;61(11):1346–50.
[38] Cohen SR, Burstein FD, Stewart MB, et al. Maxillary-midface distraction in children with cleft lip and pal-

[39] Dolanmaz D, Karman AI, Ozyesil AG. Maxillary anterior segmental advancement by using distraction osteogenesis: a case report. Angle Orthod 2003;73(2): 201–5.

[40] Guerrero CA, Bell WH, Meza LS. Intraoral distraction osteogenesis: maxillary and mandibular lengthening. Atlas Oral Maxillofac Surg Clin North Am 1999;7(1): 111–51.

[41] Yamaji KE, Gateno J, Xia JJ, et al. New internal LeFort I distractor for the treatment of midfacial hypoplasia. J Craniofac Surg 2004;15(1):124–7.

[42] Kessler P, Wiltfang J, Schultze-Mosgau S, et al. Distraction osteogenesis of the maxilla and midface using a subcutaneous device: report of four cases. Br J Oral Maxillofac Surg 2001;39(2):13–21.

[43] Haluck RS, MacKay DR, Gorman PJ, et al. A comparison of gradual distraction techniques for modification of the midface in growing sheep. Ann Plast Surg 1999;42(5):476–80.

[44] Weinzweig J, Baker SB, MacKay GJ, et al. Immediate versus delayed midface distraction in a primate model using a new intraoral device. Plast Reconstr Surg 2002;109(5):1600–10.

[45] Fearon JA. The LeFort III osteotomy: to distract or not to distract? Plast Reconstr Surg 2001;107(5): 1091–103.

[46] Marchac D, Arnaud E. Midface surgery from Tessier to distraction. Childs Nerv Syst 1999;15(11–12): 681–94.

[47] Molina F. From midface distraction to the "true monoblock". Clin Plast Surg 2004;31(3):463–79.

[48] Yu JC, Fearon J, Havlik JR, et al. Distraction osteogenesis of the craniofacial skeleton. Plast Reconstr Surg 2004;114(1):1E–20E.

[49] McCarthy JG, Hopper RA. Distraction osteogenesis of zygomatic bone grafts in a patient with Treacher Collins syndrome: a case report. J Craniofac Surg 2002;13(2):279–83.

[50] Stelmnicki EJ, Hollier L, Lee C, et al. Distraction osteogenesis of costochondral bone grafts in the mandible. Plast Reconstr Surg 2002;109(3):925–33.

[51] Talisman R, Hemmy C, Denny AD. Frontofacial osteotomies, advancement and remodeling distraction: an extended application of the technique. J Craniofac Surg 1997;8(4):308–17.

[52] Lauritzen C, Sugawara Y, Kocabalkan O, et al. Spring mediated dynamic craniofacial reshaping: case report. Scand J Plast Reconstr Surg Hand Surg 1998;32(3): 331–8.

[53] Li M, Park SG, Kang DI, et al. Introduction of a novel spring-driven craniofacial bone distraction device. J Craniofac Surg 2004;15(2):324–8.

[54] Maull DJ. Review of devices for distraction osteogenesis of the craniofacial complex. Semin Orthod 1999;5(1):64–73.

[55] Polley JW, Figueroa AA. Management of severe maxillary deficiency in childhood and adolescence through distraction osteogenesis with an external, adjustable, rigid distraction device. J Craniofac Surg 1997;8(3):181–5.

[56] Mavili ME, Vargel I, Tuncbilek G. Stoppers in RED II distraction device: is it possible to prevent pin migration. J Craniofac Surg 2004;15(3):377–83.

[57] Havlik RJ, Seelinger MJ, Feashemo DV, et al. "Cat's cradle" midfacial fixation in distraction osteogenesis after LeFort III osteotomy. J Craniofac Surg 2004; 15(6):946–52.

[58] Mavili ME, Tuncbilek G, Vargel I. Rigid external distraction of the midface with direct wiring of the distraction unit in patients with craniofacial dysplasia. J Craniofac Surg 2003;14(5):783–5.

[59] Riediger D, Poukens JM. LeFort III osteotomy: a new internal positioned distractor. J Oral Maxillofac Surg 2003;61(8):882–9.

[60] Cohen SR, Holmes RE, Amis P, et al. Internal craniofacial distraction with biodegradable device early stabilization and protected bone regeneration. J Craniofac Surg 2000;11(4):354–66.

[61] Cohen SR, Holmes RE. Internal LeFort III distraction with biodegradable devices. J Craniofac Surg 2001; 12(3):264–72.

[62] Burstein FD, Williams JK, Hudgins R, et al. Single stage craniofacial distraction using resorbable devices. J Craniofac Surg 2002;13(6):776–82.

[63] Satoh K, Mitsukawa N, Hosaka Y. Dual midfacial distraction osteogenesis: LeFort III minus and LeFort I for syndromic craniosynostosis. Plast Reconstr Surg 2003;111(3):1019–28.

[64] Belser U, Buser D, Higgenbottom F. Consensus statements and recommended clinical procedures regarding esthetics in implant dentistry. In Proceedings of the Third ITI Consensus Conference, Gstaad, Switzerland. Int J Oral Maxillofac Implants 2004; 19(Suppl):73–4.

[65] Simion M, Jovanovic SA, Tinti C, et al. Long-term evaluation of osseointegrated implants inserted at the time or after vertical ridge augmentation: a retrospective study on 123 implants with 1–5 year follow-up. Clin Oral Implants Res 2001;12(1):35–45.

[66] Clarizio LF. Vertical alveolar distraction versus bone grafting for implant cases: the clinical issues. In: Jensen OT, editor. Alveolar distraction osteogenesis. Chicago: Quintessence Publishing; 2002. p. 59–68.

[67] Jensen OT, Kuhlke L, Reed C. Prosthetic considerations and treatment planning by classification for alveolar distraction ontogenesis. In: Jensen OT, editor. Alveolar distraction osteogenesis. Chicago: Quintessence Publishing; 2002. p. 29–40.

[68] Stucki-McCormick S, Moses JL, Robinson R, et al. Alveolar distraction devices. In: Jensen OT, editors. Alveolar distraction osteogenesis. Chicago: Quintessence Publishing; 2002. p. 41–58.

[69] Chin M, Toth BA. Distraction osteogenesis in maxillofacial surgery using internal devices: review of five cases. J Oral Maxillofac Surg 1996;54(1): 45–53.

[70] Ödman J, Gröndahl K, Lekholm U, et al. The effect of osseointegrated implants on the dento-alveolar development: a clinical and radiographic study in growing pigs. Eur J Orthod 1991;13(4):279–86.

[71] Thilander B, Ödman J, Gröndahl K, et al. Osseointegrated implants in adolescents: a three year study. Ned Tijdschr Tandheelkd 1995;102(4):383–5.

[72] Kuröl J, Ödman J. Treatment alternatives in young patients with missing teeth: aspects on growth and development. In: Koch G, Bergendal T, Kvint S, et al, editors. Consensus conference on oral implants in young patients: state of the art. Jönköping, Sweden: Institute for Postgraduate Dental Research; 1996. p. 77–107.

[73] Tarlow JL. The effect of adult growth on an anterior single-tooth implant: a clinical report. J Prosthet Dent 2004;92(3):213–5.

[74] Oesterle LJ, Cronin Jr RJ. Adult growth, aging, and the single-tooth implant. Int J Oral Maxillofac Implants 2000;15(2):252–60.

[75] Bishara SE, Treder JE, Damon P, et al. Changes in the dental arches and dentition between 25 and 45 years of age. Angle Orthod 1996;66(6):417–22.

[76] Forsberg CM, Eliasson S, Westergren H. Face height and tooth eruption in adults: a 20-year follow-up investigation. Eur J Orthod 1991;12(4):249–54.

[77] Levine JP, Rowe NM, Bradley JP, et al. The combination of endoscopy and distraction osteogenesis in the development of a canine midface advancement model. J Craniofac Surg 1998;9(5):423–32.

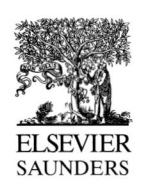

Orthognathic Surgery for Secondary Cleft and Craniofacial Deformities

Radhika Chigurupati, BDS, DMD

Department of Oral and Maxillofacial Surgery, University of California–San Francisco, 521 Parnassus Avenue, C-522, San Francisco, CA 94143-0440, USA

Children born with craniofacial anomalies can have several functional problems such as feeding, breathing, speech and hearing difficulties, visual disturbances, poor neuromuscular coordination and other organ system disturbances, in addition to the facial dysmorphology. Complete rehabilitation to achieve adequate function and an acceptable facial appearance requires correction of the primary and secondary deformities in a timely fashion by an interdisciplinary team of specialists.

Initial surgeries performed during infancy and early childhood should aim to address functional problems with morphology as a secondary goal. Most of the secondary skeletal facial deformities can be corrected by orthognathic surgery during late childhood or after skeletal maturity. The goal of orthognathic surgery is to minimize or mask the primary deformity, correct the underlying skeletal disproportion, correct associated malocclusion, optimize facial aesthetics, enhance function (breathing, mastication, speech), develop self esteem and improve social acceptability. The operations must be well planned, staged when necessary and performed in a setting where adequate nursing, anesthesia, social services and surgical skill and expertise are available.

The absence, deficiency or malposition of normal anatomic structures, presence of scar tissue from previous operations, severe functional deficits, and psychosocial problems makes orthognathic surgery more challenging in individuals with craniofacial deformities. In the last decade, applications of distraction osteogenesis in the management of craniofacial deformities have become more popular because of its advantage of bone regeneration at the osteotomy site, expansion of the soft tissue envelope, and lack of donor site morbidity; however this technique does not replace conventional orthognathic surgery that can achieve acceptable results safely and predictably in most craniofacial deformities.

A thorough preoperative evaluation is necessary to establish a surgical plan and ensure that the patient and family understand the potential benefits, risks, and difficulties and have realistic expectations. Assessment by cephalometric analysis helps in early prediction of craniofacial growth and timing for surgical correction of secondary deformities. Typical preoperative records include good facial and intraoral photographs, articulated study models with bite registration and face bow transfer, and anteroposterior, lateral cephalometric, and panoramic radiographs. Special imaging studies (eg, three-dimensional CT) and investigations (eg, sleep studies and endoscopic examination of the airway) may be necessary before orthognathic surgery in some patients to evaluate the nasal and oropharyngeal airway and velopharyngeal function.

Stereolithographic models obtained from three-dimensional CT scans offer the surgeon additional relevant information that is helpful in the correction of facial asymmetry and hypertelorism [1,2]. Chang and colleagues [3] have shown that existing skeletal defects can be constructed with stereolithographic models using mirror image templates of the normal contralateral side with digital correlation and subtraction techniques. This approach helps to carve a framework for autogenous grafts or construct allo-

E-mail address: cradhik@itsa.ucsf.edu

plastic implants during the operation. Troulis and colleagues [4] have shown that use of a three-dimensional planning system based on CT data is helpful in planning surgery. They used a CT-based software program to reconstruct virtual three-dimensional models from CT scans and then created a treatment plan for patients with mandibular deformities (eg, Treacher Collins syndrome and hemifacial microsomia). The simplicity of these systems, cost effectiveness, and the overall difference in outcome have not yet been studied [4]. Computer-based simulation methods for surgical procedures that are based on imaging data provide the ability to perform virtual surgery preoperatively. Xia and colleagues [5] have reported the use of three-dimensional virtual reality surgical planning and simulation workbench for orthognathic surgery.

Timing of surgery

The timing of surgery depends on functional problems, psychosocial factors, and the facial growth pattern. This will vary depending on the type of craniofacial anomaly and should be tailored to the needs of each individual patient. Generally, maxillomandibular deformities are corrected by combined surgical and orthodontic treatment after completion of growth or when the skeleton is mature to achieve predictable results. Facial growth in girls is completed between age 14 and 16 years and in boys by age 16 to 18 years. In selective cases, orthognathic surgery is performed during growth for psychosocial or functional reasons. In some cases, early correction can decrease the severity of the secondary skeletal deformity, as in hemifacial microsomia [6]. Conversely, early surgery has shown unpredictable results because of continued growth of the unaffected facial skeleton. Freihofer [7] evaluated patients with maxillary hypoplasia who underwent Le Fort I osteotomy and found that 71% of patients younger than 16 years and 46% between 16 and 17 years had unacceptable outcomes because of pseudo-relapse as a result of continued mandibular growth after maxillary advancement. Wolford and colleagues [8] have demonstrated similarly that early correction of the maxillary hypoplasia in growing patients does not produce predictable results because of continued mandibular and vertical maxillary growth.

Maxillary distraction in the mixed dentition phase has been shown to improve facial aesthetics and influence psychological development of adolescents who have a cleft deformity [9]. Figueroa et al [10], reviewed their results after a 3-year follow up of maxillary distraction with a rigid external device in growing cleft children with mid-face hypoplasia. They found that the maxillary position was stable in the sagittal plane with minimal antero-posterior growth, but there was continued vertical maxillary growth. Some of these patients required reoperation for correction of vertical maxillary excess after skeletal maturity. Wiltfang and colleagues [11] found that it was necessary to overcorrect the position of the midface when distracting in a growing child to compensate for further growth of the mandible. The inability to predict future growth was the most challenging aspect of preoperative planning for distraction in these children.

Performing surgery after skeletal maturity helps to avoid multiple procedures that can cause scarring and further deformation of the tissues, injury to the developing dentition, need for revision, or reoperation because of continued growth of unaffected facial skeleton and avoids unpleasant experiences of multiple surgeries in a growing child. On the other hand, the advantages of early surgery in these children are the ability to improve function in a young child, provide a functional matrix to stimulate growth and decrease the severity of secondary deformity, and improve facial appearance and psychological development. Conventional orthognathic surgery or distraction osteogenesis should be performed selectively for correction of skeletal facial deformities in growing patients, with the understanding that future surgical correction may be necessary after completion of growth.

Orthodontic considerations

Orthodontic treatment is often prolonged and can be challenging for the child and the treating doctor. These children often have delay in eruption of teeth, severe crowding of arches with impacted, malformed, and supernumerary teeth, and sometimes limited ability to open their mouth. Interceptive or phase I orthodontic treatment should include monitoring eruption status of teeth, space management, and preventing ectopic eruption of permanent teeth by removal of retained primary and impacted or unerupted permanent teeth when arch length is deficient. Functional appliances may be beneficial in selected patients who have hemifacial microsomia and cleft lip and palate (CLP) to promote growth [12,13]. Maxillary arch expansion in the early mixed dentition phase helps to correct the position of the collapsed cleft segment to some extent and facilitate alveolar bone grafting.

Presurgical or phase II orthodontic treatment can be initiated toward the end of growth before orthognathic surgery. Dental compensations should be removed, segmental leveling of the teeth in the individual arches should be completed, and divergence of roots should be adequate if segmental osteotomies are planned. Teeth can be substituted instead of replacement whenever possible, and canines can be substituted for the missing lateral incisors in patients who have a cleft. In patients who have Apert syndrome with severe maxillary arch crowding, extraction of severely impacted maxillary canines instead of first premolars can shorten the period of presurgical treatment time. It is important to limit the movement of the teeth that are adjacent to the unrepaired alveolar cleft margins to maintain good bone height and periodontal support of these teeth. The goal of presurgical orthodontic treatment is to achieve arch compatibility so that the teeth in the maxillary and mandibular arches interdigitate well after surgery [14,15]. Orthodontic treatment progress should be evaluated by obtaining a set of dental casts to check the occlusion, interference in the molar region from lingual cusps caused by lack of torque control, supraerupted second molars, and incompatible intercanine width. Postsurgical orthodontic treatment should take into account the need for dental compensation to accommodate for relapse, especially during the first year after surgery [14].

Cleft lip and palate

CLP is the most common congenital facial deformity. Embryologically, it results from failure of mesenchymal fusion between the nasofrontal and lateral facial components of the fetus between 4 and 7 weeks of gestation, and the spectrum can vary from subtle philtral marking (form fruste) to complete bilateral cleft of the nasal, lip, alveolar, and palatal structures. The cleft deformity itself and subsequent primary surgical operations affect facial growth and development, particularly maxillary growth that results in secondary deformities, including maxillary deficiency, malocclusion, and lip and nasal deformities. Orthognathic surgery can correct the maxillary deficiency and malocclusion and, to some extent, the associated upper lip and nasal deformities and mask the cleft facial appearance.

Growth in patients who have cleft lip and palate

Some degree of maxillary hypoplasia is evident in the postpubertal phase in most patients who have CLP [16–20]. The heterogeneity in cleft types, variations in surgical skill and techniques of primary repair, and differences in cleft team protocols make it difficult to evaluate large samples in multiple centers to understand the factors that contribute to maxillary hypoplasia. The cause of maxillary deficiency is attributed to the intrinsic cleft defect, primary surgical procedures, particularly surgical skill and subsequent healing, mechanical adaptations of the jaws, and the inherent racial and genetic variations in facial form and growth pattern of these individuals [21].

The typical facial morphologic characteristics of an individual who has a cleft are deficiencies in the maxillary, alveolar, paranasal, infraorbital, and zygomatic regions. These deficiencies contribute to increased scleral show, lack of normal cheek contour, inadequate nasal tip and upper lip support, acute nasolabial angle, and short upper lip. The maxilla is deficient in antero-posterior, transverse, and vertical dimensions and there is displacement of the cleft segments. In complete unilateral CLP, typically the lesser segment is hypoplastic and displaced superiorly, and medially. In patients who have bilateral CLP, the lateral segments are collapsed, which results in a narrow maxillary arch and bilateral posterior cross-bite. The premaxilla is often protruberant, inferiorly positioned, and tipped palatally. Although mandibular growth is normal, the mandibular plane angle is steep, the chin is retruded, posterior facial height is decreased, and anterior facial height is increased. These factors, combined with maxillary hypoplasia, give patients who have a cleft a pseudoprognathic appearance. Functionally, patients with clefts can have: 1. Airway obstruction secondary to hypertrophied inferior turbinates, deviated nasal septum, intranasal strictures, enlarged tonsils or adenoids, and pharyngeal flaps; 2. Speech impairment secondary to velopharyngeal insufficiency, malpositioned teeth and oro-nasal fistulae. These functional deficiencies should be taken into account while planning orthognathic surgery to correct skeletal morphology and improve facial appearance.

The incidence of maxillary deficiency and subsequent need for orthognathic surgery in individuals who have clefts vary. Ross [18], in a large Toronto-based sample of men with unilateral CLP, and DeLuke and colleagues [22], in a unilateral CLP sample, reported this incidence to be 25%, whereas Rosenstein and colleagues [23] found that 22% of their patients who had unilateral CLP and primary alveolar bone grafting required orthognathic surgery. Posnick and Ricalde [24] stated that the need for orthognathic surgery can vary from 25% to 75% of patients with this deformity, depending on the indications or criteria used. After reviewing our data at the University of California, San Francisco Center for Craniofacial Anomalies, we found that 14% of

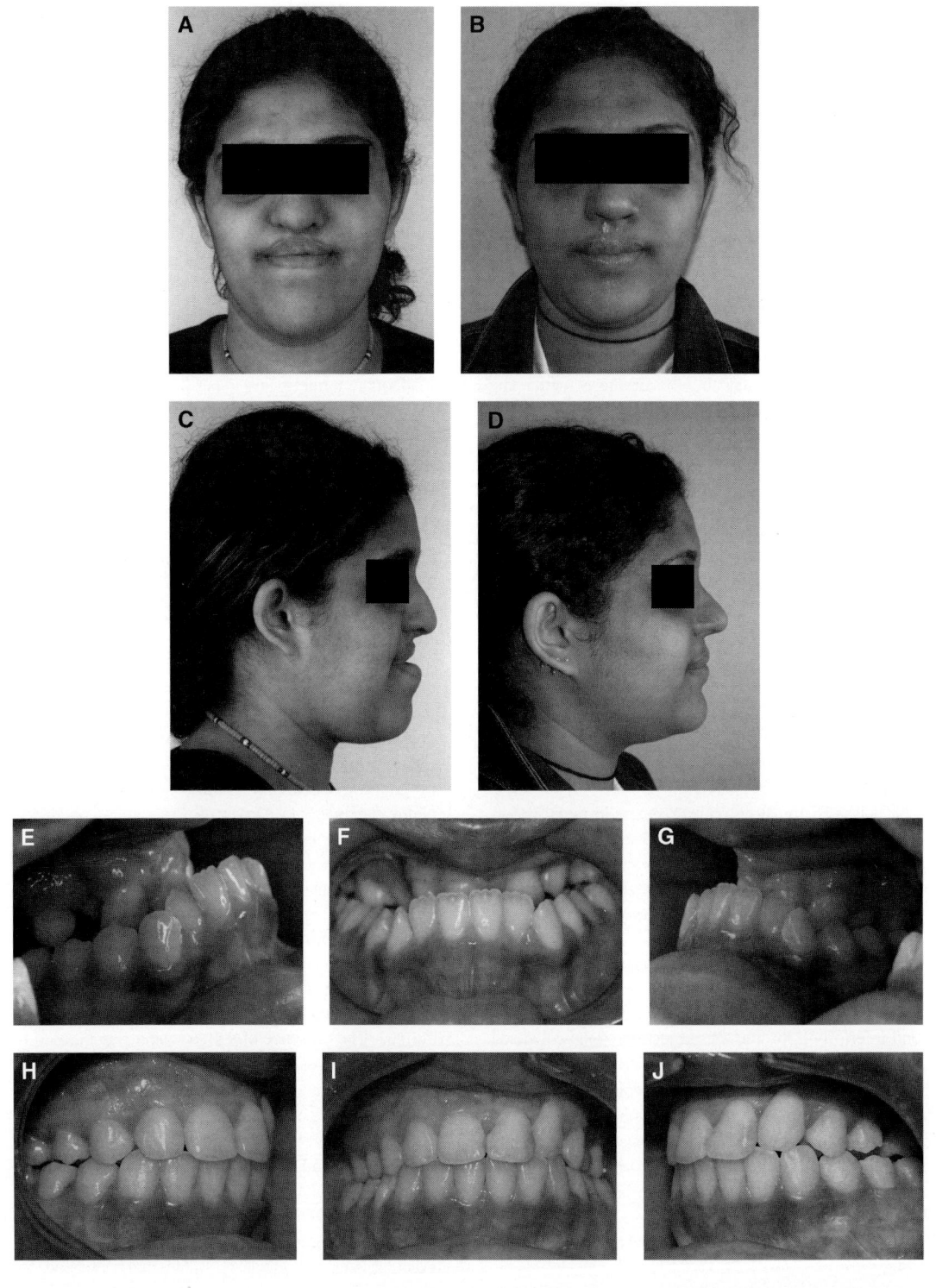

Fig. 1. 18-year-old female with secondary skeletal and soft tissue deformities of BCLP corrected with orthognathic surgery - Le Fort I maxillary osteotomy, bilateral sagittal split osteotomy, and genioplasty. (*A*) Preoperative frontal view. (*B*) Postoperative frontal view after bimaxillary osteotomy and cheilorhinoplasty. (*C*) Preoperative lateral view. (*D*) Postoperative lateral view after bimaxillary osteotomy and cheilorhinoplasty. (*E,F,G*) Preoperative occlusion reveals anterior and posterior cross bite. (*H,I,J*) Postoperative occlusion after combined orthodontic and surgical correction.

our non-syndromic UCLP patients required surgical correction for maxillary hypoplasia [25]. The need for orthognathic surgery should be based not only on occlusion and jaw relationship but also on facial proportions, midface projection, upper lip and nasal tip support, position of the cleft alveolar segments (eg, a collapsed lesser segment in unilateral CLP and abnormal position of the premaxilla in bilateral CLP), and velopharyngeal function.

Osteotomies for correction of secondary cleft deformities

The Le Fort I maxillary osteotomy initially was described by Axhausen [26] in 1932, performed by Gillies and Rowe [27] in an individual who had a cleft in 1954, and popularized by Obwegesser [28] in the 1960s. This osteotomy is the basic procedure for correction of the maxillary deficiency in patients who have cleft. Midface osteotomies at the Le Fort II level [29] and Le Fort III level also have been used depending on the aesthetic needs of the patient who has a cleft. If the maxillary deficiency is severe, then gradual distraction of the maxilla using internal or external devices can facilitate larger advancement, or the maxillary osteotomy can be combined with a mandibular osteotomy when the sagittal discrepancy is larger than 10 to 12 mm (Figs. 1 and 2) [30–32].

Many modifications of the Le Fort I osteotomy have been reported. When the alveolar cleft is already repaired before orthognathic surgery, the maxilla can be advanced and inferiorly repositioned as one unit. If an alveolar cleft is present at the time of surgery then the Le Fort I osteotomy can be combined with alveolar bone grafting to repair the oro-nasal fistula, close the cleft dental gap, correct the position of the lesser cleft segment, and advance the maxilla [33–38]. Making the Le Fort I osteotomy higher on the cleft segment and repositioning it laterally and inferiorly improves the projection of the collapsed lesser segment. In patients with severe hypoplasia of the infraorbital, maxillary, and malar region, a high Le Fort I osteotomy that includes the zygoma or a Le Fort III osteotomy would be particularly beneficial (Fig. 3) [39]. Autogenous bone grafts are frequently necessary to bridge the defect caused by asymmetric repositioning of the cleft alveolar segments or repair of the alveolar cleft or to allow bony union when the degree of skeletal movement is large. The use of distraction techniques where applicable may eliminate the need for bone grafts and decrease associated donor site morbidity. Use of modified vertical soft tissue incisions to maintain labial and buccal pedicles instead of circumvestibular incisions may not have an added benefit in the unilateral cleft cases, but they make the osteotomy and mobilization of the maxilla technically more difficult. Conversely, maintaining the premaxilla pedicled to the labial mucosa is important in patients who have bilateral cleft with an unrepaired alveolar cleft, in which most of blood flow to the premaxilla comes from the upper lip.

Skeletal stability

Advancement and postoperative stability after Le Fort I maxillary osteotomy in patients who have cleft are less favorable than in patients who do not have cleft because of tension and scarring of surrounding soft tissues (particularly the palate and upper lip), magnitude and direction of the skeletal movement, presence of multiple (two or three) alveolar segments, oronasal fistulae, and congenital absence of teeth, and presence of a pharyngeal flap. Willmar [40], Houston and colleagues [41], Posnick and Dagys [42], Cheung and colleagues [43], and Heliovaara and colleagues [44] show that there is some degree of relapse in patients who have clefts who underwent orthognathic surgery.

In 1991, Eskenazi and Schendel [45] reviewed the literature, analyzed their results, and reviewed the literature on Le Fort I osteotomy in patients who have clefts. Published evidence on skeletal stability showed that most of the relapse occurred during the first year postoperatively. Wire fixation resulted in greater relapse than plate and screw fixation. There was no need for bone grafting at the pterygomaxillary junction to improve stability. Relapse was greater in vertical dimensions in comparison to anteroposterior dimensions. The relapse was influenced by magnitude of advancement in some studies [44], whereas others reported no difference in outcome with magnitude of advancement or type of operation (ie, bimaxillary versus only maxillary osteotomy) [42,43]. The presence of a pharyngeal flap seemed to increase the possibility of relapse, although this was not statistically significant [45]. Correction of maxillary deficiency in growing patients who have cleft is not predictable because of continued mandibular growth, vertical maxillary growth, and decreased anteroposterior maxillary growth.

Houston and colleagues [41] reported that the mean horizontal relapse rate was 7% and mean vertical relapse rate was 23%. Posnick and Dagys [42] found that the vertical relapse rate was 19% and the horizontal relapse rate was 23% of the achieved advancement after a mean follow-up of 1.5 years when they evaluated skeletal stability in patients who had unilateral CLP and underwent orthognathic

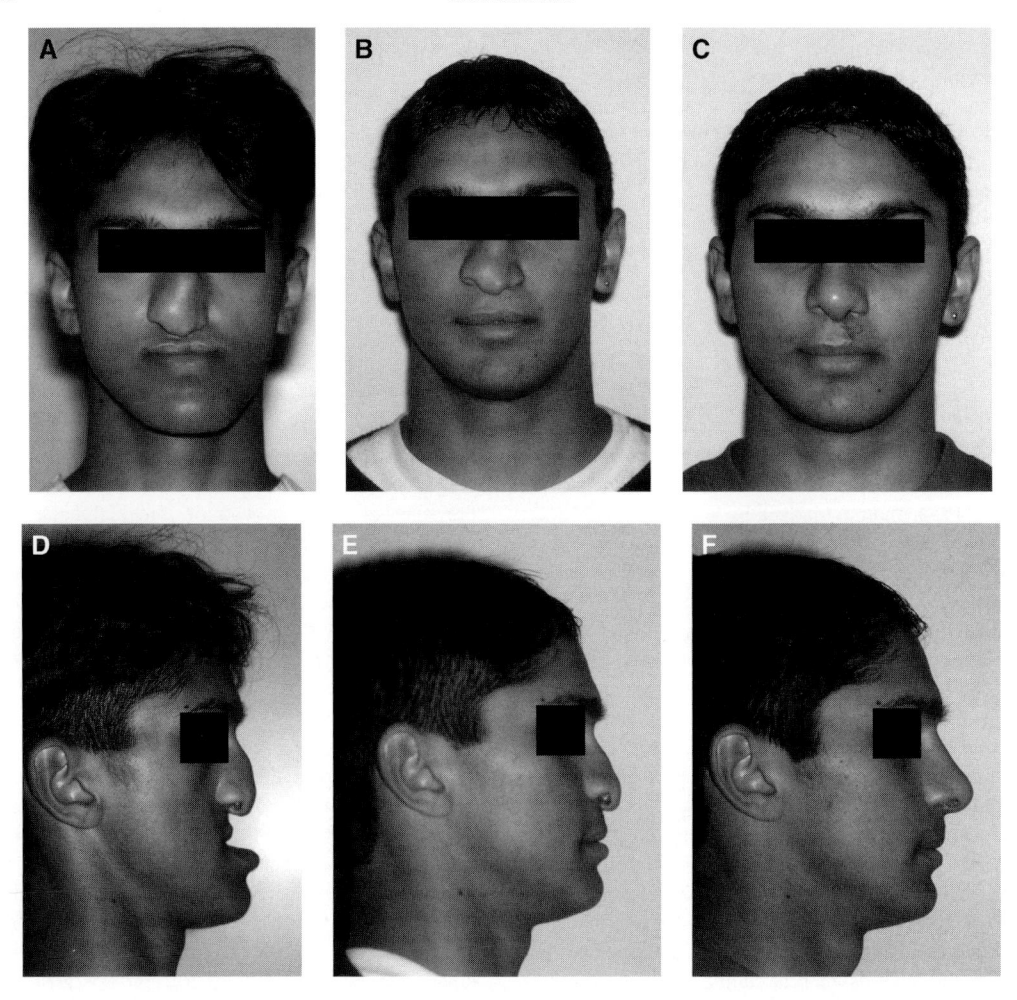

Fig. 2. 18-year-old male with UCLP and severe maxillary hypoplasia corrected by staged orthognathic surgery - Le Fort I osteotomy and bilateral sagittal split mandibular osteotomy. (*A*) Preoperative frontal view. (*B*) Postoperative frontal view after orthognathic surgery. (*C*) Postoperative frontal view after cheilorhinoplasty. (*D*) Preoperative lateral view. (*E*) Postoperative lateral view after orthognathic surgery. (*F*) Postoperative lateral view after cheilorhinoplasty. (*G*) Preoperative lateral cephalometric radiograph. (*H*) Postoperative lateral cephalometric radiograph after initial maxillary advancement. (*I*) Postoperative lateral cephalometric radiograph after maxillary advancement and mandibular setback. (*J*) Presurgical occlusion. (*K*) Postsurgical occlusion. (*L*) Postorthodontic treatment.

surgery with miniplate fixation. Cheung and colleagues [43] studied 46 consecutive patients with residual alveolar clefts and maxillary hypoplasia who underwent maxillary osteotomies and simultaneous bone grafting of the alveolar cleft prospectively. They reported a relapse rate of 22% in the horizontal plane, 22.5% in the vertical plane in unilateral CLP, and 17.5% and 7%, respectively, in bilateral CLP, with no statistically significant difference between the two groups. Relapse rate in the transverse plane ranged from 13.4% to 33.6%. Heliovaara and colleagues [44] found that the mean relapse rate in anteroposterior dimension was 20.5% (0.8 mm) and the mean vertical relapse rate was 22.2% (1 mm). There was a correlation between the degree of maxillary advancement and relapse in vertical and horizontal dimensions.

Soft tissue changes

Friehofer [46] compared soft tissue changes in cleft and non-cleft individuals with maxillary hypoplasia who underwent Le Fort I osteotomy for maxillary advancement and reported there was no major difference in the two groups. He concluded that leaving the anterior nasal spine has a favorable influence on lip support in patients with maxillary hypoplasia.

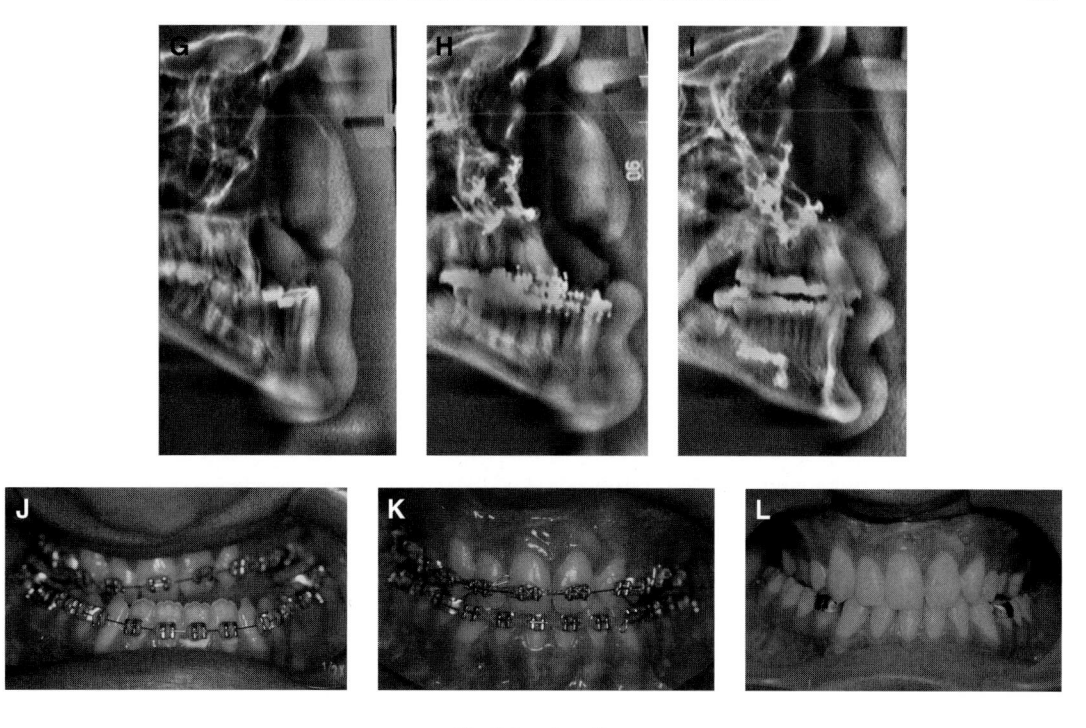

Fig. 2 (*continued*).

He also noted that thin lips follow the movement of the maxilla better than voluminous lips and to achieve a specified lip advancement the maxilla must be advanced twice this distance. Hui and colleagues [47] and Wolford [48] found that the correlation between soft and hard tissue movements is more significant in individuals who have cleft than in individuals who do not have cleft for a given maxillary advancement. This difference may be attributed to the thin upper lip, lack of nasal tip support, and decreased support at the alar base in patients who have cleft [47,48]. In general, secondary cheilorhinoplasty should be postponed until the underlying skeletal and dental corrections are completed by orthognathic surgery and orthodontic treatment, because the upper lip position and the nasal form and function are altered by changes in the maxillary position.

Velopharyngeal insufficiency

An individual who does not have a cleft can tolerate large advancements without any alteration in speech; in patients who have a repaired cleft palate, however, velopharyngeal insufficiency is an adverse effect of maxillary advancement. Patients must be warned of the risk of hypernasal speech after orthognathic surgery. A combination of speech intelligibility rating by a speech pathologist and endoscopic examination to assess soft palate and pharyngeal wall motion and static measurements, such as pharyngeal depth to velar length (need ratio), on lateral cephalometric radiographs are useful in objective assessment of velopharyngeal function before and after orthognathic surgery. Witzel and Munro [49] reported that velopharyngeal function can be compromised in patients with borderline velopharyngeal closure who undergo large maxillary advancements that exceed 10 mm. Janulewicz and colleagues [50] confirmed previous findings that patients with borderline velopharyngeal function preoperatively are more likely to have alterations in function after maxillary advancement. If function does not return to normal in 6 to 12 months, it may be necessary to perform a palate lengthening procedure. Guyette and colleagues [51] reported that maxillary distraction might decrease the likelihood of velopharyngeal insufficiency, because the palate is advanced in small increments and the patient may have time to adapt to these small, gradual changes. In their pilot study of six patients who had cleft, Harada and colleagues [52] concluded that velopharyngeal function might not be affected markedly with the maxillary distraction when the advancement is less than 15 mm.

The outcome of orthognathic surgery in patients who have cleft can be considered acceptable if a

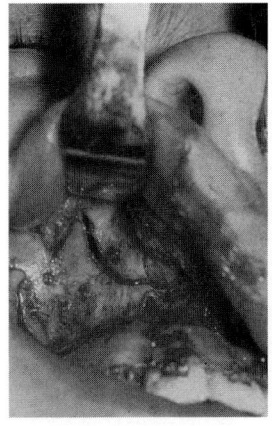

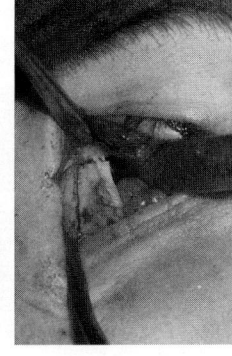

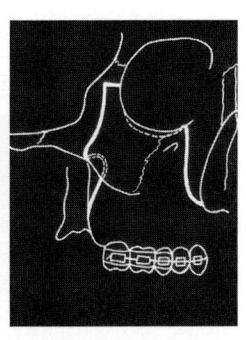

Fig. 3. A high Le Fort I osteotomy including the zygoma to correct mid-face deficiency in some cleft patients.

functional occlusion and an acceptable aesthetic result can be achieved with no deterioration of speech intelligibility, if postoperative skeletal position of the maxillary cleft segments are stable and there are no residual oronasal fistulae, if there is no loss of dentoalveolar segments or teeth, if there is adequate periodontal support of teeth adjacent to the cleft, and if there is closure of the cleft dental gap or the ability to replace the congenitally missing teeth with a fixed or implant-retained prosthesis.

Hemifacial microsomia

Hemifacial microsomia is the second most common congenital facial birth defect after CLP and has many phenotypic variations. It has an overall incidence of 1:5600 live births and primarily affects the skeletal, soft tissue, and neuromuscular derivatives of the first and second pharyngeal arches [53]. Presence of extracranial anomalies, namely cardiac, renal, skeletal (vertebral), pulmonary, and gastrointestinal anomalies, has been well documented [54]. The exact cause is not known, but theories based on experimental animal studies have been postulated by Poswillo [55] and Johnston and Bronsky [56].

Mandibular asymmetry and hypoplasia often are the earliest manifestations at birth. Hypoplasia is generally manifested unilaterally, but 5% to 15% of patients have bilateral asymmetric involvement [57]. Other facial anomalies include temporal bone abnormalities, variable degrees of orbitozygomatic hypoplasia, deficiency of the overlying soft tissues and muscles of mastication, external and middle ear deformities, abnormalities of eyelid and adnexal structures, functional deficit of facial nerve branches, facial clefts (macrostomia), and cleft of the lip and palate [58]. Several classification systems have been proposed to describe the findings, but the orbit, mandible, ear, nerve, and soft tissue (OMENS) classification, which was modified to OMENS plus to include extracranial anomalies, is the most comprehensive because it grades the orbital, mandibular, ear, facial nerve, and soft tissue defects [59].

The type of mandibular deformity, facial growth, and degree of asymmetry are factors that influence the timing and type of surgical treatment for skeletal facial deformity in patients who have hemifacial microsomia. The Pruzanky classification modified by Kaban and Mulliken [60], which helps to delineate the mandibular deformity into three types (namely, type I, type IIA, type IIB, and type III), is based on the presence of absence of structures of the temporomandibular joint and mandibular ramus. In type I, the mandible on the affected side is small or diminutive but all structures are present. In type IIA, the condyle and ramus are present, but the condyle is anterior and medially placed. In type IIB, the mandibular ramus is hypoplastic and displaced medially, anteriorly, and inferiorly without a condyle and articular fossa. Type III represents the most severe form of the deformity, with absence of the entire ramus and condyle and articular fossa of the mandible [60–62]. The deficiency of the muscles of mastication is proportionate to the degree of skeletal deformity [63].

Growth in hemifacial microsomia

The functional matrix and the structures necessary for mandibular growth are rudimentary or missing on the affected side, which results in less growth than the unaffected side and consequent facial asymmetry. Longitudinal follow-up of mandibular asymmetry by radiographic assessment in patients who have hemifacial microsomia was reported by Rune and colleagues [64], Polley and colleagues [65], and Sarnas and colleagues [66]. Radiographic stereometric analysis by Rune and colleagues [64] and Sarnas and colleagues [66] found considerable variation in mandibular growth and ensuing facial asymmetry. It is difficult to make conclusive statements based on their longitudinal assessment as to who would benefit from early surgery and in whom surgery should be postponed. Polley and colleagues [65] longitudinally followed 26 unoperated patients who had hemifacial microsomia and evaluated skeletal mandibular asymmetry using posteroanterior cephalometric radiographs. Their results showed that the vertical mandibular asymmetry measured by intergonial angle was significantly greater in the type III mandibular deformity, and the average vertical gonial height difference between the affected and unaffected sides was significant in all patients, except individuals with type I mandibular deformity. In a retrospective evaluation of 67 patients who had untreated hemifacial microsomia, Kearns and colleagues [67] examined the progression of facial asymmetry. The patients were divided into two groups (type I, IIA and type IIB, III) based on severity of mandibular deformity. Facial measurements based on clinical and radiographic observations of the occlusal plane cant and piriform rim asymmetry showed that facial asymmetry becomes worse with time as a result of continued asymmetric mandibular growth and progressive restriction of growth of the maxillary and zygomatic complex on the affected side [67].

Proponents of early surgery believe that mandibular reconstruction during childhood may limit secondary growth deformities, especially in the maxilla, avoid cant of the occlusal plane and asymmetry at oral commissure, and improve psychosocial development [6,68]. They proposed the following protocol for correction of the maxillomandibular deformity in the growing child. In type I mandibular deformity, in which the structures on the affected side are simply smaller compared with the unaffected side, use of a functional appliance (activator) in the mixed dentition phase may promote growth on the affected side. In type I or type IIA deformity, if there is an occlusal cant, then early surgical lengthening of the ramus of the mandible on the affected side is performed to create an open bite in the mixed dentition. Mandibular lengthening can be performed by a sagittal split mandibular osteotomy on the affected side; sometimes an osteotomy also may be necessary on the opposite side. This effect also can be achieved by distracting the short ramus of the mandible on the affected side. Early elongation of the mandible should result in a more symmetric growth pattern, minimize the secondary deformity, and avoid maxillary osteotomy. In individuals with type IIB and type III deformity, in which the mandibular ramus is hypoplastic or absent and the condyle is absent, reconstruction of the condyle-ramus unit with a costochondral graft is recommended in the early mixed dentition phases to elongate and rotate the mandible. Finally, maxillomandibular surgery is necessary in this group after completion of growth.

Vargervik and colleagues [69] reviewed treatment of hemifacial microsomia in 25 patients. Of these patients, 10 had surgery performed during growth. In seven of ten growing patients, postoperative growth was similar on both sides and the established symmetry was maintained. In the remaining three patients, however, the asymmetry recurred and further surgical correction was necessary.

Posnick [70] argues that the facial asymmetry in this condition is not progressive and proposes waiting until skeletal maturity is attained and performing one maxillomandibular surgical procedure if necessary for correction of facial asymmetry. The results are predictable, and stable aftergrowth is completed without exposing a child to several surgical interventions and prolonged orthodontic treatment. In type III or some type IIB cases, in which the condyle-ramus unit is not yet reconstructed, an autogenous costochondral graft can be used to reconstruct this portion simultaneously, or it can be staged with the initial phase consisting of reconstruction of congenitally missing ramus-condyle unit during the mixed dentition phase and second phase for maxillomandibular reconstruction at the end of skeletal maturity (Fig. 4) [70].

In the skeletally mature patient who has hemifacial microsomia, the facial skeletal deformity consists of a retruded asymmetric mandible with a short medially displaced ramus with or without condyle and articular fossa, with chin point deviated to the affected side, short midface with canted maxillary occlusal plane and oral commissure, and flat malar region on the affected side occasionally accompanied by orbital dystopia. The maxillomandibular reconstruction can be achieved in one stage by a Le Fort I maxillary osteotomy to level the occlusal plane cant, increase posterior facial height, correct maxillary midline, lengthen the shortened ramus with a mandibular sagittal split osteotomy, rotate and advance the retruded mandible, and perform a genioplasty to correct mandibular and chin asymmetry (Fig. 5). An inverted-L osteotomy or a C-shaped osteotomy

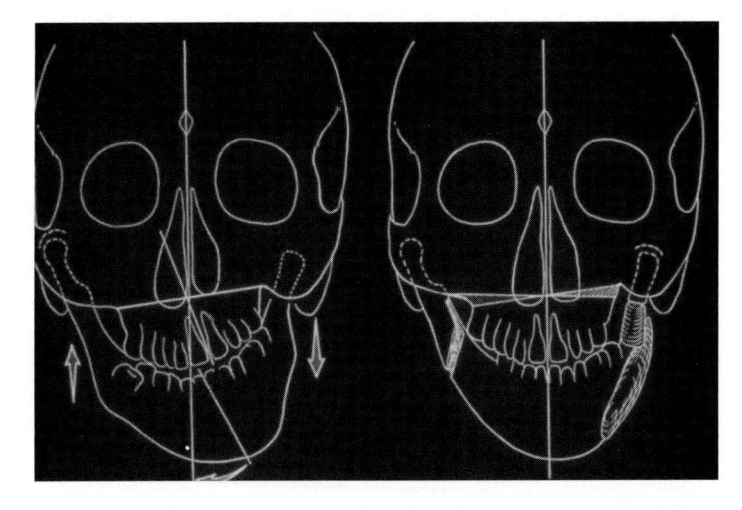

Fig. 4. Maxillo-mandibular reconstruction for hemifacial microsomia.

with interpositional bone grafts has been described instead of the sagittal split osteotomy to increase posterior facial height. Augmenting the gonial angle and malar region on the affected side by onlay with rigidly fixed autogenous cortical bone or alloplastic customized implants and soft tissue reconstruction with vascularized free flaps or fat injection at a later stage helps to mask the facial asymmetry well.

Mandibulofacial dyostosis (Treacher Collins syndrome)

This craniofacial anomaly with an autosomal dominant inheritance pattern has an incidence in the range of 1in 25,000 to 1 in 50,000 live births. The gene has been mapped to the long arm of the fifth chromosome [71]. There is bilateral involvement with varying degrees of mandibular, zygomatic, orbital, and maxillary hypoplasia. Ear abnormalities with hearing impairment, coloboma of lower eyelids, and down-slanted palpebral fissures are other characteristic features. Presence of cleft palate with or without cleft lip, choanal atresia, and tracheal abnormalities is variable [53]. Airway obstruction can occur because of choanal atresia, tracheal abnormalities, mandibular retrognathia, and decreased cranial base angle that requires early surgical intervention in these children. Mandibular distraction has been reported in these children for relief of airway obstruction and early decannulation when a tracheostomy is present [72].

Maxillomandibular reconstruction in Treacher Collins syndrome requires correction of the altered facial height, ie, increased anterior facial height, decreased posterior facial height, anteroposterior mandibular deficiency, and chin dysplasia. Serial cephalometric radiography has shown that facial convexity remains constant over time in these patients. Upper anterior facial height remains normal, but lower anterior facial height increases with increasing chin dysplasia and mandibular retrusion. The type of mandibular deformity dictates the timing and procedure required for correction of the maxillomandibular deformity. In the absence of a condyle or a short ramus, costochondral grafts to reconstruct the ramus-condyle unit or mandibular distraction to lengthen the ramus is recommended before definitive orthognathic surgery.

Posnick and colleagues [73] recommended that the orbital and zygomatic reconstruction be performed in early childhood (age 6–7 years) with a calvarial or rib onlay graft to build the lateral orbital rims and the zygomatic arch and recommended that the final maxillomandibular reconstruction be performed at early skeletal maturity (between 13 and 15 years) in conjunction with orthodontic treatment. In these patients, a Le Fort I osteotomy is necessary to correct the posterior vertical deficiency and anteroposterior and transverse deficiency. The occlusal plane requires anticlockwise rotation to lengthen the posterior maxilla and intrude the anterior maxilla to achieve a satisfactory lip-to-incisor relationship. A sagittal split mandibular osteotomy allows effective horizontal advancement and anticlockwise rotation of the mandible. With an oblique osteotomy of the inferior border, the chin can be advanced forward, which further corrects the anteroposterior deficiency

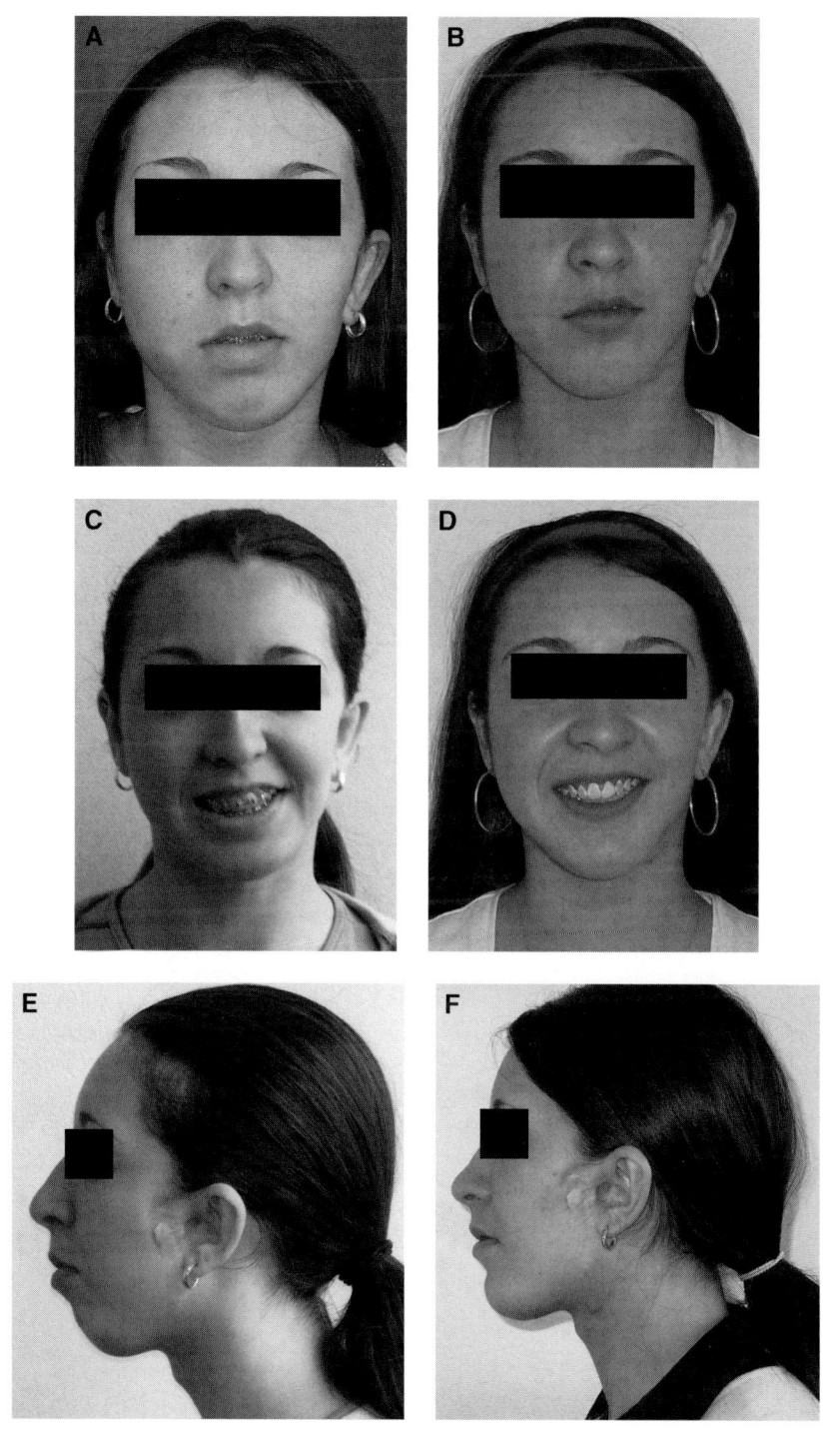

Fig. 5. 15-year-old female with left hemifacial microsomia. (*A*) Preoperative frontal repose. (*B*) Postoperative frontal repose after maxillo-mandibular reconstruction. (*C*) Preoperative frontal smiling. (*D*) Postoperative frontal smiling after maxillo-mandibular reconstruction. (*E*) Preoperative lateral view. (*F*) Postoperative lateral view after maxillo-mandibular reconstruction.

of the mandible and chin dysplasia. The vertical ramus height and angle of mandible may require augmentation with bone grafts or alloplastic materials. Traditional orthognathic surgery offers stability and predictability even in patients with severe expression of Treacher Collins syndrome [73]. Roncevic and Roncevic [74]reported that in their experience, the best results were obtained when orthognathic surgery was performed between 16 and 18 years and zygomaticomaxillary reconstruction using vascularized pericranial flaps was performed 1 year after the maxillomandibular reconstruction.

Craniofacial dysostoses

Premature fusion of the cranial vault sutures, midface, and cranial base sutures results in abnormal skull and midfacial growth, as seen in Apert, Crouzon, Pfeiffer, Carpenter, and Saethre-Chotzen syndromes [53]. Early surgical correction in these children should address the functional problems, such as headaches and visual disturbances caused by raised intracranial pressure and hydrocephalus, and allow development and growth of the brain that is restricted by the prematurely fused sutures. Reconstruction of the cranio-orbital region is performed by the age of 1 year by fronto-orbital advancement and cranial vault reshaping. By early childhood, a combination of tonsillo-adenohypertrophy and restricted midface and cranial base growth can cause upper airway obstruction. As they grow older, these children exhibit moderate to severe midfacial hypoplasia, proptosis of the globes caused by shallow orbits, mild to moderate hypertelorism, and a discrepancy in maxillomandibular relation, class III malocclusion with an anterior open bite. The mandibular growth is normal and continues through adolescence, which results in a pseudo-prognathic appearance by the completion of growth [75].

The midfacial deficiency in these children is usually corrected by a Le Fort III osteotomy. It can be corrected as early as age 6 or in late childhood, depending on the indications. Psychosocial considerations or upper airway obstruction documented by sleep studies would be the main indications for early midface advancement; otherwise surgery should be postponed until midfacial growth is completed (10–12 years). Studies by Kaban and colleagues [76] and Mc Carthy and colleagues [77]on early correction of midfacial hypoplasia in syndromic craniosynostosis showed that the midface and orbital position were stable, but recurrent class III occlusion developed in most patients because of inadequate midface growth in relation to a normal growing mandible. Mulliken and colleagues [78] recommended that correction of orbital hypertelorism be delayed until growth is near completion because they noticed significant impairment of midfacial growth in patients who underwent early correction of orbital hypertelorism.

A Le Fort III facial osteotomy can improve the globe position, correct the infraorbital, zygomatic, and maxillary deficiency, and increase nasal length. If there is deficiency of the supraorbital ridge and the frontal region along with the midface deficiency, then a monobloc procedure, which helps to advance the orbits and the midface as a unit, would be preferred [79]. In some cases where midfacial hypoplasia is associated with hypertelorism, a facial partition procedure may be indicated. Large midface advancements have been performed successfully with internal and external distraction devices after Le Fort III osteotomies. The main advantage is the possibility of advancement without bone grafts, which decreases surgical morbidity [80,81].

While advancing the midface, care must be taken to avoid the irregularities at the lateral orbital rims and the nasal root, avoid excessive nasal length, and prevent enophthalmos caused by orbital enlargement. The degree of advancement required at the infraorbital level and maxillary occlusal level is different. Obwegesser [28] described the versatility of the combined Le Fort I and Le Fort III level osteotomy to correct the occlusion and midface deficiency simultaneously. These operations can be staged so that midface advancement by a Le Fort III osteotomy can be completed by the age of 10 to 12 years and the maxillomandibular relationship and class III malocclusion can be corrected at the end of skeletal maturity by a Le Fort I level osteotomy. The Le Fort I osteotomy is performed to advance, inferiorly reposition, and expand the maxilla when necessary and may be combined with a genioplasty and a mandibular ramus osteotomy in some cases.

Summary

Orthognathic surgery is a critical component of surgical management of craniofacial deformities such as CLP, craniofacial dysostoses, and mandibulofacial dysostoses. These operations can correct discrepancy in jaw relationship and malocclusion, relieve airway obstruction, correct facial asymmetry, optimize facial aesthetics, improve speech articulation, improve ability to masticate, and enhance psychological development and social interaction. It is generally performed after completion of growth; however, in selective cases it may be considered earlier to address functional and psychosocial problems. Oral and maxillofacial surgeons who treat these deformities should be part of a craniofacial team to provide interdisciplinary care for the patient. Distraction osteogenesis is a useful technique in the management of severe craniofacial deformities but does not replace conventional orthognathic surgery, which is safe and predictable. Recent advances in three-dimensional imaging and planning tools have made it possible to plan surgery more accurately and predictably.

References

[1] Binaghi S, Gudinchet F, Rilliet B. Three-dimensional spiral CT of craniofacial malformations in children. Pediatr Radiol 2000;30:856.

[2] Sailer HF, Haers PE, Zollikofer CP, et al. The value of stereolithographic models for preoperative diagnosis of craniofacial deformities and planning of surgical corrections. Int J Oral Maxillofac Surg 1998;27:327–33.

[3] Chang SC, Liao YF, Hung LM, et al. Prefabricated implants or grafts with reverse models of three-dimensional mirror-image templates for reconstruction of craniofacial abnormalities. Plast Reconstr Surg 1999;104:1413.

[4] Troulis MJ, Everett P, Seldin EB, et al. Development of a three-dimensional treatment planning system based on computed tomographic data. Int J Oral Maxillofac Surg 2002;31:349.

[5] Xia J, Samman N, Yeung RW, et al. Three-dimensional virtual reality surgical planning and simulation work bench for orthognathic surgery. Int J Adult Orthodon Orthognath Surg 2000;15:265.

[6] Kaban LB, Moses MH, Mulliken JB. Surgical correction of hemifacial microsomia in the growing child. Plast Reconstr Surg 1988;82:9.

[7] Freihofer Jr HP. Results of osteotomies of the facial skeleton in adolescence. J Maxillofac Surg 1977;5:267.

[8] Wolford LM, Karras SC, Mehra P. Considerations for orthognathic surgery during growth, Part 2. Maxillary deformities. Am J Orthod Dentofacial Orthop 2001; 119:102.

[9] Molina F, Ortiz-Monasterio F, de La Paz Aguilar M. Maxillary distraction: aesthetic and functional benefits in cleft lip–palate and prognathic patients during mixed dentition. Plast Reconstr Surg 1998;101(4):951–63.

[10] Figueroa AA, Polley JW, Friede H, et al. Long-term skeletal stability after maxillary advancement with distraction osteogenesis using a rigid external distraction device in cleft maxillary deformities. Plast Reconstr Surg 2004;114:1382.

[11] Wiltfang J, Hirschfelder U, Neukam FW, et al. Long-term results of distraction osteogenesis of the maxilla and midface. Br J Oral Maxillofac Surg 2002; 40:473.

[12] Silvestri A, Natali G, Iannetti G. Functional therapy in hemifacial microsomia: therapeutic protocol for growing children. J Oral Maxillofac Surg 1996;54:278.

[13] Tindlund RS. Skeletal response to maxillary protraction in patients with cleft lip and palate before the age 10 years. Cleft Palate Craniofac J 1994;31:295–308.

[14] Vig K, Turvey TA. Orthodontic-surgical interaction in the management of cleft lip and palate. Clin Plast Surg 1985;12:735–48.

[15] Evans CA. Orthodontic treatment for patients with clefts. Clin Plast Surg 2004;31:271–90.

[16] Friede H. Growth sites and growth mechanisms at risk in cleft lip and palate. Acta Odontol Scand 1998; 56:346.

[17] Horswell BB, Levant BA. Craniofacial growth in unilateral cleft lip and palate: skeletal growth from eight to eighteen years. Cleft Palate J 1988;25:114.

[18] Ross RB. Treatment variables affecting facial growth in complete unilateral cleft lip and palate. Cleft Palate J 1987;24:5.

[19] Shetye PR. Facial growth of adults with unoperated clefts. Clin Plast Surg 2004;31:361.

[20] Smahel Z, Betincova L, Mullerova Z, et al. Facial growth and development in unilateral complete cleft lip and palate from palate surgery up to adulthood. J Craniofac Genet Dev Biol 1993;13:57.

[21] Facial growth in orofacial clefting disorders. In: Vig K, Turvey T, Fonseca RJ, editors. Facial clefts and craniosynostosis: priniciples and management. Philadelphia: WB Saunders; 1996. p. 28–56.

[22] DeLuke DM, Marchand A, Robles EC, et al. Facial growth and the need for orthognathic surgery after cleft palate repair: literature review and report of 28 cases. J Oral Maxillofac Surg 1997;55:694.

[23] Rosenstein S, Kernahan D, Dado D, et al. Orthognathic surgery in cleft patients treated by early bone grafting. Plast Reconstr Surg 1991;87:835.

[24] Posnick JC, Ricalde P. Cleft-orthognathic surgery. Clin Plast Surg 2004;31:315.

[25] Oberoi SL, Chigurupati R, Vargervik K. Morphologic and management characteristics of UCLP patients who required maxillary advancement surgery. Presented at the 62nd Annual Meeting of the ACPA. Myrtle Beach, SC, April 4–9, 2005

[26] Axhausen G. Zur behandlung veralteter disloziert geheilter oberkieferbruche. Dtsch Zahn Mund n Kieferheilk 1934;1:334.

[27] Gilles H, Rowe NL. L'osteotomie du maxillaire superieur envisagee essentiellement dans les cas de bec-de-lievre total. Rev Stomatol Chir Maxillofac 1954;55:545.

[28] Obwegesser H. Surgical correction of small or retro-displaced maxillae: the dish face deformity. Plast Reconstr Surg 1969;43:351.

[29] Henderson D, Jackson IT. Naso-maxillary hypoplasia: the Le Fort II osteotomy. Br J Oral Surg 1973;11:77.

[30] Chin M, Toth BA. Distraction osteogenesis in maxil-

[30] lofacial surgery using internal devices: review of five cases. J Oral Maxillofac Surg 1996;54:45.
[31] Polley JW, Figueroa AA. Rigid external distraction: its application in cleft maxillary deformities. Plast Reconstr Surg 1998;102:1360.
[32] Herber SC, Lehman JA. Orthognathic surgery in the cleft lip and palate patient. Clin Plast Surg 1993;20:755.
[33] Tideman H, Stoelinga P, Gallia L. Le Fort I advancement with segmental palatal osteotomies in patients with cleft palates. J Oral Surg 1980;38:196.
[34] Poole MD, Robinson PP, Nunn ME. Maxillary advancement in cleft palate patients: a modification of the Le Fort I osteotomy and preliminary results. J Maxillofac Surg 1986;14:123.
[35] James D, Brook K. Maxillary hypoplasia in patients with cleft lip and palate deformity: the alternative surgical approach. Eur J Orthop 1985;7:231.
[36] Westbrook Jr MT, West RA, Mc Neil RW. Simultaneous maxillary advancement and closure of alveolar clefts and oro-nasal fistulas. J Oral Maxillofac Surg 1983;41:257.
[37] Posnick JC, Tompson B. Modification of the maxillary Le Fort I osteotomy in cleft-orthognathic surgery: the unilateral cleft lip and palate deformity. J Oral Maxillofac Surg 1992;50:666.
[38] Posnick JC, Tompson B. Modification of the maxillary Le Fort I osteotomy in cleft-orthognathic surgery: the bilateral cleft lip and palate deformity. J Oral Maxillofac Surg 1993;51:2.
[39] Norholdt SE, Sindet-Pedersen S, Jensen J. An extended Le Fort I osteotomy for correction of midface hypoplasia. J Oral Maxillofac Surg 1996;54:1297–304.
[40] Willmar K. On Le Fort I osteotomy: a follow up study of 106 operated patients with maxillofacial deformity. Scand J Plast Reconstr Surg 1974;12(Suppl):1.
[41] Houston WJ, James DR, Jones E, et al. Le Fort I maxillary osteotomies in cleft palate cases: surgical changes and stability. J Craniomaxillofac Surg 1989;17:9.
[42] Posnick JC, Dagys AP. Skeletal stability and relapse patterns after Le Fort I maxillary osteotomy fixed with miniplates: the unilateral cleft lip and palate deformity. Plast Reconstr Surg 1994;94:924–32.
[43] Cheung LK, Samman N, Hui E, et al. The 3-dimensional stability of maxillary osteotomies in cleft palate patients with residual alveolar clefts. Br J Oral Maxillofac Surg 1994;32(1):6–12.
[44] Heliovaara A, Ranta R, Hukki J, et al. Skeletal stability of Le Fort I osteotomy in patients with unilateral cleft lip and palate. Scand J Plast Reconstr Surg Hand Surg 2001;35:43.
[45] Eskenazi LB, Schendel SA. Analysis of Le Fort I maxillary advancement in cleft lip and palate patients. Plast Reconstr Surg 1992;90:779–86.
[46] Freihofer Jr HP. The lip profile after correction of retromaxillism in cleft and non-cleft patients. J Maxillofac Surg 1976;4:136.

[47] Hui E, Hagg EU, Tideman H. Soft tissue changes following maxillary osteotomies in cleft lip and palate and non-cleft patients. J Craniomaxillofac Surg 1994;22(3):182–6.
[48] Wolford LM. Effects of orthognathic surgery on nasal form and function in the cleft patient. Cleft Palate Craniofac J 1992;29:546.
[49] Witzel MA, Munro IR. Velopharyngeal insufficiency after maxillary advancement. Cleft Palate J 1977;14:176–80.
[50] Janulewicz J, Costello BJ, Buckley MJ, et al. The effects of Le Fort I osteotomies on velopharyngeal and speech functions in cleft patients. J Oral Maxillofac Surg 2004;62(3):308–14.
[51] Guyette TW, Polley JW, Figueroa A, et al. Changes in speech following maxillary distraction osteogenesis. Cleft Palate Craniofac J 2001;38:199–205.
[52] Harada K, Ishii Y, Ishii M, et al. Effect of maxillary distraction osteogenesis on velopharyngeal function: a pilot study. Oral Surg Oral Med Oral Pathol Oral Radiol Endod 2002;93:538.
[53] Gorlin RJ, Cohen MM, Hennekam RC. Syndromes of the head and neck. 4th edition. New York: Oxford University Press; 1990.
[54] Cohen MM, Rollnick BR, Kaye CI. Occulo-auriculo-vertebral spectrum: an updated critique. Cleft Palate J 1989;26:276.
[55] Poswillo DE. The pathogenesis of first and second branchial arch syndrome. Oral Surg 1973;35:302.
[56] Johnston MC, Bronsky PT. Animal models for human craniofacial malformations. J Craniofac Genet Dev Biol 1991;11:277.
[57] Cohen Jr MM. Variability vs "incidental findings" in the first and the second branchial arch syndrome: unilateral variants with anophthalmia. Birth Defects 1989;7:103.
[58] Pruzansky S. The external ear, mandible and other components of HFM. J Maxillofac Surg 1982;10:200.
[59] Horgan JE, Padwa BL, La Brie RA, et al. OMENS-Plus: analysis of craniofacial and extracranial anomalies in HFM. Cleft Palate Craniofac J 1995;32:405–12.
[60] Kaban LB, Mulliken JB, Murray JE. Three dimensional approach to analysis and treatment of HFM. Cleft Palate J 1981;18:90–9.
[61] Pruzansky S. Not all dwarfed mandibles are alike. Birth Defects 1969;1:120.
[62] Murray JE, Kaban LB, Mulliken JB. Analysis and treatment of hemifacial microsomia. Plast Reconstr Surg 1984;74:186–99.
[63] Kane AA, Lo IJ, Christensen GE, et al. Relationship between bone and muscles of mastication in hemifacial microsomia. Plast Reconstr Surg 1997;99:990.
[64] Rune B, Selvik G, Sarnas K-V, et al. Growth in hemifacial microsomia studied with the aid of roentgen stereophotogrammetry and metallic implants. Cleft Palate J 1981;17:128–46.
[65] Polley JW, Figueroa AA, Liou EJ, et al. Longitudinal analysis of mandibular asymmetry in hemifacial microsomia. Plast Reconstr Surg 1997;99:328.

[66] Sarnas K-V, Rune B, Aberg M. Maxillary and mandibular displacement in hemifacial microsomia: a longitudinal roentgen stereometric study of 21 patients with the aid of metallic implants. Cleft Palate Craniofac J 2004;41(3):290–303.

[67] Kearns GJ, Padwa BL, Mulliken JB, et al. Progression of facial asymmetry in hemifacial microsomia. Plast Reconstr Surg 2000;105:492.

[68] Kaban LB, Padwa BL, Mulliken JB. Surgical correction of mandibular hypoplasia in hemifacial microsomia: the case for treatment in early childhood. J Oral Maxillofac Surg 1998;56:628.

[69] Vargervik K, Ousterhout DK, Farias M. Factors affecting long-term results in hemifacial microsomia. Cleft Palate J 1986;23(Suppl 1):53.

[70] Posnick JC. Surgical correction of mandibular hypoplasia in hemifacial microsomia: a personal perspective. J Oral Maxillofac Surg 1998;56:639.

[71] Jabs EW, Li X, Lovett M. Genetic and physical mapping of the Treacher Collins syndrome locus with respect to loci in the chromosome 5q3 region. Genomics 1993;18:7.

[72] Anderson PJ, Netherway DJ, Abbott A, et al. Mandibular lengthening by distraction for airway obstruction in Treacher Collins syndrome: long term results. J Craniofac Surg 2004;15(1):47–50.

[73] Posnick JC, Tiwana PS, Costello BJ. Treacher Collins syndrome: comprehensive evaluation and treatment. Oral Maxillofacial Surg Clin N Am 2004;16:503–23.

[74] Roncevic R, Roncevic D. Mandibulofacial dysostosis: surgical treatment. J Craniofac Surg 1996;7(4):280–3.

[75] Posnick JC. The craniofacial dysostosis syndromes: staging of reconstruction and management of secondary deformities. Clin Plast Surg 1997;24:429.

[76] Kaban LB, West B, Conover M, et al. Midface position after Le Fort III advancement. Plast Reconstr Surg 1984;73:758.

[77] McCarthy JG, Grayson B, Bookstein F, et al. Le Fort III advancement osteotomy in the growing child. Plast Reconstr Surg 1984;74:343.

[78] Mulliken JB, Kaban LB, Evans CA, et al. Facial skeletal changes following hypertelorbitism correction. Plast Reconstr Surg 1986;77:7.

[79] Ortiz-Monasterio F, del Campo AF, Carrillo A. Advancement of the orbits and the midface in one piece, combined with frontal repositioning, for the correction of Crouzon's deformities. Plast Reconstr Surg 1978;61:507.

[80] Chin M, Toth BA. Le Fort III advancement with gradual distraction using internal devices. Plast Reconstr Surg 1997;100:819–32.

[81] Holmes AD, Wright GW, Meara JG, et al. Le Fort III internal distraction in syndromic craniosynostosis. J Craniofac Surg 2002;13:262–72.

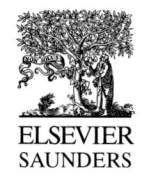

Cumulative Index 2005

Note: Page numbers of article titles are in **boldface** type.

A

Abdominal injuries, in child abuse and neglect, 439–440

Acral lentiginous malignant melanoma, growth patterns in, 137, 199

Actinic keratoses, and squamous cell carcinoma, 134, 147–151
　management of
　　chemical peels in, 148
　　cryotherapy in, 147–148
　　curettage with or without electrodesiccation in, 148
　　dermabrasion in, 148
　　diclofenac sodium in, 151
　　5-fluorouracil in, 149–150
　　imiquimod in, 150
　　laser therapy in, 148–149
　　photodynamic therapy in, 149
　　retinoids in, 150

Adenomas, pleomorphic, in children, 392–393

Adhesions, submentoplasty and, 96

Adipocytes, harvesting of, for autologous fat transplantation, 101

Advancement flaps, in surgical management, of skin cancer, 210–211

Airway management
　in battlefield injuries, 331–332, 336
　in facial burns, 269–270
　in maxillofacial injuries, due to improvised explosive devices, 283

Airway problems, mandibular hypomobility and, in children, 456, 462

Alar subunit defects, skin cancer and, reconstruction of, 217, 221

Alpha viruses, in biologic warfare. *See* Bioterrorism.

Alveolar distraction osteogenesis, in children, 493–496

Amelanotic melanoma, growth patterns in, 199

Ameloblastoma in situ, in children, 405

Amifostine, for radiation injuries, due to terrorist attacks, 295

Aminolevulinic acid, in photodynamic therapy
　for actinic keratoses, 149
　for basal cell carcinoma, 153

Anchoring filaments, in suture suspension lifts, 69–70, 75

Anesthesia
　in autologous fat transplantation, 101
　in children, rheumatoid arthritis and, 470
　with facial fillers, 21–23

Aneurysmal bone cysts, in children, 403

Angiogenesis, in wound healing, 243

Ankylosis, and mandibular hypomobility, in children, 464

Anthrax, in bioterrorism. *See* Bioterrorism.

Antibiotics
　for plague, 312–313
　for Q fever, 320
　for tularemia, 317
　in surgical management, of skin cancer, 229, 232
　in wound management, of skin cancer, 182

Antimetabolites, in scar management, 186

Antiptosis suture threads, in suture suspension lifts. *See* Suture suspension lifts.

Antisepsis, in surgical management, of skin cancer, 229, 231

Arenavirus. *See* Bioterrorism, viral hemorrhagic fevers in.

Argentine hemorrhagic fever. *See* Bioterrorism, viral hemorrhagic fevers in.

Arthritis, rheumatoid, in children. *See* Rheumatoid arthritis.

Arthrogryposis, and mandibular hypomobility, in children, 460–461

Arthrotomy, gap, for mandibular hypomobility, in children, 463–464

Asphyxiation, in inhalation burns, 268–269

Auricularis muscles, anatomy and function of, 7–8

Autologous fat augmentation, in scar management, 187

Autologous fat transplantation, for facial volume loss. *See* Facial volume loss.

Avanta facial implants, **29–39**
    complications of, 36–37
    for glabellar lines, 36
    for mandibulolabial folds, 36
    for nasolabial folds, 35–36
    Gore-Tex in, 29–30
    measurement of, 32–33
    patient selection for, 31–32
    placement of, 32
    postoperative care for, 34–35
    technique for, 33–34

Avulsive gunshot wounds, healing of, 247

B

Baby bottle decay, child neglect and, 442

Bacillus anthracis. See Bioterrorism, anthrax in.

Ballistic injuries, **251–259**
    at close range versus distance, 257–258
    caliber of projectile in, 251–252
    exit versus entrance wounds in, 258
    full metal jacketed bullets in, 254–255
    high-velocity projectiles in, 255–256
        versus low-velocity projectiles, 252–254
        yaw in, 256–257
    magnum cartridges in, 252
    sterility of projectiles in, 258

Basal cell carcinoma. *See also* Skin cancer.
    etiology of, 134
    management of
        cryotherapy in, 152
        electrodesiccation and curettage in, 152
        excision in, 151
        5-fluorouracil in, 153
        imiquimod in, 154
        interferons in, 153–154
        laser therapy in, 152–153
        Mohs' micrographic surgery in, 151–152
        photodynamic therapy in, 153
        radiation therapy in, 153
        retinoids in, 154
        surgical. *See* Skin cancer, surgical management of.
    metastatic rate of, 138
    pathology and histopathology of, 136
    risk factors for, 138

Bicarbonate
    for radiation injuries, due to terrorist attacks, 295
    in facial liposuction, 87–88

Bilobe flaps, in surgical management, of skin cancer, 221

Biologic warfare. *See* Bioterrorism.

Biopsy
    of fibrous dysplasia, in children, 418
    of skin cancer, **143–146**
        incisional and excisional biopsy, 143, 145–146, 199–200
        punch biopsy, 143, 144–145
        shave biopsy, 143–144
    sentinel lymph node, of malignant melanoma, 139, 157, 200–201

Bioterrorism, **299–330**
    alpha viruses in, 324
        clinical features of, 324
        diagnosis of, 324
        infection control and prevention in, 324
        management of, 324
        virology of, 324
    and oral and maxillofacial surgeon, 324–325
    anthrax in, 306–311
        anthrax meningitis, 308
        cutaneous, 307, 308, 309
        diagnosis of, 308–309
        differential diagnosis of, 308–309
        epidemiology of, 306–307
        gastrointestinal, 307–308
        historical aspects of, 300, 306
        infection control and prevention in, 309–311
        inhalational, 308, 309–311
        management of, 309
        microbiology of, 307–308
    biologic weapons proliferation in, 300–301
    botulinum toxin in, 313–315
        diagnosis of, 315
        differential diagnosis of, 315
        epidemiology of, 313–314
        historical aspects of, 313
        infection control and prevention in, 315
        management of, 315

microbiology of, 314
pathogenesis and clinical features of, 314
brucellosis in, 320–321
diagnosis of, 321
epidemiology of, 321
historical aspects of, 320
management of, 321
microbiology of, 321
pathogenesis and clinical features of, 321
future directions in, 325–326
future threats of, assessment of, 326
historical aspects of, 299–300
Internet resources on, 326
plague in, 311–313
bubonic, 312
diagnosis of, 312
epidemiology of, 311
historical aspects of, 311
infection control and prevention in, 313
management of, 312–313
microbiology of, 311
pathogenesis and clinical features of, 311–312
plague meningitis, 312
pneumonic, 312
septicemic, 312
public health issues in, 325
Q fever in, 319–320
diagnosis of, 320
epidemiology of, 319
historical aspects of, 319
infection control and prevention in, 320
management of, 320
microbiology of, 319–320
pathogenesis and clinical features of, 320
ricin in, 321–323
diagnosis of, 323
historical aspects of, 300
infection control and prevention in, 323
management of, 323
pathogenesis and clinical features of, 323
toxicology of, 321–323
smallpox in, 301–306
diagnosis of, 303–304
differential diagnosis of, 304
epidemiology of, 301–302
historical aspects of, 299, 301
infection control and prevention in, 304–306
management of, 304
microbiology of, 302
otologic, nasal, and ocular complications of, 303
pathogenesis and clinical features of, 302–303
post-event sequelae of, 306
vaccination for, 305–306

staphylococcal enterotoxin B in, 323–324
clinical features of, 323
diagnosis of, 323
historical aspects of, 323
infection control and prevention in, 323
management of, 323
toxicology of, 323
tularemia in, 315–318
diagnosis of, 317
differential diagnosis of, 317
epidemiology of, 316
historical aspects of, 315
infection control and prevention in, 317–318
management of, 317
microbiology of, 316
pathogenesis and clinical features of, 316
viral hemorrhagic fevers in, 318–319
diagnosis of, 318
differential diagnosis of, 318
historical aspects of, 318
infection control and prevention in, 319
management of, 318–319
pathogenesis and clinical features of, 318
virology of, 318

Bisphosphonates, for fibrous dysplasia, in children, 421

Bite marks, in child abuse and neglect, 438

Blast injuries
healing of, 245–246
radiation and, due to terrorist attacks, 293

Bleomycin, in scar management, 186

Blood loss, intraoperative, hemoglobin-based oxygen carriers for, 264

Blood substitutes, hemoglobin-based oxygen carriers as. *See* Hemoglobin-based oxygen carriers.

Bolivian hemorrhagic fever. *See* Bioterrorism, viral hemorrhagic fevers in.

Bombings, suicide
in terrorist attacks, 277–279
maxillofacial injuries due to, 282

Bone cavities, idiopathic, in children, 405–406

Bone cysts, aneurysmal, in children, 403

Bone scans, of mandibular hypomobility, in children, 458

Bones, battlefield injuries of, 338

Botox injections, **41–49**
for nasolabial folds, 42–44
for perioral rhytids, 44–45

in depressor anguli oris muscle, 48
in mentalis muscle, 45–48

Botulinum toxin, in bioterrorism. *See* Bioterrorism.

Botulinum toxin A injections. *See* Botox injections.

Bovine collagen, for facial rhytids, 17–19

Bowen's disease
and squamous cell carcinoma, 134
management of
5-fluorouracil in, 155–156
imiquimod in, 156
laser therapy in, 155
photodynamic therapy in, 155

Brazilian hemorrhagic fever. *See* Bioterrorism, viral hemorrhagic fevers in.

Brucellosis, in bioterrorism. *See* Bioterrorism.

Bruises, in child abuse and neglect, 437

Bubonic plague, in bioterrorism, 312

Buccinator muscle, anatomy and function of, 10–12

Burn-related injuries, due to improvised explosive devices, 284

Burns
facial. *See* Facial burns.
in child abuse and neglect, 438–439

C

Calcifying odontogenic cysts, in children, 403–404

Calcium channel blockers, in scar management, 186

Camouflage therapy, in scar management, 187–188

Canine smile pattern, Botox injections for, 42

Canines, maxillary, impacted, in children, 366–367

Capillary hemangiomas, in children, 388

Carac, for actinic keratoses, 150

Carbon dioxide laser therapy
for actinic keratoses, 149
for basal cell carcinoma, 152–153

Carnoy's solution, for odontogenic keratocysts, in children, 409

Cheek defects, skin cancer and, reconstruction of, 212–216

Cheeks
autologous fat transplantation in, 104–105
facial implants for, 78–82
suture suspension lifts of, 72–74

Chemical injuries, in inhalation burns, 269

Chemical peels, for actinic keratoses, 148

Chemicals, and skin cancer, 134

Chemotherapy, for malignant melanoma, 157

Cherubism, in children. *See* Fibro-osseous lesions.

Chickenpox, versus smallpox, 304

Child abuse and neglect
abdominal injuries in, 439–440
baby bottle decay in, 442
behavioral signs of, 441–442
child protective services for, 443
fractures in, 440–441
head injuries in, 439
oral aspects of, **435–445**
bite marks, 438
burns, 438–439
cutaneous injuries, 437
epidemiology of, 436
initial evaluation of, 435–436
lacerations of upper labial frenulum, 438
missed injuries, 436–437
tooth luxations and avulsions, 438
oral surgeon's legal issues in, 443–444
psychological neglect in, 442–443
sexual abuse in, 441

Chin, facial implants for, 82–83

Choristomas, in children, 391

Cleft lip and palate, in children
and distraction osteogenesis, 488, 489–491
impacted teeth with, 369–370
orthognathic surgery for. *See* Orthognathic surgery.

Cleidocranial dysostosis, in children, impacted teeth with, 372

Clostridium botulinum. *See* Bioterrorism, botulinum toxin in.

Collagen
for facial rhytids, 17–19
percutaneous. *See* Percutaneous collagen induction.

Collagen augmentation, in scar management, 187

Colony-stimulating factors, for radiation injuries, due to terrorist attacks, 295

Compression injuries, healing of, 245

Computed tomography, in children
of fibrous dysplasia, 418
of juvenile ossifying fibromas, 429

of mandibular hypomobility, 458
of ramus-condyle unit fractures, 448

Condyloma acuminatum, in children, 395–396
sexual abuse and, 441

Cone beam computed tomography, of impacted teeth, in children, 370–371

Congenital epulis, of newborns, 386–387

Congenital nevi, and malignant melanoma, 135

Contact burns, in child abuse and neglect, 438

Contour excision, of fibrous dysplasia, in children, 419–420

Coronal flaps, for maxillofacial fractures, 350–351

Coronoid process, hypertrophy of, and mandibular hypomobility, in children, 458

Corrugator supercilii muscle, anatomy and function of, 3–4

Cosmetic surgery
for posttraumatic scars, 353–354
hemoglobin-based oxygen carriers in, 264
legal issues in, **123–127**
documentation, 124–125
informed consent, 124
past patient history, 123–124
patient preparation, 124
patient refunds and releases, 126
postoperative communication, 125
surgical complications, 125–126

Cosmetic tattooing, in scar management, 187–188

Cosmoderm, for facial rhytids, 19

Cosmoplex, for facial rhytids, 19

Costochondral grafts, in children
for craniofacial microsomia, 483
for mandibular hypomobility, 464
for rheumatoid arthritis, 471

Coxiella burnetii. See Bioterrorism, Q fever in.

Craniofacial dysostosis, in children, orthognathic surgery for, 514

Craniofacial microsomia, in children, distraction osteogenesis for, 481–483

Craniofacial plates, for maxillary fractures, due to battlefield injuries, 334–335

Craniofacial syndromes, in children, impacted teeth with, 371–372

Crimean Congo hemorrhagic fever. See Bioterrorism, viral hemorrhagic fevers in.

Cryopreservation, of fat, for autologous transplantation, 108

Cryotherapy
for actinic keratoses, 147–148
for basal cell carcinoma, 152
for squamous cell carcinoma, 155

Curettage, with electrodesiccation. See Electrodesiccation and curettage.

Cutaneous anthrax, in bioterrorism, 307, 308, 309

Cutaneous injuries, in child abuse and neglect, 437

Cystic hygromas, in children, 390

Cysts, of jaws, in children. See Jaws.

Cytokines, for radiation injuries, due to terrorist attacks, 295

D

Deer fly fever. See Bioterrorism, tularemia in.

Dengue fever. See Bioterrorism, viral hemorrhagic fevers in.

Dental implants. See Endosseous implants.

Dentigerous cysts, in children, 404–405

Depressor and adductor muscle of brow, anatomy and function of, 3–4

Depressor anguli oris muscle
anatomy and function of, 12
Botox injections in, 48

Depressor labii inferioris muscle, anatomy and function of, 12

Depressor muscle of angle of mouth
anatomy and function of, 12
Botox injections in, 48

Depressor muscle of brow, anatomy and function of, 3

Depressor muscle of brow and eyelid, anatomy and function of, 4–5

Depressor muscle of lip, anatomy and function of, 12, 13–14

Depressor muscle of nose, anatomy and function of, 9

Depressor septi muscle, anatomy and function of, 9

Dermabrasion
for actinic keratoses, 148
in skin resurfacing, 184–185

Dermatology, maxillofacial.
   See Maxillofacial dermatology.

Diclofenac sodium, for actinic keratoses, 151

Diethyleneaminepenta-acetate, for radiation injuries, due to terrorist attacks, 295

Dilator and compressor muscle of nares, anatomy and function of, 8–9

Dilator muscle of nares
   anatomy and function of, 9
   Botox injections in, 42, 44

Distraction osteogenesis, in children, **475–484**
   activation phase in, 476
   biological basis of, 475–476
   consolidation phase in, 476
   control of skeletal movements in, 477
   effects on soft tissue structures, 477
   for mandibular hypomobility, 464–465
   for rheumatoid arthritis, 471–472
   historical aspects of, 475
   indications for, 476–483
      craniofacial microsomia, 481–483
      mandibular hypoplasia/micrognathia, 480–481
   latency phase in, 476
   of midface, **485–501**
      across midpalatal suture, 488–489
      alveolar distraction in, 493–496
      endosseous implants in, 496–498
      future directions in, 498
      high level Le Fort I osteogenesis in, 491–493
      historical aspects of, 485–486
      indications for, 487–488
      irregularly shaped membranous bones in, 486–487
      risks of, 488
      tubular long bones in, 486
      with cleft lip and palate, 488, 489–491
   postoperative care for, 479

Drool lines, Avanta facial implants for, 36

Dysplastic nevi, and malignant melanoma, 135

E

Ear defects, skin cancer and, surgical management of, 229

Eastern equine encephalitis. *See* Bioterrorism, staphylococcal enterotoxin B in.

Ebola virus. *See* Bioterrorism, viral hemorrhagic fevers in.

Ectodermal dysplasia, in children, and endosseous implants, 379–380

Electrodesiccation and curettage
   for actinic keratoses, 148
   for basal cell carcinoma, 152
   for skin cancer, 138
   for squamous cell carcinoma, 155

Elevator muscle of angle of mouth, anatomy and function of, 9

Elevator muscle of brow, anatomy and function of, 3

Elevator muscle of lip
   anatomy and function of, 9
   Botox injections in, 42, 44

Elevator muscle of lower lip and chin
   anatomy and function of, 13
   Botox injections in, 45–48

Elevator muscle of mouth, anatomy and function of, 9–10

Elevator muscle of upper eyelid, anatomy and function of, 5–7

Embolization, autologous fat transplantation and, 108

Endosseous implants, in children, **375–381**
   animal studies of, 377–379
   facial growth and, 375–376
      mandibular, 376
      maxillary, 375–376
   in distraction osteogenesis, 496–498
   indications for, 380
   results of, 380–381
   with ectodermal dysplasia, 379–380

Enucleation, of odontogenic keratocysts, in children, 409

Epinephrine, in facial liposuction, 87

Epithelialization, in wound healing, 243–244

Epulis, congenital, of newborns, 386–387

Eruption cysts, in children, 405

Er:YAG laser therapy, for actinic keratoses, 149

Excisional biopsy, of skin cancer, 143, 145–146, 199–200

Expanded polytetrafluoroethylene, in facial implants, 29–30

Extracapsular tissues, tumors of, and mandibular hypomobility, in children, 459–460

Extracorporeal membrane oxygenation, hemoglobin-based oxygen carriers in, 264

Extravasation mucoceles, in children, 392

Eyebrows, suture suspension lifts of, 70–72

Eyelids, facial implants for, 77

F

Face-lift
 S-Lift technique for. See S-Lift rhytidectomy.
 suture suspension technique for. See Suture suspension lifts.
 with submentoplasty, 93–95

Facial burns
 acute management of, **267–272**
  airway in, 269–270
  classification in, 267–268
  fluid loss and, 271
  inhalation injuries, 268–271
   asphyxiation in, 268–269
   chemical injuries in, 269
   thermal injuries in, 269
  initial evaluation of, 269
  ocular injuries, 270, 271
  pain control in, 271
  soft tissue injuries, 267–268
 due to battlefield injuries, 332

Facial defects, skin cancer and, reconstruction of. See Skin cancer.

Facial fillers, **17–28**
 anesthesia with, 21–23
 bovine collagen, 17–19
 complications of, 26–27
 Cosmoderm, 19
 Cosmoplast, 19
 for nasolabial folds, 25–26
 for oral commissures, 23–24
 for perioral rhytids, 25
 human cell cultured products, 19–20
 hyaluronic acid, 19, 24–25
 hydroxyapatite products, 19, 24
 patient expectations for, 20–21
 serial puncture technique for, 21
 threading technique for, 21

Facial growth, and endosseous implants, in children. See Endosseous implants.

Facial implants, **77–84**
 Avanta. See Avanta facial implants.
 for chin, 82–83
 for eyelids, 77
 for midface and malar regions, 78–79
 for perioral region, 79
 for periorbital region, 78
 for submalar region, 80–82
 for suborbital region, 78

Facial liposuction, 85–90
 complications of, 89–90
 patient assessment for, 85–86
 postoperative care for, 89
 technique for, 88–89
 tumescent solution in, 87–88
  drug interactions with, 88

Facial musculature, **1–15**
 lower third, 10–14
  buccinator, 10–12
  depressor anguli oris, 12
  depressor labii inferioris, 12
  mentalis, 13
  orbicularis oris, 12–13
  platysma, 13–14
  risorius, 10
 middle third, 7–10
  auricularis, 7–8
  depressor septi, 9
  levator anguli oris, 9
  levator labii superioris, 9
  levator labii superioris alaeque nasii, 9
  nasalis, 8–9
  zygomaticus major, 9–10
  zygomaticus minor, 10
 modiolus, 4–15
 upper third, 2–7
  corrugator supercilii, 3–4
  frontalis, 3
  in Asians versus Caucasians, 6–7
  levator palpebrae superioris, 5–7
  orbicularis oculi, 4–5
  procerus, 3

Facial volume loss
 aging and, 99–101
 autologous fat transplantation for, **99–109**
  complications of, 106–108
   cryopreservation, 108
   embolization, 108
   infections, 106–108
   weight loss/gain, 108
  fat infiltration technique for, 102–104
  fat processing for, 101–102
  future trends in, 108–109
  graft placement site in, 102
  harvesting technique for, 101
  in cheeks, 104–105

in periorbital region, 104
in temples, 105
repeat procedures in, 106

Fat transplantation, autologous, for facial volume loss. *See* Facial volume loss.

Feather Lift, technique for, 67–68

Feeding problems, mandibular hypomobility and, in children, 456

Fibroblasts, in wound healing, 243

Fibromas
in children, 383, 384–385
juvenile ossifying, in children. *See* Fibro-osseous lesions.

Fibromatosis, in children. *See* Soft tissue lesions.

Fibro-osseous lesions, in children, **415–434**
cherubism, 421–426
diagnosis of, 424–425
genetics of, 422–423
grading of, 424
histopathology of, 425
historical aspects of, 421–422
management of, 425–426
molecular analysis of, 425
molecular biology of, 424
plain films of, 425
with Noonan syndrome, 423–424
fibrous dysplasia and McCune-Albright syndrome, 415–421
biopsy of, 418
bisphosphonates for, 421
computed tomography of, 418
contour excision of, 419–420
diagnosis of, 417–419
forms of, 416
genetic tests for, 418–419
historical aspects of, 415
laboratory tests for, 418
magnetic resonance imaging of, 418
management of, 419–421
molecular biology of, 416–417
optic nerve decompression for, 420–421
plain films of, 417–418
juvenile ossifying fibromas, 426–429
computed tomography of, 429
diagnosis of, 426, 429
historical aspects of, 426
magnetic resonance imaging of, 429
management of, 429
molecular biology of, 426
plain films of, 429

osteoblastomas, 429–431
diagnosis of, 430
management of, 431

Fibrosarcomas, infantile, 399

Fibrosis, of hard and soft tissues, avoidance of, in maxillofacial trauma, 351, 353

Fibrous dysplasia, in children. *See* Fibro-osseous lesions.

Firearm injuries
healing of, 246–249
in terrorist attacks, 276–277

Flail mandibular segment, due to improvised explosive devices, 285

Flaps
coronal, for maxillofacial fractures, 350–351
for cleft lip and palate, in children, 369
in maxillofacial dermatology, 180–181
in surgical management, of skin cancer, 207, 210–212, 213, 221, 224, 225, 227, 229

Flashlamp-pumped pulse-dye lasers, in skin resurfacing, 184

Fluid loss, in facial burns, 271

5-Fluorouracil
for actinic keratoses, 149–150
for basal cell carcinoma, 153
for Bowen's disease, 155–156
for squamous cell carcinoma, 155–156
in scar management, 186

Focal epithelial hyperplasia, in children, 395

Follicular cysts, in children, 404–405

Forehead defects, skin cancer and, reconstruction of. *See* Skin cancer.

Fractures
in child abuse and neglect, 440–441
mandibular, due to battlefield injuries, 333
maxillary, due to battlefield injuries, 333–335
of ramus-condyle unit, in children. *See* Ramus-condyle unit fractures.
traumatic maxillofacial, management of, 348–351
zygomaticomaxillary complex, due to battlefield injuries, 334

Fragmentation injuries, contaminated, due to improvised explosive devices, 283–284, 286

Francisella tularensis. *See* Bioterrorism, tularemia in.

Frontalis muscle, anatomy and function of, 3

Fusiform technique, in scar excision, 177, 179

G

Gap arthrotomy, for mandibular hypomobility, in children, 463–464

Gastrointestinal anthrax, in bioterrorism, 307–308

Gastrointestinal syndrome, radiation and, due to terrorist attacks, 294

Genetic tests, for fibrous dysplasia, in children, 418–419

Genioplasty, for rheumatoid arthritis, in children, 471

Geometric designs, in scar excision, 179–180

Giant cell fibromas, in children, 383

Gingival cysts, in children, 405

Gingival fibromatosis, hereditary, in children, 387

Glabellar lines, Avanta facial implants for, 36

Glandular tularemia, in bioterrorism, 316

Gore-Tex, in facial implants, 29–30

Gorlin-Goltz syndrome. See Nevoid basal cell carcinoma syndrome.

Grafts
costochondral, in children. See Costochondral grafts.
skin, in surgical management, of skin cancer, 225, 229

Granulomas
peripheral giant cell, in children, 385–386
pyogenic, in children, 383–384

Growth factors, in wound healing, 242

Gummy smile pattern, Botox injections for, 42

Gunshot wounds
healing of. See Wound healing.
in terrorist attacks, 276–277

H

Hanta virus. See Bioterrorism, viral hemorrhagic fevers in.

Hard tissue fibrosis, avoidance of, in maxillofacial trauma, 351, 353

HBOC-201, indications for, 261–264

Head injuries, in child abuse and neglect, 439

Healing, wound. See Wound healing.

Hearing loss, due to battlefield injuries, 335

Heck's disease, in children, 395

Hemangiomas, in children, 388, 389

Hematomas
septal, due to battlefield injuries, 334
submentoplasty and, 96

Hematopoietic syndrome, radiation and, due to terrorist attacks, 294

Hemifacial microsomia, in children, orthognathic surgery for, 511–513

Hemoglobin-based oxygen carriers, **261–266**
after hemodilution, 264
and increase in vascular resistance, 262
for intraoperative blood loss, 264
for septic shock, 262
HBOC-201, 261–264
immune response to, 263
immunomodulatory effects of, 263
in elective surgery, 263–264
in extracorporeal membrane oxygenation, 264
in military versus civilian settings, 261
in patients with religious objections, 264
in plastic surgery, 264
PolyHeme, 262, 263
versus lactated Ringer's solution, 262, 263
versus standard resuscitation regimens, 262

Hemorrhagic fevers, viral, in bioterrorism. See Bioterrorism.

Hemostasis, in wound healing, 242–243

Hereditary gingival fibromatosis, in children, 387

Herpes simplex infections, in children, sexual abuse and, 441

Human cell cultured products, for facial rhytids, 19–20

Human papillomavirus infections, in children, sexual abuse and, 441

Hyaluronic acid, for facial rhytids, 19, 24–25

Hypertrophic scars, versus keloids, 177, 184

I

Idiopathic bone cavities, in children, 405–406

Imiquimod
for actinic keratoses, 150
for basal cell carcinoma, 154
for Bowen's disease, 156
for squamous cell carcinoma, 156

Immunocompromised patients, Mohs' micrographic surgery in, 163

Impacted teeth, in children, **365–373**
    cone beam computed tomography of, 370–371
    etiology of, 365
    incidence of, 365–366
    mandibular premolars, 367
    maxillary canines, 366–367
    maxillary incisors, 368
    molars, 368
    supernumerary teeth, 368–369
    with cleft lip and palate, 369–370
    with craniofacial syndromes, 371–372

Implants, endosseous. See Endosseous implants.

Improvised explosive devices, maxillofacial injuries due to, **281–287**
    airway management in, 283
    burn-related injuries, 284
    classes of injuries, 283
    contaminated fragmentation injuries, 283–284, 286
    flail mandibular segment, 285
    imaging of, 283
    ophthalmologic consultation for, 285
    package-type devices, 281
    suicide bombs, 282
    vehicle-borne devices, 281

Incisional biopsy, of skin cancer, 143, 145–146, 199–200

Incisors, maxillary, impacted, in children, 368

Infections, autologous fat transplantation and, 106–108

Infectious disease consultations, in treatment planning, for maxillofacial trauma, 343, 345–346

Inflammation, in wound healing, 242–243

Inhalation burns, management of. See Facial burns.

Inhalational anthrax, in bioterrorism, 308, 309–311

Interferons, for basal cell carcinoma, 153–154

Interleukins, for malignant melanoma, 157

Inverted L-osteotomy, for rheumatoid arthritis, in children, 471

J

Jaw components, fusion of, and mandibular hypomobility, in children, 460

Jaws, cysts of, in children, 403–411
    aneurysmal bone cysts, 403
    calcifying odontogenic cysts, 403–404
    classification of, 404
    dentigerous cysts, 404–405
    eruption cysts, 405
    gingival cysts, 405
    idiopathic bone cavities, 405–406
    lateral periodontal cysts, 406–407
    nasopalatine duct cysts, 407–408
    odontogenic keratocysts.
        See Odontogenic keratocysts.
    paradental cysts, 411
    radicular cysts, 411

Jowls, suture suspension lifts of, 74–75

Junin virus. See Bioterrorism, viral hemorrhagic fevers in.

Juvenile ossifying fibromas, in children. See Fibro-osseous lesions.

K

Keloids, versus hypertrophic scars, 177, 184

Keratoacanthoma, pathology of, 139, 154

L

Labial frenulum, lacerations of, in child abuse and neglect, 438

Lacerations, healing of, 245

Lactated Ringer's solution, versus hemoglobin-based oxygen carriers, 262, 263

Laser therapy
    for actinic keratoses, 148–149
    for basal cell carcinoma, 152–152
    for Bowen's disease, 155
    for skin tattooing, after maxillofacial trauma, 354
    for squamous cell carcinoma, 155

Lasers, in skin resurfacing, 184–185

Lassa fever. See Bioterrorism, viral hemorrhagic fevers in.

Lateral periodontal cysts, in children, 406–407

Le Fort I osteogenesis, in children, 491–493

Le Fort I osteotomy, for cleft lip and palate, in children, 506, 509

Le Fort III osteotomy, for craniofacial dysostosis, in children, 514

Lentigo maligna
    growth patterns in, 137–138
    Mohs' micrographic surgery for, 168

Levator anguli oris muscle, anatomy and function of, 9

Levator labii superioris alaeque nasii muscle
 anatomy and function of, 9
 Botox injections in, 42, 44

Levator labii superioris muscle, anatomy and function of, 9

Levator palpebrae superioris muscle, anatomy and function of, 5–7

Lidocaine, in facial liposuction, 87

Light radiation injuries, due to terrorist attacks, 292

Lip fillers. *See* Facial fillers.

Liposuction, facial. *See* Facial liposuction.

Lips, muscles of. *See* Facial musculature.

Lobed flaps, in maxillofacial dermatology, 181

Lymph node dissection, for malignant melanoma, 139, 157, 200–201

Lymphangiomas, in children, 388, 389–390

M

Machupa virus. *See* Bioterrorism, viral hemorrhagic fevers in.

Macrophages, in wound healing, 243

Magnetic resonance imaging, in children
 of fibrous dysplasia, 418
 of juvenile ossifying fibromas, 429
 of mandibular hypomobility, 458
 of rheumatoid arthritis, 468

Malignant melanoma, **191–204**. *See also* Skin cancer.
 diagnosis of, 199
  sentinel lymph node biopsy in, 139, 157, 200–201
 etiology of, 195
  sun exposure in, 135, 195
 growth patterns in, 137, 199
 incidence of, 191–192
 management of, 138
  adjuvant chemotherapy in, 157
  cytotoxic chemotherapy in, 157
  excision in, 156–157, 199–200
  for regional lymphatics, 200–201
  for unknown primary, 201
  interleukins in, 157
  lymph node dissection in, 157
  Mohs' micrographic surgery in, 168

 nevi and, 135, 199
 pathology and histopathology of, 136–137
 prevention of, sunscreen in, 135
 prognosis for, 138
 risk factors for, 195, 199
 staging of, 139, 201–203

Mandibular fractures, due to battlefield injuries, 333

Mandibular growth, and endosseous implants, in children, 376

Mandibular hypomobility, in children, **455–466**
 anatomy and pathophysiology of, 456
 consequences of, 455–456
  airway obstruction, 456
  feeding difficulties, 456
  restriction of mandibular growth, 456
  speech and language problems, 456
 extracapsular pathology in, 458–461
  arthrogryposis, 460–461
  contracture of temporalis tendons, 458–459
  fusion of jaw components, 460
  hypertrophy of coronoid process, 458
  trauma to zygomatic complex, 459
  tumors of extracapsular tissues, 459
 history and physical examination for, 456–457
 imaging of, 457–458
 intracapsular pathology in, 461–462
  internal derangement of temporomandibular joint, 461
 management of, 462–465
  costochondral grafts for, 464
  distraction osteogenesis in, 464–465
  for airway problems, 462
  for ankylosis, 464
  for poor oral hygiene, 463
  gap arthrotomy in, 463–464
  physical therapy in, 463
  temporomandibular joint reconstruction in, 464
 nomenclature in, 455

Mandibular hypoplasia, in children, distraction osteogenesis for, 480–481

Mandibular micrognathia, in children, distraction osteogenesis for, 480–481

Mandibular premolars, impacted, in children, 367

Mandibulofacial dysostosis, in children, orthognathic surgery for, 513–514

Mandibulofacial folds, Avanta facial implants for, 36

Marburg virus. *See* Bioterrorism, viral hemorrhagic fevers in.

Marionette lines, Botox injections for, 48

Marsupialization, of odontogenic keratocysts, in children, 409

Maxillary canines, impacted, in children, 366–367

Maxillary fractures, due to battlefield injuries, 333–335

Maxillary growth, and endosseous implants, in children, 375–376

Maxillary incisors, impacted, in children, 368

Maxillofacial dermatology, secondary procedures in, **173–189**
 camouflage therapy, 187–188
 excision of scars, 177, 179–180
  fusiform and Z-plasty techniques in, 177, 179
  geometric designs in, 179–180
 flaps in, 180–181
 immediate postoperative wound management, 182–184
  antibiotics in, 182
 late postoperative wound management, 184
 medications in, 185–186
  antimetabolites, 186
  calcium channel blockers, 186
  steroids, 185
  topical, 185–186
 pressure therapy, 187
 prevention of scars, 175–176
 resurfacing, 184–185
 revision of scars, 176–177
  nature of injury and, 177
  scar location and, 176–177
  scar morphology and, 177
  timing and, 176
  wound healing history and, 177
 silicone gel sheeting, 186–187
 soft-tissue augmentation, 187
 tissue expansion, 181–182
 wound healing, 173–175
  dermatologic conditions and, 175
  host and local factors in, 174–175

Maxillofacial trauma, treatment protocol for, **341–355**
 aggressive physical and occupational therapy in, 351, 353
 coronal flaps in, 350–351
 for panfacial trauma, 350
 hard tissue base stabilization in, 347
 historical aspects of, 341
 imaging in, 342–343, 347–348
 infectious disease consultations in, 343
  cultures and sensitivities in, 345–346
 injury identification in, 342
 nutrition and speech therapy consultations in, 343
 pain management services in, 345
 patient stabilization in, 342
 physical therapy consultations in, 344–345
 posttraumatic scarring and cosmetic management in, 353–354
 primary reconstruction and fracture management in, 348–351
 psychiatric consultations in, 344
 replacement of missing soft tissue components in, 348
 secondary reconstruction in, 353
 serial debridement in, 346–347
 stereolithographic models in, 342–343, 347–348

Maxillomandibular fixation, for ramus-condyle unit fractures, in children, 448

McCune-Albright syndrome, in children. See Fibro-osseous lesions.

Melanocytic lesions, benign, and malignant melanoma, 199

Melanotic neuroectodermal tumors, of infancy, 387–388

Meningitis
 anthrax, in bioterrorism, 308
 plague, in bioterrorism, 312

Mentalis muscle
 anatomy and function of, 13
 Botox injections in, 45–48

Merkel cell tumors, pathology of, 139

Methyl aminolevulinic acid, in photodynamic therapy
 for actinic keratoses, 149
 for basal cell carcinoma, 153

Micrognathia, mandibular, in children, distraction osteogenesis for, 480–481

Microinvasive ameloblastomas, in children, 405

Micropigmentation, in scar management, 187–188

Microsomia
 craniofacial, in children, distraction osteogenesis for, 481–483
 hemifacial, in children, orthognathic surgery for, 511–513

Mixed tumors, of salivary glands, in children, 392–393

Modiolus, musculature of, anatomy and function of, 14–15

Mohs' micrographic surgery, **161–171**
  completion of, 165
  efficacy of, 169–170
  first laboratory stage in, 164–165
  first surgical stage in, 164
  for basal cell carcinoma, 151–152
  for lentigo maligna, 168
  for malignant melanoma, 168
  for squamous cell carcinoma, 155
  historical aspects of, 161–162
  in immunocompromised patients, 163
  incomplete, 165–166
  microscopic examination in, 165
  on previously radiated skin, 163–164, 166
  patient selection for, 163–164, 166
  preoperative preparation for, 164
  subsequent stages in, 165
  technique for, 162–163
  tumor location and, 168–169
  tumor type and characteristics in, 166, 168

Molars, impacted, in children, 368

Mona Lisa smile pattern, Botox injections for, 42

Morpheaform basal cell carcinoma
  pathology and histopathology of, 136
  surgical management of, 205–206

Mouth, muscles of. See Facial musculature.

Mucoceles, in children, 391–392

Mucoepidermoid carcinoma, in children, 398

Multiple endocrine neoplasia type 2b, in children, 393

Myofibromatosis, infantile, 397–398

N

Nairovirus. See Bioterrorism, viral hemorrhagic fevers in.

Nasal defects, skin cancer and, reconstruction of, 216–217, 221

Nasalis muscle, anatomy and function of, 8–9

Nasolabial folds
  Avanta facial implants for, 35–36
  Botox injections for, 42–44
  facial fillers for, 25–26

Nasopalatine duct cysts, in children, 407–408

Neuroectodermal tumors, melanotic, of infancy, 387–388

Neurovascular syndrome, radiation and, due to terrorist attacks, 294

Neutrophils, in wound healing, 242–243

Nevi, and malignant melanoma, 135, 199

Nevoid basal cell carcinoma syndrome, in children, 411–413
  diagnosis of, 412
  genetics of, 412
  historical aspects of, 411
  odontogenic keratocysts with, 412–413

Nodular basal cell carcinoma, pathology and histopathology of, 136

Nodular malignant melanoma, growth patterns in, 137, 199

Noonan syndrome, in children, cherubism with, 423–424

Nuclear terrorist attacks, radiation injuries due to. See Radiation injuries.

Nutrition consultations, in treatment planning, for maxillofacial trauma, 344

O

Occupational therapy, for maxillofacial trauma, 351, 353

Oculoglandular tularemia, in bioterrorism, 316

Odontogenic cysts, calcifying, in children, 403–404

Odontogenic keratocysts, in children, 408–411
  Carnoy's solution for, 409
  diagnosis of, 408
  enucleation of, 409
  histology of, 408–409
  immunocytochemistry of, 409–410
  marsupialization for, 409
  recurrent, 409
  with nevoid basal cell carcinoma, 412–413

OMENS classification, of hemifacial microsomia, 512

Open reduction, for ramus-condyle unit fractures, in children, 448

Operation Iraqi Freedom, injuries sustained in, **331–339**
  airway management in, 331–332, 336
  avoidance of scar contracture in, 338
  bony injuries in, 338
  craniofacial plates for, 334–335
  facial burns, 332
  imaging of, 331

initial management of: days 1 to 3, 335–336
mandibular fractures, 333
maxillary fractures, 333–335
mechanisms of, 331
otologic injuries, 335
septal hematomas, 334
soft tissue injuries, 332, 336–337
treatment planning for, 336–338
  stereolithographic model in, 336
  three-dimensional computerized reconstruction in, 336
zygomaticomaxillary complex fractures, 334

Ophthalmologic consultations, for maxillofacial injuries, due to improvised explosive devices, 285

Optic nerve decompression, for fibrous dysplasia, in children, 420–421

Oral commissures, facial fillers for, 23–24

Orbicularis oculi muscle, anatomy and function of, 4–5

Orbicularis oris muscle, anatomy and function of, 12–13

Oropharyngeal tularemia, in bioterrorism, 316

Orthodontically assisted eruption, of impacted teeth, in children with cleidocranial dysostosis, 372

Orthognathic surgery, in children, **503–517**
for cleft lip and palate, 505–511
  maxillary growth in, 505–506
  osteotomies in, 505, 509
  skeletal stability in, 509, 511
  soft tissue changes in, 511
  velopharyngeal insufficiency in, 511
for craniofacial dysostosis, 514
for hemifacial microsomia, 511–513
for mandibulofacial dysostosis, 513–514
orthodontic issues in, 504–505
preoperative planning for, 503–504
timing of, 504

Osteoblastomas, in children. *See* Fibro-osseous lesions.

Osteotomy
in children
  for cleft lip and palate, 505, 509
  for craniofacial dysostosis, 514
  for rheumatoid arthritis, 471

Otologic disorders, due to battlefield injuries, 335

P

Package-type improvised explosive devices, maxillofacial injuries due to, 281

Pain control, in facial burns, 271

Pain management services, in treatment planning, for maxillofacial trauma, 345

Pamidronate, for fibrous dysplasia, in children, 421

Panfacial trauma, maxillofacial, management of, 350

Panoramic radiographs, of impacted maxillary canines, in children, 366

Panoramic tomography, of mandibular hypomobility, in children, 457

Papillomas, in children, 395

Paradental cysts, in children, 411

Paramedian forehead flaps, in surgical management, of skin cancer, 221, 224

Penetrating gunshot wounds, healing of, 247

Penetrating radiation injuries, due to terrorist attacks, 293–294

Percutaneous collagen induction, **51–65**
advantages of, 62
appearance after, 61–62
  in darker pigmented skin, 61–62
contraindications to, 53
disadvantages of, 62
indications for, 53
mechanism of action of, 57–60
  initial injury, 57–58
  tissue proliferation, 58–59
  tissue remodeling, 59–60
postoperative care for, 60–61
results of, 62
skin preparation for, 53–55
technique for, 55–57
  needling in, 52–53

Periodontal cysts, lateral, in children, 406–407

Perioral region
Botox injections for, 44–45
facial fillers for, 25
facial implants for, 79

Periorbital defects, skin cancer and, reconstruction of. *See* Skin cancer.

Periorbital region
autologous fat transplantation in, 104
facial implants for, 78

Peripheral giant cell granulomas, in children, 385–386

Peripheral ossifying fibromas, in children, 384–385

Perlane, for facial rhytids, 24

Phlebovirus. See Bioterrorism, viral hemorrhagic fevers in.

Photodynamic therapy
 for actinic keratoses, 149
 for basal cell carcinoma, 153
 for Bowen's disease, 155
 for squamous cell carcinoma, 155

Physical therapy
 for mandibular hypomobility, in children, 463
 for maxillofacial trauma, 351, 353

Physical therapy consultations, in treatment planning, for maxillofacial trauma, 344–345

Pigmentary changes, dermabrasion and, 184

Pigmented basal cell carcinoma, pathology and histopathology of, 136

Pigmented cutaneous lesions, and malignant melanoma, 199

Plague, in bioterrorism. See Bioterrorism.

Plain films, in children
 of cherubism, 425
 of fibrous dysplasia, 417–418
 of juvenile ossifying fibromas, 429

Platysma muscle, anatomy and function of, 13–14

Pleomorphic adenomas, in children, 392–393

Plunging ranulas, in children, 392

Pneumonic plague, in bioterrorism, 312

Pneumonic tularemia, in bioterrorism, 316

PolyHeme, indications for, 262, 263

Potassium iodide, for radiation injuries, due to terrorist attacks, 296

Premalignant cutaneous tumors. See Actinic keratoses.

Premolars, mandibular, impacted, in children, 367

Pressure therapy, in scar management, 187

Procerus muscle, anatomy and function of, 3

Proliferation phase, in wound healing, 243–244

Prussian blue, for radiation injuries, due to terrorist attacks, 296

Pruzansky classification, of hemifacial microsomia, 512

Psychiatric consultations, in treatment planning, for maxillofacial trauma, 344

Pulsed dye laser therapy, for skin tattooing, after maxillofacial trauma, 354

Punch biopsy, of skin cancer, 143, 144–145

Pyogenic granulomas, in children, 383–384

Q

Q fever, in bioterrorism. See Bioterrorism.

R

Rabbit fever. See Bioterrorism, tularemia in.

Radiance FN, for facial rhytids, 19, 24

Radiation injuries, due to terrorist attacks, **289–298**
 blast injuries, 293
 fall out, 294
 from dirty bombs, 289–290
 from inside our borders, 289
 from outside our borders, 289
 gastrointestinal syndrome, 294
 hematopoietic syndrome, 294
 light radiation injuries, 292
 management of, 294–296
  amifostine in, 295
  bicarbonate in, 295
  colony-stimulating factors in, 295
  cytokines in, 295
  diethyleneaminepenta-acetate in, 295
  potassium iodide in, 296
  Prussian blue in, 296
  stem cell transplantation in, 296
 neurovascular syndrome, 294
 patient decontamination in, 290–291
 patient triage in, 291–292
 penetrating radiation injuries, 293–294
 radiation exposure in, 290
 radioactive contamination, 294
 risks for health care providers in, 290
 shock wave injuries, 293
 thermal injuries, 292

Radiation therapy
 for basal cell carcinoma, 153
 for squamous cell carcinoma, 155
 previous
  and Mohs' micrographic surgery, 163–164, 166
  and wound healing, 175

Radicular cysts, in children, 411

Ramus-condyle unit fractures, in children, **447–453**
    clinical features of, 447–448
    history and physical examination for, 447
    imaging of, 448
    management of, 448
    outcomes of, 449–452
        developmental, 449
        functional, 449
        radiographic, 449, 452

Ranulas, in children, 391–392

Relaxed skin tension lines
    in maxillofacial dermatology, 177, 179, 181
    in surgical management, of skin cancer, 207, 209–210

Remodeling phase, in wound healing, 244

Restylane, for facial rhytids, 19, 24–25

Restylane Fine Line, for facial rhytids, 24–25

Retinal hemorrhage, in child abuse and neglect, 439

Retinoids
    for actinic keratoses, 150
    for basal cell carcinoma, 154
    for squamous cell carcinoma, 156

Retractor muscle of angle of mouth, anatomy and function of, 10

Rhabdomyomas, fetal, 390–391

Rhabdomyosarcomas, in children, 398–399

Rheumatoid arthritis, in children, **467–473**
    and anesthesia, 470
    and condylar ramus height, 468–469
    and masticatory muscles, 469
    imaging of, 468
    subtypes of, 467
    surgical management of, 470–472
        mandibular, 471–472
        maxillary, 472
    temporomandibular joint therapy for, 469–470

Rhomboid flaps
    in maxillofacial dermatology, 181
    in surgical management, of skin cancer, 211–212

Rhytidectomy
    S-Lift technique for. See S-Lift rhytidectomy.
    suture suspension technique for. See Suture suspension lift.
    with submentoplasty, 93–95

Rhytids, facial fillers for. See Facial fillers.

Ricin, in bioterrorism. See Bioterrorism.

Rift Valley fever. See Bioterrorism, viral hemorrhagic fevers in.

Risorius muscle, anatomy and function of, 10

Rotation flaps, in maxillofacial dermatology, 181

S

Sabia virus. See Bioterrorism, viral hemorrhagic fevers in.

Sagittal split osteotomy, for rheumatoid arthritis, in children, 471

Scald burns, in child abuse and neglect, 438–439

Scalp defects, skin cancer and, surgical management of, 227, 229

Scar contracture, avoidance of
    in battlefield injuries, 338
    in maxillofacial trauma, 347, 351

Scars
    management of, in maxillofacial dermatology. See Maxillofacial dermatology.
    maxillofacial trauma and, cosmetic management of, 353–354

Sentinel lymph node biopsy, of malignant melanoma, 139, 157, 200–201

Septal hematomas, due to battlefield injuries, 334

Septic shock, hemoglobin-based oxygen carriers for, 262

Septicemic plague, in bioterrorism, 312

Sexual abuse, in children, 441

Sexually transmitted diseases, in children, sexual abuse and, 441

Shave biopsy, of skin cancer, 143–144

Shock wave injuries, radiation and, due to terrorist attacks, 293

Shotgun wounds, healing of, 248–249

Sialoceles, submentoplasty and, 96

Silicone gel sheeting, in scar management, 186–187

Skin cancer. See also Basal cell carcinoma; Malignant melanoma; Squamous cell carcinoma.
    biopsy of. See Biopsy.
    etiology of, 134–135
        chemicals in, 134
        sun exposure in, 134

incidence of, 133–134
keratoacanthoma, 139, 154
management of, 138–139
   Mohs' micrographic surgery in. See Mohs' micrographic surgery.
Merkel cell tumors, 139
pathology and histopathology of, 136–138
prognosis for, 138–139
surgical management of, **205–233**
   alar subunit reconstruction in, 217, 221
   antibiotics in, 229
   antisepsis in, 229, 231
   cheek reconstruction in, 212–216
      flaps in, 213
      skin grafts in, 213
   complications of, 229
   ear reconstruction in, 229
   facial reconstruction in, 206–209
      flaps in, 207
      relaxed skin tension lines in, 207
   forehead and temporal reconstruction in, 209–212, 221, 224
      flaps in, 210–212, 221, 224
      relaxed skin tension lines in, 209–210
   lateral nasal wall subunit reconstruction in, 221
   nasal dorsum reconstruction in, 221
   nasal reconstruction in, 216–217
   nasal tip reconstruction in, 221
   periorbital reconstruction in, 224–227
      flaps in, 225, 227
      skin grafts in, 225
   scalp reconstruction in, 227, 229
   wound care in, 231–232

Skin grafts, in surgical management, of skin cancer, 225, 229

Skin resurfacing, in scar management, 184–185

S-Lift rhytidectomy, **111–121**
   advantages of, 113–115
      excellent neck and jowl rejuvenation, 114
      limited incisions and scars, 113
      minimal risk, 113–114
      reduced surgical and anesthesia time, 114
      short recovery period, 114–115
      SMAS procedure, 114
      vertical vector rejuvenation, 114
   case series of, 118
   disadvantages of, 115–116
      extrusion of suture through skin, 116
      limited access to neck, 115
      limited improvement on ptotic midface, 116
      limited improvement on severely ptotic or aged neck, 116
      pain over zygomatic arch, 116
      palpability of "knot," 116
      posterior "dog-ear," 115–116
   indications for, 117–118
   patient selection for, 119–120
   technique for, 116–117

Smallpox, in bioterrorism. See Bioterrorism.

Soft tissue augmentation, in scar management, 187

Soft tissue fibrosis, avoidance of, in maxillofacial trauma, 351

Soft tissue lesions, in children, **383–402**
   aggressive fibromatosis, 396–397
   choristomas, 391
   condyloma acuminatum, 395–396
   congenital epulis of newborns, 386–387
   cystic hygromas, 390
   fetal rhabdomyomas, 390–391
   fibromas, 383, 384–385
   focal epithelial hyperplasia, 395
   giant cell fibromas, 383
   hemangiomas, 388, 389
   hereditary gingival fibromatosis, 387
   infantile fibrosarcomas, 399
   infantile myofibromatosis, 397–398
   lymphangiomas, 388, 389–390
   melanotic neuroectodermal tumor of infancy, 387–388
   mixed tumors, 392–393
   mucoceles/ranulas, 391–392
   mucoepidermoid carcinoma, 398
   multiple endocrine neoplasia type 2b, 393
   neurofibromatosis, 393–394
   papillomas, 395
   peripheral giant cell granulomas, 385–386
   peripheral ossifying fibromas, 384–385
   pyogenic granulomas, 383–384
   rhabdomyosarcomas, 398–399
   Sturge-Weber syndrome, 388–389
   verruca vulgaris, 394–395

Soft tissues
   battlefield injuries of, 332, 336–337
   facial, burns of, 267–268
   missing, replacement of, in maxillofacial trauma, 348

Speech and language problems, in children
   cleft lip and palate and, 511
   mandibular hypomobility and, 456

Speech therapy consultations, in treatment planning, for maxillofacial trauma, 344

Sphincter muscle of mouth, anatomy and function of, 12–13

Squamous cell carcinoma. *See also* Skin cancer.
  etiology of, 134
  management of, 138
    cryotherapy in, 155
    electrodesiccation and curettage in, 155
    excision in, 154–155
    5-fluorouracil in, 155–156
    imiquimod in, 156
    laser therapy in, 155
    Mohs' micrographic surgery in, 155
    photodynamic therapy in, 155
    radiation therapy in, 155
    retinoids in, 156
  metastatic rate of, 138
  pathology and histopathology of, 136
  precursors to. *See* Actinic keratoses.
  prognosis for, 138
  surgical management of. *See* Skin cancer, surgical management of.
  versus keratoacanthoma, 154

Squamous cell carcinoma in situ. *See* Bowen's disease.

Stab wounds, in terrorist attacks, 275–276

Staphylococcal enterotoxin B, in bioterrorism. *See* Bioterrorism.

Stem cell transplantation, for radiation injuries, due to terrorist attacks, 296

Stereolithographic models, in treatment planning
  for battlefield injuries, 336
  for maxillofacial trauma, 342–343, 347–348

Steroid injections, for rheumatoid arthritis, in children, 469–470

Steroids, in scar management, 185

Stitch lift, technique for, 68–69, 72

Stoning injuries, in terrorist attacks, 273–275

Sturge-Weber syndrome, in children, 388–389

Submalar region, facial implants for, 80–82

Submandibular gland resection, technique for, 95–96

Submentoplasty, 85–86, 90–96
  anatomy in, 90–91
  complications of, 96
  patient assessment for, 85–86
  technique for, 91–96
    partial submandibular gland resection, 95–96
    with face-lift, 93–95

Suborbital region, facial implants for, 78

Subungual malignant melanoma, growth patterns in, 137

Suicide bombings, in terrorist attacks, 277–279
  maxillofacial injuries due to, 282

Sun exposure
  and skin cancer, 134, 135, 195
  and wound healing, 175

Sunscreen, in prevention, of malignant melanoma, 135

Superficial spreading melanoma, growth patterns in, 137, 199

Supernumerary teeth, impacted, in children, 368–369

Suture suspension lifts, **65–76**
  antiptosis suture threads in, 66–70, 72, 74–75
    Feather Lift, 67–68
    secure anchoring filaments, 68–70, 75
    stitch lift, 68–69, 74
  combination procedures in, 75
  definition of, 65–66
  of cheeks, 72–74
  of eyebrows, 70–72
    complications of, 71–72
  of jowls, 74–75
  patient selection for, 66

T

Tattooing
  cosmetic, in scar management, 187–188
  of skin, maxillofacial trauma and, cosmetic management of, 354

Teeth, impacted, in children. *See* Impacted teeth.

Temples, autologous fat transplantation in, 105

Temporal defects, skin cancer and, reconstruction of. *See* Skin cancer.

Temporalis tendons, contracture of, and mandibular hypomobility, in children, 458–459

Temporomandibular joint derangement, and mandibular hypomobility, in children, 461

Temporomandibular joint function, ramus-condyle unit fractures and, in children, 449

Temporomandibular joint reconstruction, for mandibular hypomobility, in children, 464

Temporomandibular joint therapy, for rheumatoid arthritis, in children, 469–470

Tendon injuries, healing of, 245

Terrorist attacks
  bioterrorism in. *See* Bioterrorism.

maxillofacial injuries due to, **273–280**
  gunshot wounds, 276–277
  stab wounds, 275–276
  stoning injuries, 273–275
  suicide bombings, 277–279
nuclear, radiation injuries due to.
  See Radiation injuries.

Tetanus immunization status, in maxillofacial trauma, 345

Therabite device, for maxillofacial trauma, 351

Thermal injuries
  in inhalation burns, 269
  radiation and, due to terrorist attacks, 292

Three-dimensional computerized reconstruction, in treatment planning, for battlefield injuries, 336

Tinnitus, due to battlefield injuries, 335

Tissue expansion, in maxillofacial dermatology, 181–182

Tissue healing. See Wound healing.

Tooth luxations and avulsions, in child abuse and neglect, 438

Trauma, maxillofacial. See Maxillofacial trauma.

Treacher Collins syndrome, in children, orthognathic surgery for, 513

Tube shift technique, in panoramic radiographs, of impacted maxillary canines, in children, 366

Tularemia, in bioterrorism. See Bioterrorism.

Tumescent solution, in facial liposuction, 87–88

Tympanic membrane perforation, due to battlefield injuries, 335

Typhoidal tularemia, in bioterrorism, 316

U

Ulceroglandular tularemia, in bioterrorism, 316

Ultraviolet radiation, and skin cancer, 134, 135

Unicystic ameloblastomas, in children, 405

Upper labial frenulum, lacerations of, in child abuse and neglect, 438

V

Vaccination, for smallpox, 305–306

Varicella, versus smallpox, 304

Vehicle-borne improvised explosive devices, maxillofacial injuries due to, 281

Velopharyngeal insufficiency, in children, cleft lip and palate and, 511

Venezuelan equine encephalitis. See Bioterrorism, staphylococcal enterotoxin B in.

Verruca vulgaris, in children, 394–395

Vertigo, due to battlefield injuries, 335

Viral hemorrhagic fevers, in bioterrorism. See Bioterrorism.

Viral infections, dermabrasion and, 184

Vitamin E, in scar management, 186

W

Warts, in children, 394–395

Weight loss/gain, autologous fat transplantation and, 108

Western equine encephalitis. See Bioterrorism, staphylococcal enterotoxin B in.

Whiplash acceleration injuries, in child abuse and neglect, 439

Wound healing, **241–250**
  acute versus chronic, 241
  angiogenesis in, 243
  biomechanical factors in, 244–245
  epithelialization in, 243–244
  fibroblasts in, 243
  growth factors in, 242
  hemostasis and inflammation in, 242–243
  in maxillofacial dermatology, 173–175
    host and local factors in, 174–175
  in surgical management, of skin cancer, 229, 231–232
  macrophages in, 243
  neutrophils in, 242–243
  of blast injuries, 245–246
  of compression injuries, 245
  of gunshot wounds, 246–248
    avulsive, 247
    penetrating, 247
  of lacerations, 245
  of shotgun wounds, 248–249
  of tendon injuries, 245
  primary closure in, 241
  proliferation phase in, 243–244
  remodeling phase in, 244

secondary closure in, 241
   tertiary closure in, 242
   wounding mechanisms and, 244
Wrinkles, fillers for. *See* Facial fillers.

Y

Yellow fever. *See* Bioterrorism, viral hemorrhagic fevers in.

Yersinia pestis. *See* Bioterrorism, plague in.

Z

Z-plasty technique, in scar excision, 177, 179

Zygomatic complex, trauma to, and mandibular hypomobility, in children, 459

Zygomaticomaxillary complex fractures, due to battlefield injuries, 334

Zygomaticus major muscle, anatomy and function of, 9–10

Zygomaticus minor muscle, anatomy and function of, 10

United States Postal Service
Statement of Ownership, Management, and Circulation

1. Publication Title	2. Publication Number	3. Filing Date
Oral and Maxillofacial Surgery Clinics	1 0 4 2 - 3 6 9 9	9/15/05

4. Issue Frequency	5. Number of Issues Published Annually	6. Annual Subscription Price
Feb, May, Aug, Nov	4	$180.00

7. Complete Mailing Address of Known Office of Publication (Not printer) (Street, city, county, state, and ZIP+4)

Elsevier Inc.
6277 Sea Harbor Drive
Orlando, FL 32887-4800

Contact Person: Gwen C. Campbell
Telephone: 215-239-3685

8. Complete Mailing Address of Headquarters or General Business Office of Publisher (Not printer)

Elsevier Inc., 360 Park Avenue South, New York, NY 10010-1710

9. Full Names and Complete Mailing Addresses of Publisher, Editor, and Managing Editor (Do not leave blank)

Publisher (Name and complete mailing address)
Tim Griswold, Elsevier Inc., 1600 John F. Kennedy Blvd., Suite 1800, Philadelphia, PA 19103-2899

Editor (Name and complete mailing address)
John Vassallo, Elsevier Inc., 1600 John F. Kennedy Blvd., Suite 1800, Philadelphia, PA 19103-2899

Managing Editor (Name and complete mailing address)
Heather Cullen, Elsevier, 1600 John F. Kennedy Blvd., Suite 1800, Philadelphia, PA 19103-2899

10. Owner (Do not leave blank. If the publication is owned by a corporation, give the name and address of the corporation immediately followed by the names and addresses of all stockholders owning or holding 1 percent or more of the total amount of stock. If not owned by a corporation, give the names and addresses of the individual owners. If owned by a partnership or other unincorporated firm, give its name and address as well as those of each individual owner. If the publication is published by a nonprofit organization, give its name and address.)

Full Name	Complete Mailing Address
Wholly owned subsidiary of	4520 East-West Highway
Reed/Elsevier Inc., US holdings	Bethesda, MD 20814

11. Known Bondholders, Mortgagees, and Other Security Holders Owning or Holding 1 Percent or More of Total Amount of Bonds, Mortgages, or Other Securities. If none, check box ▶ ☐ None

Full Name	Complete Mailing Address
N/A	

12. Tax Status (For completion by nonprofit organizations authorized to mail at nonprofit rates) (Check one)
The purpose, function, and nonprofit status of this organization and the exempt status for federal income tax purposes:
☐ Has Not Changed During Preceding 12 Months
☐ Has Changed During Preceding 12 Months (Publisher must submit explanation of change with this statement)

(See Instructions on Reverse)

PS Form 3526, October 1999

13. Publication Title	14. Issue Date for Circulation Data Below
Oral and Maxillofacial Surgery Clinics	August 2005

15. Extent and Nature of Circulation	Average No. Copies Each Issue During Preceding 12 Months	No. Copies of Single Issue Published Nearest to Filing Date
a. Total Number of Copies (Net press run)	3650	3400
b. Paid and/or Requested Circulation (1) Paid/Requested Outside-County Mail Subscriptions Stated on Form 3541. (Include advertiser's proof and exchange copies)	2368	2378
(2) Paid In-County Subscriptions Stated on Form 3541 (Include advertiser's proof and exchange copies)		
(3) Sales Through Dealers and Carriers, Street Vendors, Counter Sales, and Other Non-USPS Paid Distribution	284	310
(4) Other Classes Mailed Through the USPS		
c. Total Paid and/or Requested Circulation [Sum of 15b. (1), (2), (3), and (4)] ▶	2652	2688
d. Free Distribution by Mail (Samples, complimentary, and other free) (1) Outside-County as Stated on Form 3541	150	116
(2) In-County as Stated on Form 3541		
(3) Other Classes Mailed Through the USPS		
e. Free Distribution Outside the Mail (Carriers or other means)		
f. Total Free Distribution (Sum of 15d. and 15e.) ▶	150	116
g. Total Distribution (Sum of 15c. and 15f) ▶	2802	2804
h. Copies not Distributed	848	596
i. Total (Sum of 15g. and h.) ▶	3650	3400
j. Percent Paid and/or Requested Circulation (15c. divided by 15g. times 100)	95%	96%

16. Publication of Statement of Ownership
☐ Publication required. Will be printed in the November 2005 issue of this publication. ☐ Publication not required

17. Signature and Title of Editor, Publisher, Business Manager, or Owner

Sean Fanucci — Executive Director of Subscription Services   Date: 9/15/05

I certify that all information furnished on this form is true and complete. I understand that anyone who furnishes false or misleading information on this form or who omits material or information requested on the form may be subject to criminal sanctions (including fines and imprisonment) and/or civil sanctions (including civil penalties).

Instructions to Publishers

1. Complete and file one copy of this form with your postmaster annually on or before October 1. Keep a copy of the completed form for your records.
2. In cases where the stockholder or security holder is a trustee, include in items 10 and 11 the name of the person or corporation for whom the trustee is acting. Also include the names and addresses of individuals who are stockholders who own or hold 1 percent or more of the total amount of bonds, mortgages, or other securities of the publishing corporation. In item 11, if none, check the box. Use blank sheets if more space is required.
3. Be sure to furnish all circulation information called for in item 15. Free circulation must be shown in items 15d, e, and f.
4. Item 15h, Copies not Distributed, must include (1) newsstand copies originally stated on Form 3541, and returned to the publisher, (2) estimated returns from news agents, and (3), copies for office use, leftovers, spoiled, and all other copies not distributed.
5. If the publication had Periodicals authorization as a general or requester publication, this Statement of Ownership, Management, and Circulation must be published; it must be printed in any issue in October or, if the publication is not published during October, the first issue printed after October.
6. In item 16, indicate the date of the issue in which this Statement of Ownership will be published.
7. Item 17 must be signed.

Failure to file or publish a statement of ownership may lead to suspension of Periodicals authorization.

PS Form 3526, October 1999 (Reverse)

Changing Your Address?

Make sure your subscription changes too! When you notify us of your new address, you can help make our job easier by including an exact copy of your Clinics label number with your old address (see illustration below.) This number identifies you to our computer system and will speed the processing of your address change. Please be sure this label number accompanies your old address and your corrected address—you can send an old Clinics label with your number on it or just copy it exactly and send it to the address listed below.

We appreciate your help in our attempt to give you continuous coverage. Thank you.

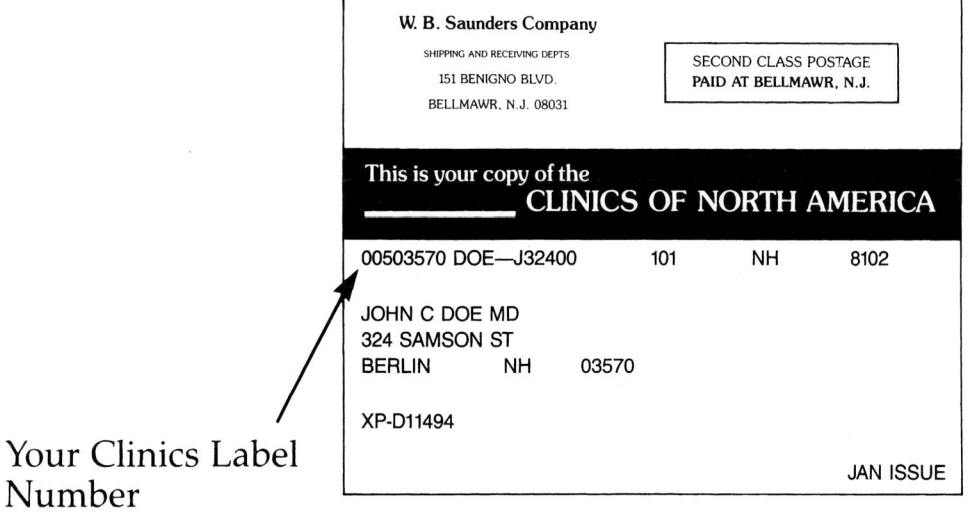

```
W. B. Saunders Company
SHIPPING AND RECEIVING DEPTS.
151 BENIGNO BLVD.
BELLMAWR, N.J. 08031

SECOND CLASS POSTAGE
PAID AT BELLMAWR, N.J.

This is your copy of the
_____ CLINICS OF NORTH AMERICA

00503570 DOE—J32400      101      NH      8102

JOHN C DOE MD
324 SAMSON ST
BERLIN      NH      03570

XP-D11494

JAN ISSUE
```

Your Clinics Label Number
Copy it exactly or send your label along with your address to:
W.B. Saunders Company, Customer Service
Orlando, FL 32887-4800
Call Toll Free 1-800-654-2452

Please allow four to six weeks for delivery of new subscriptions and for processing address changes.